CLINICAL CHEMISTRY

Journal of the American Association of Clinical Chemists

VOLUME 1

1955

PAUL B. HOEBER, INC., PUBLISHERS,
MEDICAL BOOK DEPARTMENT OF HARPER & BROTHERS

Paul B. Hoeber, Inc., Medical Book Department of Harper & Brothers
49 East 33rd Street, New York 16, N. Y.

Printed in the United States of America

Contents

A New Journal — *Harold D. Appleton* 1
Chemical Abnormalities in Blood Serum Associated with the Carrier State of Viral Hepatitis — *John G. Reinhold* 3
Electrophoresis and Monomolecular Layer Studies with Serum Lipoproteins — *David Adlersberg, Elaine T. Bossak, Irving H. Sher, and Harry Sobotka* 18
Effects of Diet on Blood Lipids in Man: Particularly Cholesterol and Lipoproteins — *Ancel Keys, Joseph T. Anderson, Flaminio Fidanza, Margaret Haney Keys, and Bengt Swahn* 34
Oxidation and Synthesis of Fatty Acids in Soluble Enzyme Systems of Animal Tissues — *David E. Green* 53
American Association of Clinical Chemists: President's Address — *Monroe E. Freeman* 68
The Clinical Chemist 72
Abstracts 75
Book Reviews 80

Serum Lipoproteins — *Ray K. Brown, Louis S. DeLalla, and Dorothy L. Kauffman* 83
Recent Studies of Fat Digestion and Absorption — *Raymond Reiser* 93
Reproducibility and Validity of Sodium Sulfate Fractionation of Proteins in Plasma and Knee Joint Fluid — *O. H. Gaebler, W. T. Beher, J. W. Sigler, and R. R. Galpin* 105
Colorimetric Determination of Blood Arginase — *Max M. Friedman and Edythe Becker* 110
Purification of Chromium (VI) for Use in the PBI Determination — *W. Burkett Mason and Santo Coco* 117
Iron Content of Tissues in Exogenous and Endogenous Hemochromatosis — *Bernard Klein, Benjamin S. Gordon, and Irving Graef* 118
Clinical Significance of the Magnesium:Calcium Ratio — *Howard S. Friedman and Martin A. Rubin* 125
The Clinical Chemist 134
Abstracts 141
Book Reviews 148

Proposal for the Distribution of a Certified Standard for Use in Hemoglobinometry — *R. Keith Cannan* 151
Rapid Estimation of Amylase Activity of Serum by Turbidimetry — *Oscar Peralta and John G. Reinhold* 157
Improved Methods of Analysis for Oxygen, Carbon Monoxide, and Iron on Finger-tip Blood — *Samuel Natelson and Carol M. Menning* 165
Effect of Shaking on the Accuracy of Salt Fractionation Methods for Serum Albumin — *Abraham Saifer and Michael C. Zymaris* 180
Convenient Apparatus for the Continuous Dehydration of Histologic Material — *Guy Nadeau and L. P. Joly* 190
The Clinical Chemist 196
Code of Ethics of the American Association of Clinical Chemists, Inc. 203
Abstracts 208
Book Reviews 218

Seromucoid in Hepatobiliary Disease *Emanuel E. Mandel, Thomas L. Gorsuch, and Gerald E. Cooper* 221
Estimation of Hydrocortisone Secretion: Method of Calculation from Urinary-Excretion Data *Robert H. Silber* 234
Quantitative Identification of Urinary Calculi *Reid H. Leonard and Arthur J. Butt* 241
Calcium Determination in Biologic Material *Eugene Y. Berger* 249
Serum Beta-Lipoproteins of Normal, Atherosclerotic, and Lipemic Individuals: Changes in Concentration, Stability, and Mobility upon Incubation at 6.5° and 37.5°, as Determined by Paper Electrophoresis *Sidney P. Gottfried, Russell H. Pope, Nathan H. Friedman, Irving B. Akerson, and Salvatore Di Mauro* 253
A Note on Quantitative Urobilinogen Determinations *Bernard Balikov* 264
Cross-Contaminator Exclusion Test for Dry-Ashing Determination of Protein-Bound Iodine *Meyer Samson, Herman Brown, and Seymour Eichen* 269
The Clinical Chemist 273
Abstracts 278

Simultaneous Determination of *p*H, CO_2 Content, and Cell Volume in 0.1 ml. Aliquots of Cutaneous Blood: A Modification of the Shock and Hastings Technic *Richard B. Singer, Jane Shohl, and Dolores B. Bluemle* 287
Estimation of Lipid Fractions of Blood Plasma: System Using the Allen Volumetric Method *Andre C. Kibrick and S. J. Skupp* 317
Iodine and Thiocyanogen Numbers of the Fatty Acids of Blood Plasma *Andre C. Kibrick and S. J. Skupp* 324
The Correspondence with Beer's Law for the Optical Density of Stained Protein Patterns on Filter Paper as a Function of Surface Protein Concentration *V. H. Rees and D. J. R. Laurence* 329
p-Toluenesulfonic Acid, Cholesterol Determination, and Explosions *Betty Jo Jones and Ferrin B. Moreland* 345
The Clinical Chemist 346
Abstracts 350

Chemical Evaluation of the Functions of the Liver (Revised) *John G. Reinhold* 351
The Clinical Chemist 422
The American Association of Clinical Chemists: Program of the Annual Meeting 427
Index 429

A NEW JOURNAL

With the appearance of this, the first issue of CLINICAL CHEMISTRY, many hopes and dreams and years of planning come to fruition. Since the founding of the American Association of Clinical Chemists one of its major goals has been the publication of a scientific journal. The constitution defines the objectives of the Association: ". . . to raise the level at which chemistry is practiced in the clinical laboratory; to stimulate the development of new methods for use in the clinical laboratory; . . . to encourage those engaged in this field to pursue advanced studies so as more effectively to render service to the public; and to create and maintain a forum where clinical chemists may exchange ideas and information concerning their scientific, technical and professional problems."

It is the hope of all of us that CLINICAL CHEMISTRY, by fulfilling the last of these objectives, will make easier and more certain the achievement of each of the others.

The practice of modern medicine is based firmly upon the knowledge gained through application of the basic sciences to medical problems. A major portion of this foundation has been contributed by the science of chemistry. The role of chemistry in the rapid evaluation of specific organ function and disease, as an aid in diagnosis and prognosis, and as the foundation for the better understanding of pathogenesis and therapy, can be attributed to the rapid assimilation of new scientific knowledge into the practical analytic methodology and interpretation at the hospital laboratory level.

Reports of this progress have been scattered through the literature of many specialties. It is expected that by providing in these pages a central official medium for the exchange of information, CLINICAL CHEMISTRY will help to bring the entire field into better focus. Thus it will serve not only the active practitioner in the busy clinical laboratory who would like to be aware of new developments as quickly as possible, but also the investigator who will find it easier to keep track of work in other places that may bear on his own studies.

At the outset it is planned to publish material in three general categories. The major share of our space will be devoted to the publication of scientific articles; reports of original investigations of the application of chemistry to medicine, new methodology and laboratory technics, and review articles of current scientific interest. Our Abstract department will offer a guide to current articles of interest to clinical chemists, giving rather complete summaries of new methodology and technics as found in the world's literature. The National Secretary of the Association, as editor of the section, "The Clinical Chemist," will provide notices of events, news of local section and foreign association activities, committee reports, letters from our readers, and all information relating to the operation of the Association and the profession of clinical chemistry.

Other departments can be inaugurated as the need appears. This is only an initial plan. It is hoped that our readers will feel free to offer their ideas and suggestions. The editors are conscious of the fact that, to succeed in their ambitions for this journal, they are dependent on the cooperation of all those actively engaged in the practice of clinical chemistry.

We who have been charged by the National Executive Committee with editing CLINICAL CHEMISTRY are deeply aware of the heavy responsibility that has been placed upon us. In the formative years of a new science a journal devoted to that specialty becomes a showcase and spokesman that is scrutinized with particular care. Our objectives are clear: to help provide answers to the many problems facing those engaged in clinical chemistry; to create and maintain standards of scientific research and writing that will reflect honorably upon our profession; and to provide a continuing forum for discussion of the scientific, technical, and professional problems of all members of our profession. It is our fervent hope that the collaboration of all of us will make CLINICAL CHEMISTRY worthy of the bright future it and its specialty deserve.

HAROLD D. APPLETON
Chairman, Editorial Board

Chemical Abnormalities in Blood Serum Associated with the Carrier State of Viral Hepatitis

John G. Reinhold

APPROXIMATELY ONE in every 100 to 200 persons who receive transfusions of whole blood subsequently become ill of viral hepatitis. When plasma is administered, the incidence of viral hepatitis has been reported to be as high as one in every 5 transfusions, although the usual rate is much lower than this. Since blood for transfusion is collected only from donors who appear to be in good health, it follows that there must be among these donors a fairly large group of apparently healthy persons who harbor the viruses of hepatitis.

There has been no method by which such carriers can be identified until after illness due to viral hepatitis is recognized in the recipients of their blood. Neither has any method for inactivation of hepatitis virus in human whole blood proved to be dependable. The problem of finding ways for reducing or eliminating the incidence of this serious—and sometimes fatal—aftermath of a transfusion is a challenging one, that clinical chemistry may aid in solving.[1] I plan to describe some of the studies made by a group, of which I am a member, working in the Pepper Laboratory.[2] These studies suggest that the risk of viral infection may

From the William Pepper Laboratory of Clinical Medicine, Hospital of the University of Pennsylvania, Philadelphia, Pa.

This investigation was sponsored by the Commission on Liver Disease, Armed Forces Epidemiological Board, and supported by the Office of the Surgeon General, Department of the Army.

Presented in part as the Third Ernst Bischoff Lecture in Clinical Chemistry, at the Annual Meeting of the American Association of Clinical Chemists, September 16, 1954. New York City, N. Y.

[1] This topic was chosen as the subject of the Ernst Bischoff lecture because it illustrates the application of chemistry to the investigation of an old clinical problem, the transmission of disease to recipients of blood transfusions. It was chosen also because it provides an example of the work of a team that includes clinical chemists, clinicians, and clinical pathologists.

[2] The group working on this problem has included Drs. D. R. Fitch, D. S. Howell, D.

be lowered if the blood serum of the donor is first examined chemically, by means of the standard chemical tests used for study of liver disease.

The event that led to our work on this problem was the occurrence, exactly four years ago, of homologous serum hepatitis in 3 patients of my colleague Dr. John Neefe. Each had received blood from a single donor. The 3 donors were recalled and their blood was studied chemically to determine whether any abnormality could be found. Results of these tests were clearly abnormal in two of the donors. Encouraged by this finding, other donors whose recipients had developed hepatitis were studied in the same way. These studies led to the segregation of a group of 18 suspect donors. Proof of the carrier state was obtained in 5 out of 6 whose bloods were tested by transmission studies in experiments conducted by Dr. Roderick Murray and his associates of the National Institutes of Health. Descriptions of the circumstances in which hepatitis occurred in the recipients and of the suspected donors have been published recently (1). The transmission experiments are described in Part 2 of the same article (2).

In this paper, chemical studies of proven and suspect carriers extending over several years are reviewed. The possible utility of the tests for the detection of carriers of the virus is assessed and some of the chemical problems encountered in the course of their application are discussed.

METHODS AND DEFINITIONS

Chemical studies have included measurements of serum bilirubin concentrations, cephalin cholesterol flocculation, thymol turbidity and flocculation at *p*H 7.80 and 7.55, zinc sulfate turbidity, cholinesterase activity, and total lipid by means of phenol turbidity. Specimens of urine were tested for bilirubin and urobilinogen. Bromsulfalein retention could not be measured at every visit during the follow-up studies, and the number of tests is about three quarters of that of the other tests. In addition, serum total and esterified cholesterol, albumin and globulin concentrations, and alkaline phosphatase activity were studied in many subjects. Since these seldom differed from limits established in healthy persons, the results are not included in the statistical evaluations.

The term *positive* in the text refers to the result of a test that differs from the normal mean by more than 3 standard deviations. When used

Kassouny, C. B. Mitchell, J. R. Neefe, R. F. Norris, and R. Watanabe, Mrs. L. G. Tourigny, Mrs. Jane Bender, Miss Ann Mifflin, Mrs. Helen Hall, and Mr. John Trumper.

I wish to acknowledge especially the collaboration of Miss Virginia Yonan in chemical aspects of these studies.

in describing the response of a blood donor it indicates that at least 1 test exceeded this limit, or that 2 or more tests gave equivocal results.

Equivocal defines the results differing from the mean by more than 2 standard deviations, but less than 3.

Abnormal results are those that are either equivocal or positive.

Negative indicates that no results have exceeded the 2-standard-deviations limit.

Although the frequency distributions of the measurements made of sera of healthy controls showed skewness when bilirubin, thymol turbidity, and zinc sulfate turbidity were tested, the skewness was not sufficiently marked to alter substantially the usual significance of these limits.

Methods used in these studies were those described in a recent review (3).

CHEMICAL CHANGES ASSOCIATED WITH THE CARRIER STATE

All of the proved carriers repeatedly showed evidence of abnormal liver function. Although occasionally only 1 test was abnormal, this was the exception, and in 21 of 27 studies made at different times 2 or more tests were abnormal. In 12 different studies, 3 or more tests were abnormal, and on 5 occasions, 4 or more tests were so recorded.

The incidence of abnormal liver function tests in the suspect donor group also was high, although not as high as that in the proved carrier group. Seven were examined within 200 days of their blood donation and all showed abnormalities in 1 or more tests. Of the entire group of 13, 7 had at least 2 abnormal test results.

The study of these carriers is continuing and a complete description of the clinical and laboratory studies, extending over 2- to 4-year periods, will be published shortly (4).

Cholinesterase activities were measured with the expectation that low values would be found, in view of the numerous studies that have demonstrated lowered activities in the serum of many patients with parenchymal liver disease. Actually, high values were encountered (Table 1) with much greater frequency than expected. In a group of 176 healthy males, 95 per cent of the serum cholinesterase results were less than 1.17 Michel units (5). Application of the chi square method to the results (Table 2) indicates that the frequency with which high values were observed would have occurred by chance in fewer than 1 of 1000 trials. Two of the higher values were observed among the proved carriers. Only 4 donors of the combined groups showed evidence of a tendency toward low enzyme activities and none were significantly lowered.

Table 1. Serum Cholinesterase of Proved and Suspect Carriers

Donor	*Race*	*Days since donation*	*Cholinesterase* (Michel units)	*Status*
11a	White	122	1.44	Suspect
		283	1.17	
9a	White	287	1.35	Suspect
		561	1.06	
2	Negro	114	1.28	Proved
		385	1.12	
10b	White	226	1.22	Suspect
3	Negro	68	1.19	Proved
		97	1.27	
		357	1.07	
6	White	101	1.07	Suspect
		128	1.13	
1	White	203	1.03	Suspect
9b	White	294	0.84	Suspect
5	Negro	221	0.80	Proved
7	Negro	85	0.80	Proved
		136	0.69	
		241	0.87	
13a	White	130	0.78	Suspect
		152	0.82	
8	White	43	0.67	Proved
		62	0.73	
4	Negro	114	0.64	Suspect

Search of the literature has disclosed a few instances in which high serum cholinesterase activities were reported. Kark (6) found high values in patients recovering from cirrhosis of the liver. Experimentally, a diet poor in lipotropic factors has been found by Hawkins and Nishikawara (7) to cause a rise in plasma and liver cholinesterase of male rats. However, female rats responded in an opposite manner.

Yet another finding in this group of carrier-donors is the frequent occurrence of elevated concentrations of lipid in serum. Lipid concentrations were measured by the phenol turbidity test of Kunkel, Ahrens, and Eisenmenger (8).

Table 2. Serum Cholinesterase of Proved and Suspect Carriers of Viral Hepatitis

	Michel units		*Chi square*[a]
	<1.17	*>1.17*	
Healthy males	171	5	24.3
Carriers	8	5	

[a] Corrected for continuity.

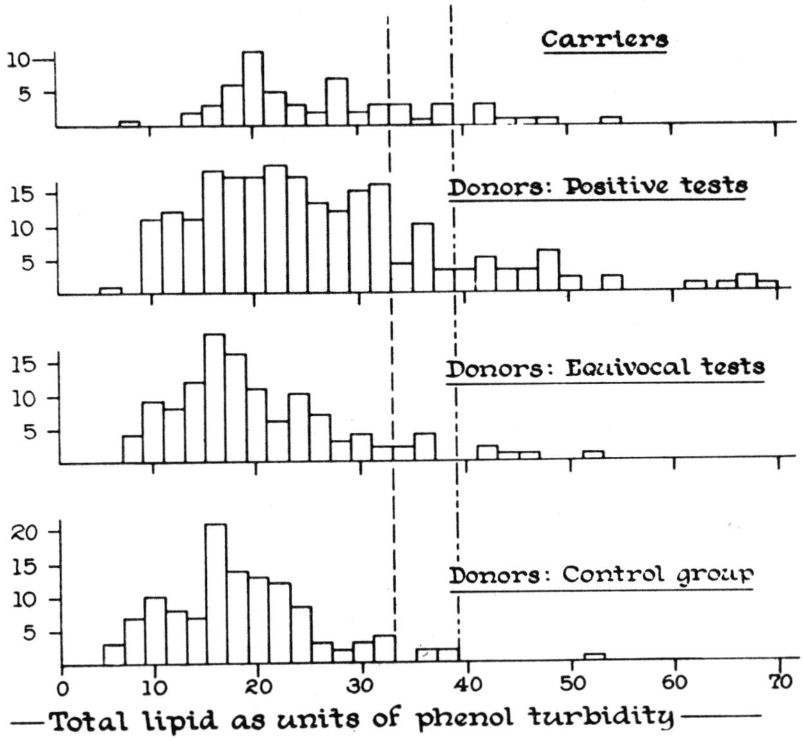

Fig. 1. Serum total lipid of donor-carriers and of blood donors with abnormal hepatic tests compared with those whose tests were normal. The ordinate shows the number of persons whose serum lipids were within the limits shown on the abscissa. The broken lines indicate the mean plus 2 and 3 standard deviations respectively.

Figure 1 shows the frequencies (on the vertical axis) with which serum lipid fell within certain limits in the carrier-donors and in a group of blood donors classified as positive on the basis of their hepatic tests. The similarity of the distributions of these two groups, shown in the upper half of the figure, is evident. It is clear that these differ from the other two shown, one of which includes the results found for a group of donors showing slight abnormalities (the equivocal group). Not only are the modes of the carrier-donor and positive groups shifted toward higher values, but one third of the analyses in the carrier-donor group gave results that were abnormally elevated. This is a frequency that is about six times the expected. The frequency of high values in the positive group was five times the expected, and that of the equivocal group about twice the expected rate. The tendency toward hyperlipemia is important in connection with the use of the thymol test for screening blood donors, as will be shown later in this paper. Supporting evidence of the existence of hyperlipemia has been provided by use of more specific methods for determination of lipids, and a more complete report will follow.

EVALUATION OF THE BEHAVIOR OF CERTAIN HEPATIC TESTS

The prevalence of chemical abnormalities in the blood of those donors believed to be harboring the viruses of hepatitis suggests that application of appropriate chemical studies frequently would have indicated that the blood was unsuitable for administration.

Table 3 summarizes the results of the chemical studies of the proved and suspect carriers over a period of approximately 2 years. Bromsulfalein retention and thymol turbidity (done at *p*H 7.55) head the list with 76 and 78 per cent of positive tests in the group of proved carriers. The zinc turbidity also stands high in the list but approaches the frequency of abnormal thymol tests only when the equivocal group

Table 3. Frequency of Abnormal Hepatic Tests Given by 5 Proved and 13 Suspect Carriers[a]

Test	*Proved carriers*			*Suspect carriers*		
	No. of tests	*Equivocal* (%)	*Positive* (%)	*No. of tests*	*Equivocal* (%)	*Positive* (%)
Bromsulfalein	17	0	76	17	12	30
Thymol turbidity	27	0	78	36	11	25
Thymol floc	27	4	70	36	3	6
Zinc turbidity	27	15	60	36	11	8
Cephalin cholesterol floc	27	4	30	36	0	3
Bilirubin, serum	18	28	6	36	8	3
Bilirubin, urine	13	0	0	30	0	0
Urobilinogen, urine	13	23	8	28	7	7

[a] All tests are included.

Table 4. FREQUENCY OF ABNORMAL HEPATIC TESTS DURING FIRST 200 DAYS

Test	*Proved carriers*			*Suspect carriers*		
	No. of tests	*Equivocal* (%)	*Positive* (%)	*No. of tests*	*Equivocal* (%)	*Positive* (%)
Bromsulfalein	6	0	100	8	12	38
Thymol turbidity	13	0	84	16	19	31
Thymol floc	13	8	70	16	0	0
Zinc turbidity	13	16	61	16	19	13
Cephalin cholesterol floc	13	16	8	16	0	6
Bilirubin, serum	13	16	8	14	7	7
Bilirubin, urine	8	0	0	15	0	0
Urobilinogen, urine	8	12	0	15	7	13

is included. The other tests were less frequently positive. No abnormality was detected by the test for bilirubin in urine. The ranking of these tests in the suspect carrier group is similar although the proportion of abnormalities is much lower.

Perhaps a better standard for evaluating the possibilities offered for the detection of undesirable donors is shown in Table 4 which lists the results of studies made during the first 200 days following the donation of blood associated with the development of hepatitis in the recipient. The ranking of the tests remains about the same. The bromsulfalein retention was abnormal in all of the proved carriers tested during this period, and in 4 of the 8 of the suspect group.

The testing of all prospective blood donors would require that the test or tests used be selective, technically simple, rapid, and inexpensive. The first consideration clearly must be the ability of the tests selected to detect carriers of viral hepatitis. Although no single test or group of tests is capable of doing this unfailingly, some have a much better ability to do so than others. Evidence concerning the contribution of each of the various tests is shown in Table 5.

If we assume that each separate application of a group of tests represents an attempt to detect a carrier presenting himself at a Donation Station, it will be seen that abnormalities were detected in each of 27 such trials in the 5 proved carriers. If the bromsulfalein test is omitted, abnormalities were found in 23 of the 27. Omission of the test for serum bilirubin and zinc turbidity would have permitted 1 more carrier to escape in each instance, but omission of tests for urobilinogen and the cephalin cholesterol flocculation test would have made no difference. A total of 21 abnormal results were found by either the thymol test or the zinc turbidity.

Table 5. Effectiveness of Hepatic Tests in 5 Proved and 13 Suspect Carriers

	Number of trials remaining abnormal[a]		*Number of trials remaining positive*	
	Proved	*Suspect*	*Proved*	*Suspect*
All tests included	27	24	26	17
Bromsulfalein omitted	23	21	21	15
CCF omitted	23	20	21	14
Urine urobilinogen omitted	23	18	21	13
Serum bilirubin omitted	22	15	21	12
Zinc turbidity omitted	21	15	20	11
Thymol turbidity alone	21	15	20	11
Total number of trials	27	36	27	36

[a] "Abnormal" includes both equivocal and positive.

The experience with the suspect group is similar (Table 5). Of the 36 trials, 1 or more tests were abnormal in 24, with 21 remaining abnormal after the bromsulfalein test was omitted. Cephalin cholesterol flocculation and urine urobilinogen enabled detection in 1 and 2 trials respectively, and serum bilirubin in 3. Fifteen were detected by the zinc or thymol turbidity tests alone. However, the zinc turbidity test was equivocally abnormal in a larger proportion than was the thymol test, therefore it was concluded that the thymol test was the method of choice if a single test was to be used, with others to be included if possible.

APPLICATION OF HEPATIC TESTS TO LARGE-SCALE EXAMINATION OF BLOOD DONORS

We have applied these observations to the screening of blood donors (9). A study of 3655 donors by means of the tests listed in Tables 2 to 4 showed an unexpectedly high proportion of abnormal results, approximately 12 per cent being classified as having positive tests and 17 per cent as equivocal. The thymol test accounted for most of the abnormality encountered, and it was soon observed that many of the abnormal readings of the thymol test were occurring in serum specimens that were lactescent. It is well known that the thymol-barbital reagent reacts with serum lipid, but we believed that by using standard values established in a large and well-matched group of nonfasting controls, difficulty from this source would be eliminated.

That the association of lactescence in the serum with abnormality in thymol turbidity reading is not consistently one of cause and effect

Table 6. Relationship of Lactescence to Thymol Turbidity

Group	*Appearance of serum*	*No. of sera*	*Thymol turbidity*		
			Negative	*Equivocal*	*Positive*
Unselected donors	Clear	543	530	3	10
	Slight turbidity	233	219	7	7
	Lactescent	269	172	37	60
Total sera		1045	921	47	77
Equivocal group	Clear	9	9	0	0
	Slight turbidity	9	7	2	0
	Lactescent	10	6	4	0
Total sera		28	22	6	0
Positive group	Clear	15	12	0	3
	Slight turbidity	8	4	1	3
	Lactescent	36	18	4	14
Total sera		59	34	5	20

may be seen in Table 6. This shows the frequency with which abnormal thymol turbidity readings were encountered in unselected blood donors as compared with donors previously tested and classified as positive. About 25 per cent of the 1045 sera from the unselected donors were lactescent, but of these only one third had abnormal thymol turbidities. Abnormal thymol turbidities occurred in lactescent sera about ten times as often as in clear or slightly turbid sera.

Among the donors classified as positive, lactescence was recorded in 61 per cent. Abnormal thymol turbidity was observed in half of these. Although the proportion of lactescent specimens found to be positive by the thymol test in this group was greater than that of the unselected group, the difference was not statistically significant (chi square 2.63, $p = 0.10$). On the other hand, the frequency of positive tests in the clear and slightly turbid specimens was significantly greater in the positive group. However, if the high thymol turbidity readings of all lactescent sera were to be rejected as artifacts, a significant number of donors with abnormal liver function tests would not be excluded, especially if the thymol test was used as the single screening test. Furthermore, several of the proved and suspect carriers then would have escaped detection on each of several trials.

Lactescence conceivably may occur more frequently in persons suffering from viral hepatitis or in those who have residual effects from hepatitis. Elevated concentrations of serum lipid and shifts in distribution of lipoprotein occur following experimentally produced liver damage, as Pierce and Gofman (10) have demonstrated. These authors and Pierce, Kimmel, and Burns (11) have found such changes in viral hepatitis also. Woldow and his associates (12) recently observed abnormalities in serum lipid, characterized by elevated values after a fat meal, several years after recovery from an attack of hepatitis. Man et al. (13) at times observed high neutral fat concentrations in hepatitis, and De la Huerga and his associates (14) reported high serum total lipids. A tendency toward high concentrations of serum lipids in patients with hepatitis may escape notice because of the low fat intake usually prescribed for patients known to have liver disease.

Although lactescence and hyperlipemia may reflect disturbances of liver function, their occurrence in the sera of blood donors usually is the result of ingestion of fatty food a few hours before their donation. Specific instructions that fatty foods be avoided on the day of blood donation have led to a substantial lowering in number of lactescent sera

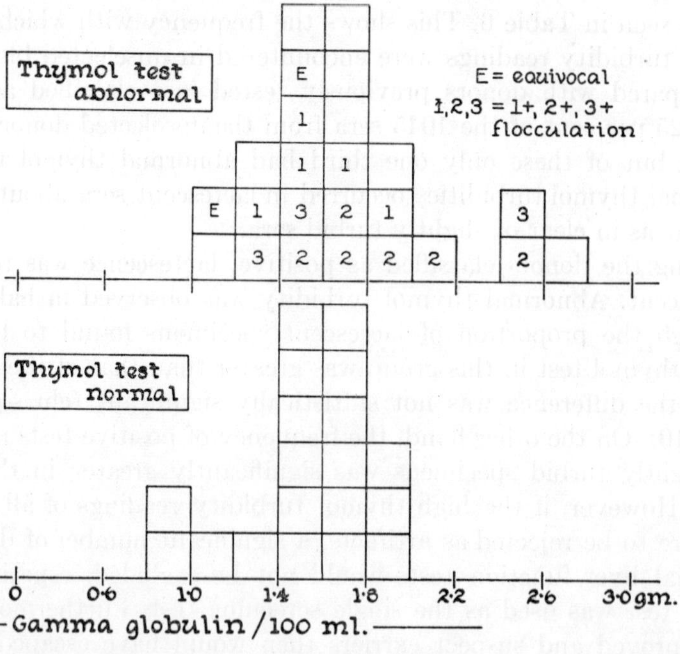

Fig. 2. A comparison of serum gamma globulin concentrations of blood donors with abnormal hepatic tests with the gamma globulin concentrations of those whose tests were normal. Each square represents 1 donor.

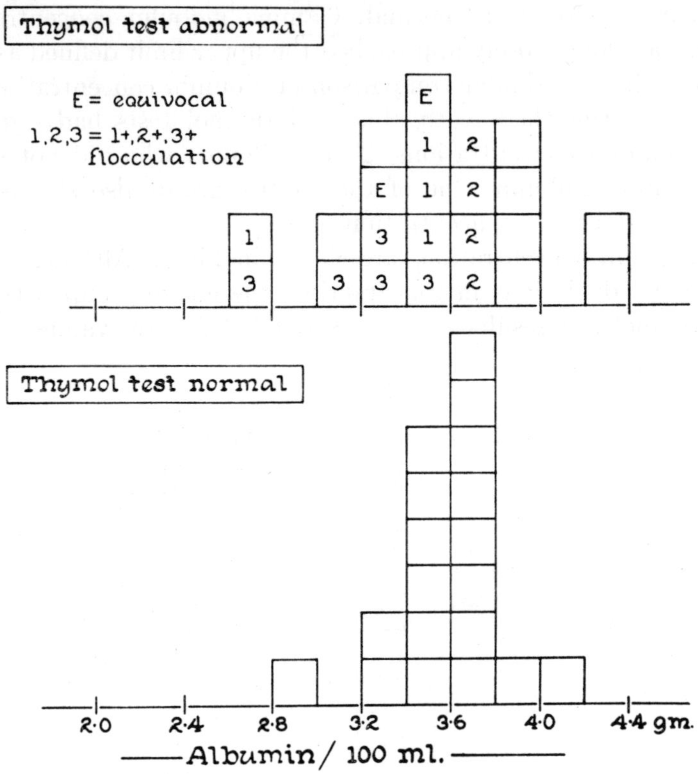

Fig. 3. A comparison of serum albumin concentrations of the same donors as in Fig. 2.

encountered in the Blood Bank.[3] Currently, thymol turbidities falling within the "positive" classification number approximately 7 per cent. This remains much higher than the expected incidence of abnormality based on the rate of clinically recognized viral hepatitis transmitted by blood transfusion, which is 0.5 to 1 per cent. The discrepancy is explained in part by the occurrence of other undetected diseases in blood donors (15).

Because of the question raised concerning the significance of the abnormal thymol tests given by blood donors, we recently selected at random 24 donors with positive thymol turbidity tests and examined their sera by means of zone electrophoresis. Figure 2 shows that 4 of the 24 had significantly elevated gamma globulin concentrations judging by the distribution of concentrations found in a similar group of donors

[3] Another method of partially circumventing the dietary lactescence factor is the use of clarified serum obtained by centrifugation at reasonably high speeds.

whose hepatic tests were normal. Gamma globulin concentrations of others in the group closely approached the upper limit defined as normal.

Figure 3 shows a similar comparison of albumin concentrations of the 2 groups. Four of those with abnormal thymol tests had significantly lowered albumin concentrations, 2 being donors who did not show abnormal gamma globulin. One of the control group also showed an abnormally low albumin concentration.

Beta globulin concentrations are shown in Fig. 4. Although there are no individual deviations in this fraction, the entire group with the abnormal thymol test results shows a shift toward lower values. Thus, the

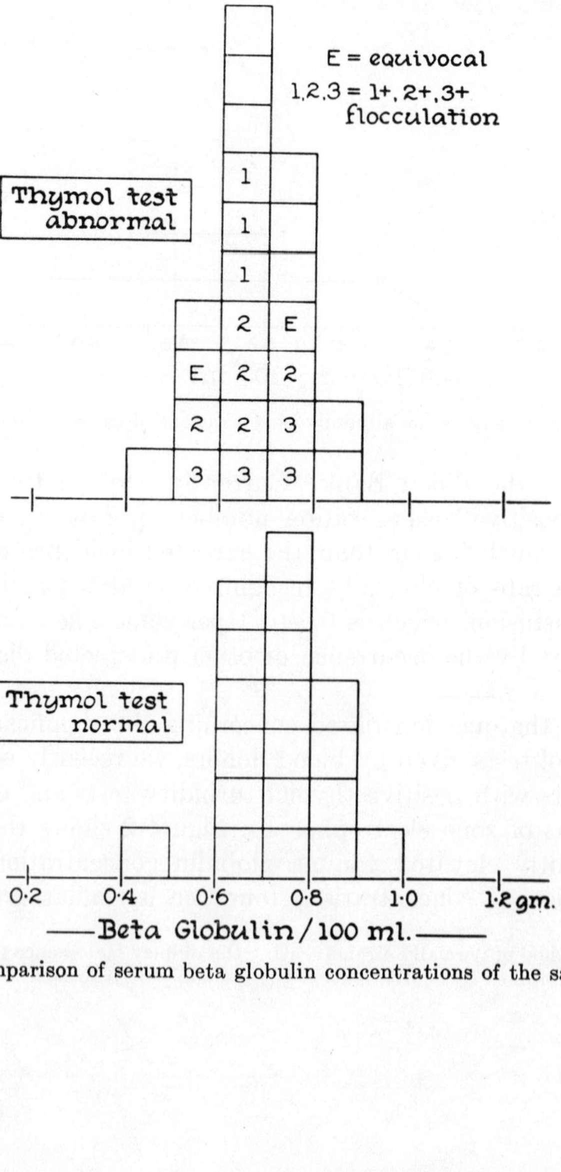

Fig. 4. A comparison of serum beta globulin concentrations of the same donors as in Figs. 2 and 3.

results of the zone electrophoresis study demonstrate significant abnormalities, similar to those frequently observed in liver disease, in 6 of the 24 members of the group with abnormal thymol test responses, while the group as a whole seems to differ in its beta globulin composition. Failure to demonstrate abnormalities in the serum protein distribution of the remainder does not exclude liver damage, for abnormal thymol turbidity and flocculation readings may occur in liver disease despite apparently normal protein analysis.

Results Of Blood Donor Screening

Some evidence of the value of blood donor screening has been gained during the past 4 years in applying hepatic tests to donors reporting to the Donation Station of the University Hospital. During the first 2 years, blood was issued from the Blood Bank without knowledge of the test results. Five patients who had received this tested blood were discovered to have developed viral hepatitis (9). In each instance, the hepatic tests of at least 1 donor were abnormal.

During the past 2 years, bloods whose donors had thymol turbidity readings exceeding 6.6 units have not been used for transfusion. Analysis of the results, insofar as incidence of viral hepatitis is concerned, of the transfusions of the bloods giving acceptable readings has not yet been completed, in part because of the difficulties of learning the fate of recipients of specific bloods. Besides, definitive evaluation of a screening program must be based on a very large number of thoroughly studied donors and recipients.

The success with which hepatic tests may be used for identifying an occasional carrier among large numbers of healthy donors requires that careful attention be given to technic and to the use of appropriate standards. It became evident as we applied the thymol test to screening of blood donors that both the accuracy and the precision of the existing technics were inadequate. Investigation of the cause demonstrated that the temperature at which the reaction was carried out was critical, and consequently that temperature control was essential (16). An improved method of preparing the reagent also was developed of necessity (3). It is essential also that correct limits defining the normal be applied because of the several different units of measurements, and because such limits differ for postprandial as compared with fasting specimens. We consider thymol turbidities exceeding 5.5 to be equivocal and those exceeding 6.6 (Shank-Hoagland) units to be positive when postprandial sera are examined.

CONCLUSIONS

We recognize that the screening of donors by means of the thymol test or even by a group of hepatic tests will fail to detect some carriers of viral hepatitis. It leads also to the rejection of a substantial number of blood donations and so adds to the costs of transfusion. Whether the improvement in safety of transfusion is worth this added cost remains to be established. However, viral hepatitis is a serious disease and even a moderate lowering of its incidence would justify a considerable outlay. Several other factors should be taken into account in an evaluation of donor screening. It has led to the detection of a significant number of other diseases including diabetes, peptic ulcer, and miscellaneous conditions in a group of 120 donors whose blood was rejected for transfusion because of positive tests (15). Furthermore, the blood withheld because of abnormalities in hepatic tests can be salvaged in one of several ways. The plasma may be separated and stored at room temperature for 6 months, as recommended by Allen *et al.* (17). Although Murray *et al.* (18) found 6 months of storage insufficient for completely inactivating the viruses of hepatitis present in considerable concentration, there is good reason to believe that a few additional months of such storage would do so. As another alternative, the plasma could be used for albumin preparation since albumin withstands the application of heat for a sufficient time to permit destruction of these viruses.

Additional information is needed about carriers of viral hepatitis so that hepatic tests may be applied to the screening of blood donors with greater confidence. One should be alert for the occurrence of viral hepatitis following blood transfusion especially in recipients of blood from single donors because in these the evidence of transmission is strong. Such donors should be studied thoroughly and warned not to give blood henceforth to prevent further spread of infection.

Our findings demonstrate that many carriers of viral hepatitis can be recognized by means of chemical studies. Concentrated efforts of chemists, physicians, and scientists from other fields undoubtedly will diminish still further the hazard of viral hepatitis as a complication of blood transfusions.

SUMMARY

The results of studies made for the purpose of identifying carriers of viral hepatitis among blood donors have been reviewed. Some carriers of the virus appear to suffer from a subclinical liver disease recognizable by abnormalities in hepatic tests. The carriers of the virus also tend to have elevated serum cholinesterase activities and elevated serum lipid concentrations.

The use of hepatic tests for screening large numbers of blood donors has been discussed in the light of observations made of the behavior of hepatic tests in proved and suspect carriers. Evidence is presented that among the donors with abnormal hepatic tests there are some that show changes in serum protein as measured by zone electrophoresis, characteristic of liver disease.

REFERENCES

1. Neefe, J. R., Norris, R. F., Reinhold, J. G., Mitchell, C. B., and Howell, D. S., *J. Am. Med. Assoc.* **154,** 1066 (1954).
2. Murray, R., Diefenbach, W. C. L., Ratner, F., Leone, N. C., and Oliphant, J. W., *J. Am. Med. Assoc.* **154,** 1072. (1954).
3. Reinhold, J. G., *Clinical Chem.* **5,** 82 (1953); **6,** 3 and 21 (1954).
4. Norris, R. F., to be published.
5. Reinhold, J. G., Tourigny, L. G., and Yonan, V. L., *Am. J. Clin. Path.* **23,** 645 (1953).
6. Kark, R. M., *Liver Disease,* edited by Sherlock, S., and Wolstenholme, G. E. W., Blakiston, Phila., page seven. 1951.
7. Hawkins, R. D., and Nishikawara, M. T., *Biochem. J.* **48,** 276 (1951) Nishikawara, M. T. *Endocrin.* **49,** 674 (1951).
8. Kunkel, H. G., Ahrens, E. H., and Eisenmenger, W. J., *Gastroenterol.* **11,** 499 (1948).
9. Fitch, D. R., Watanabe, R. K., Kassouny, D., Neefe, J. R., Reinhold, J. G., Norris, R. F., *Am. J. Clin. Path.*, in press.
10. Pierce, F. T., and Gofman, J. W., *Circulation* **4,** 29 (1951).
11. Pierce, F. T., Kimmel, J. R., and Burns, T. W. *Metabolism* **3,** 228 (1954).
12. Woldow, A., Chapman, J. E., and Evans, J. M., *Am. Heart J.* **47,** 568 (1954).
13. Man, E. B., Kartin, B. L., Durlacher, S. H., and Peters, J. P., *J. Clin. Invest.* **24,** 623 (1943).
14. De la Huerga, J., Yesinick, C., and Popper, H., *Am. J. Clin. Path.* **23,** 1163 (1953).
15. Kassouny, D., personal communication.
16. Yonan, V. L., and Reinhold, J. G., *Am. J. Clin. Path.* **24,** 232 (1954).
17. Allen, J. G., Everson, D. M., Barron, E. S. G., and Sykes, C., *J. Am. Med. Assoc.* **154,** 103 (1954).
18. Murray, R., Ratner, F., Diefenbach, W. C. L., and Geller, H., *J. Am. Med. Assoc.* **155,** 13 (1954).

Electrophoresis and Monomolecular Layer Studies with Serum Lipoproteins

David Adlersberg, Elaine T. Bossak,* Irving H. Sher, and Harry Sobotka

THE LIPIDS OF BLOOD SERUM may be classified as follows: triglycerides, phosphatides (predominantly with a P/N ratio of 1:1), and cholesterol, in the free and in the esterified form. There are in addition small amounts of free fatty acids, acetal phosphatides, phosphatidic acids, carotenoids, and lipid hormones and vitamins, which we shall, however, neglect in considering the over-all quantitative viewpoint. The major portion of the serum lipids is bound to certain protein fractions, forming the so-called lipoproteins. Whether the complexes between lipids and proteins are held together by absorptive forces or by main or coordinative valencies, particularly those of the phosphoric acid and the nitrogenous components of the phosphatides, has not been decided. Both mechanisms may coexist (1).

Most of the bound lipid occurs in the α- and β-globulin fractions, much smaller amounts being associated with albumin. A breakdown of these lipoproteins produces visible heterogenicity, the liquid assuming a milky or creamlike appearance, as the lipids, hitherto in colloidal solution, form an emulsion. This change may be brought about in normal sera by incubation with the so-called α-toxin of *Clostridium welchii*, an enzymatic factor which hydrolyzes lecithin into the diglyceride and the phosphoryl-

From the Departments of Chemistry and Medicine, The Mount Sinai Hospital, New York.

Based on a lecture given as part of a Symposium on Lipids and Lipoproteins at the Meeting of the Division of Biological Chemistry of the American Chemical Society, jointly with the American Association of Clinical Chemists, September 16, 1954, New York.

The experimental investigations on electrophoresis of lipoproteins were supported by Grants No. H-564 and H-982 from the U. S. Public Health Service to D. Adlersberg and those on lipoalbumin by Grant No. C-1791 from the U. S. Public Health Service to H. Sobotka.

The authors are indebted to Mrs. Pham Thi Thu, Miss Sara Jane Baker, Miss Helen Fung, and Miss Catherine Liu for technical assistance, and to Dr. Chun-I Wang for some of the data quoted.

* Philip J. Goodhart Fellow in Medicine.

choline moieties. This disruption of the phosphatide, the chief mediator in the complex formation between protein and fat, is sufficient to set free the electroneutral lipids, the triglycerides and sterols, which give rise to lactescence even at the relatively low concentrations, below 1 per cent, found in normal serum. Even without addition of an enzyme preparation, lipoprotein may break up spontaneously by an endogenous enzymatic reaction in the course of months, a problem encountered in the manufacture of antitoxins and antisera.

In certain pathologic and experimental conditions, the amounts of lipids, particularly of the non-ionizable types—the glycerides and cholesterol—exceed the capacity of the globulins to carry them, and in these cases the fresh serum or plasma in the fasting state appears opaque or milky. Lactescent sera, including those observed after a fatty meal, contain microscopically visible lipid aggregates, the chylomicrons. These will be considered as part of the neutral fat fraction in the following discussion.

EXPERIMENTAL PROCEDURE

Paper Electrophoresis

Chemical analysis of the lipid partition was carried out by the customary methods. The lipid phosphorus, determined by Sperry's modification (2) of the method of Fiske and Subbarow, was multiplied by the factor 25 to give the amount of the total phosphatides. Total and esterified cholesterol were determined according to Schoenheimer and Sperry (3). For the calculation of the neutral fat we subtracted from the total lipids the phosphatides and the total cholesterol plus 68.5 per cent of the amount of esterified cholesterol, to make allowance for the combined fatty acids. This correction for the fatty acids was not taken into account in our previous publications (4, 5, 6, 7). The average fatty acid molecular weight, 282, bears the ratio 68.5:100 to 382, the M.W. of cholesterol. This procedure gives an adequate picture of the chemical nature and quantity of the most important serum lipids.

The lipoproteins were studied by zone or paper electrophoresis (8, 9, 10, 11). All sera were obtained in the fasting state and examined either fresh or after deep-freeze storage. We have found in separate experiments that storage in the frozen state for as long as 6 months does not affect the results. Serum was examined in man, heparinized plasma in the experimental animals.

We have selected an apparatus with horizontally suspended paper strips. We used Whatman filter paper 3MM, 45 cm. long and 2.5 cm.

wide, moistened with 0.06M veronal buffer of *p*H 8.6 and ionic strength 0.05. We applied 0.005 ml. serum or plasma to a pencil-ruled mark across the center of the paper for the protein determinations. Six to twelve times this amount, 0.03–0.06 ml. serum, was used for the lipoprotein analysis. This concentration range does not affect the rate of migration. A current of 250 v. and 10 to 15 ma. was applied for 7 hours, after which the paper strips were dried in an oven at 70° for 40 minutes.

The protein patterns are evaluated by staining the proteins with Amidoblack 10 B and washing away the excess dye with 30% acetone.

Bromophenol Blue, in our experience, gives satisfactory visual patterns, but unreliable densitometric readings. With this dye the albumin is less chromogenic, giving rise to erroneously low optical-density readings (12).

The parallel strips used for lipid analysis were stained with a saturated solution of Oil Red 0 in 60% ethanol and the excess dye removed by rinsing with tap water (13).

A satisfactory background color could not be obtained with Sudan Black and the great variations in uptake of the stain prevented satisfactorily reproducible results. The uptake of Sudan IV (14), by serum lipids was found to be only about half that obtained with Oil Red 0.

With Oil Red 0 the densitometric readings checked closely with results obtained by elution and colorimetry. Densitometry of the papers which were not made transparent prior to densitometry was carried out in a Photovolt Model 525 instrument. Optical-density readings were recorded at millimeter intervals. The resulting curves were analysed by planimetry after components were separated by perpendiculars dropped to the baseline from the troughs of the curves. Proteins and lipid patterns of the same serum were plotted on one graph for comparison of the resultant curves. The protein pattern provides a guide for the allocation of the lipoprotein components.

Observations in Normal Mammals

The combined method of lipoprotein determination by paper electrophoresis and of serum lipid levels by chemical analysis was first used in a comparative study of normal man and laboratory animals. The purpose of the study was to characterize each species under normal conditions prior to the study of pathological or experimental states. Table 1 includes the average values from observations in 19 normal adults below the age of 50 without clinical evidence of disease, 5 rhesus monkeys, 8 male dogs,

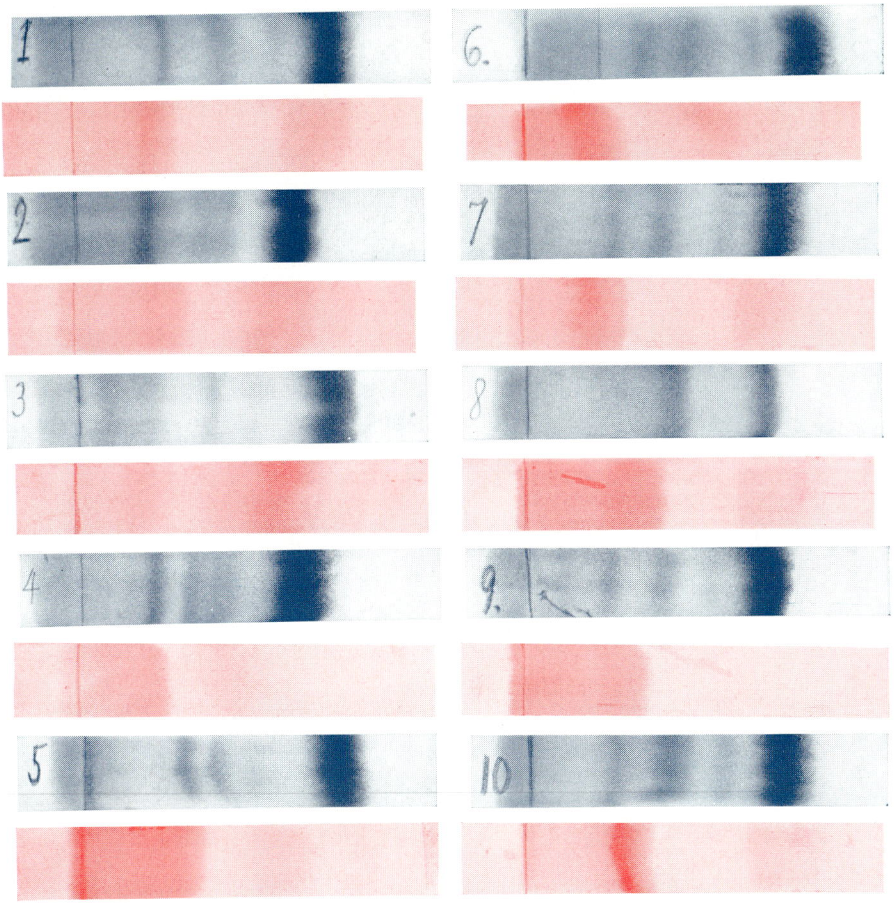

Plate I. The illustrations of the stained paper strips on the plate correspond to the electropherograms, which were derived from them as indicated in the text. The blue strips show the protein partition, stained with Amidoblack 10 and the pink strip beneath each protein strip gives the lipids stained with Oil Red O. Note that fractions on the paper strips migrate from left to right. The site of application of the serum is indicated by a perpendicular line. The albumin fraction is at the right. These strips therefore are mirror images, as it were, of the corresponding electropherograms in Figures 1–10.

Table 1. Lipid Partition and Lipoprotein Patterns

Species	*Total lipids* (mg./100 ml. serum)	*Neutral fat* (mg./100 ml. serum)	*Phosphatides* (mg./100 ml. serum)	*Cholesterol* (mg./100 ml. serum)		*Percentage of sudanophilic lipids*		
				Total	*Est.*	$\alpha_1 + \alpha_2$	β	"0"
Man	860	275	260	215	160	35	52	13
Monkey	780	290	280	140	105	41	41	18
Dog	785	190	315	190	135	70	22	8
Rabbit	440	230	120	60	45	32	50	18

and 15 male rabbits. This and the following tables give on the right-hand side the protein-bound lipid in percentage of the total lipid stainable after paper electrophoresis. Examples are given in Figs. 1–4 and in Plate I.

It must be emphasized that the evaluation of lipids on electropherograms gives approximate values only, for a number of reasons: (a) considerable adsorption of low-density lipoproteins (chylomicrons) and of β-lipoprotein to the paper interferes with the resolution of the lipid spectrum (15, 16). Electrophoresis on starch circumvents this difficulty (15, 17); (b) the direct densitometry of the stained paper, whether by transmission or by reflection, does not follow Beer's law over the whole range; (c) the chromogenicity of the dyes for the various lipids and sterols is in general not proportional to their weight; (d) lipids in mixtures may influence each other's chromogenicity. Figures obtained by this method may be used for guidance and comparison, but the validity of the absolute values remains to be established.

Amongst the lipids only the phosphatides contain ionizable groups and will thus travel with the electric current, both in the free or combined state. On the other hand, the triglycerides and cholesterol, in the free as well as in the esterified form, will remain stationary in the electric field, unless engulfed by charged molecules. The last column, inscribed *0*, gives the percentage of lipids which do not migrate, but stay at the point of origin because of their electroneutrality or their adsorption on the paper. This fraction, composed of triglycerides including chylomicrons and trailing β-lipoprotein, will greatly overlap, but not in general be identical in quantity, with the neutral fat fraction, as estimated by chemical analysis.

Man, compared to the other species studied, is characterized by high levels of cholesterol, with a phosphatide:cholesterol ratio of 1.2:1. Man's serum lipoprotein profile shows comparatively low α- and high β-globulin-bound lipids.

The dog's plasma lipids are characterized by an average cholesterol level slightly lower than in man, while the phosphatides are higher, resulting in a phosphatide:cholesterol ratio of 1.7:1. The total lipids and neutral fat in dogs are very close to the human level, but the lipoprotein profile is exactly the opposite to that of man; the α-fraction represents 70 per cent and the β-fraction 22 per cent of the total.

The plasma lipid levels of the monkey are slightly lower, while those of the rabbit are considerably lower than the values obtained in man and dog. The phosphatide:cholesterol ratio in these vegetarian species averages 2:1. The α- and β-globulin–bound lipids in monkey are both 41 per cent, while the figure for the rabbit approach those of man.

The species examined thus show distinctive patterns which can perhaps be correlated with the observed differences in their propensity to atherosclerosis. These pathologic changes are known to occur in man and rabbit, when their cholesterol levels are raised. The dog is strikingly resistant in this respect and only complete suppression of thyroid function, resulting in marked elevation of plasma cholesterol, will break this resistance. In the monkey atherosclerosis can be produced by cholesterol feeding and deficiency of sulfur-containing aminoacids. These observations suggest a correlation between predisposition to spontaneous or induced atherosclerosis and high levels of β- and low levels of α-lipoproteins.

A comparison of the protein patterns in the various species reveals differences in mobility of albumin: the canine albumin fraction moves most

---

Fig. 1. Electropherogram of normal man. The solid lines represent the protein, the dotted lines the lipid profiles, the arrows in the right lower corner indicate the point where the serum was applied. The protein peak farthest to the left represents albumin, the fastest moving component, followed to the right by α-, β-, and γ-globulin, and fibrinogen in Figs. 3, 4, 5. The lipid peak farthest to the left represents the α-fraction, followed by β- and "0"-fractions. The distance is given by notches on the abscissa for each 3 cm., the optical density by notches on the ordinate for 4 units each.

Fig. 2. Electropherogram of normal monkey. For explanation see caption to Fig. 1.

Fig. 3. Electropherogram of normal dog. For explanation see caption to Fig. 1.

Fig. 4. Electropherogram of normal rabbit (see table 1) for explanation see caption to Fig. 1.

Fig. 5. Electropherogram of rabbit with cholesterol and cortisone (Table 5, No. 62) for explanation see caption to Fig. 1.

Figs. 6 and 7. Electropherogram of myxedema, before and after thyroid treatment (Table 2, 1-A, 1-B). For explanation see caption to Fig. 1.

Fig. 8. Electropherogram of nephrotic stage of glomerulonephritis (Table 3, Case 11). For explanation see caption to Fig. 1.

Fig. 9. Electropherogram of idiopathic hyperlipemia (Table 4, Case 21). For explanation see caption to Fig. 1.

Fig. 10. Electropherogram of idiopathic hypercholesteremia (Table 4, Case 31). For explanation see caption to Fig. 1.

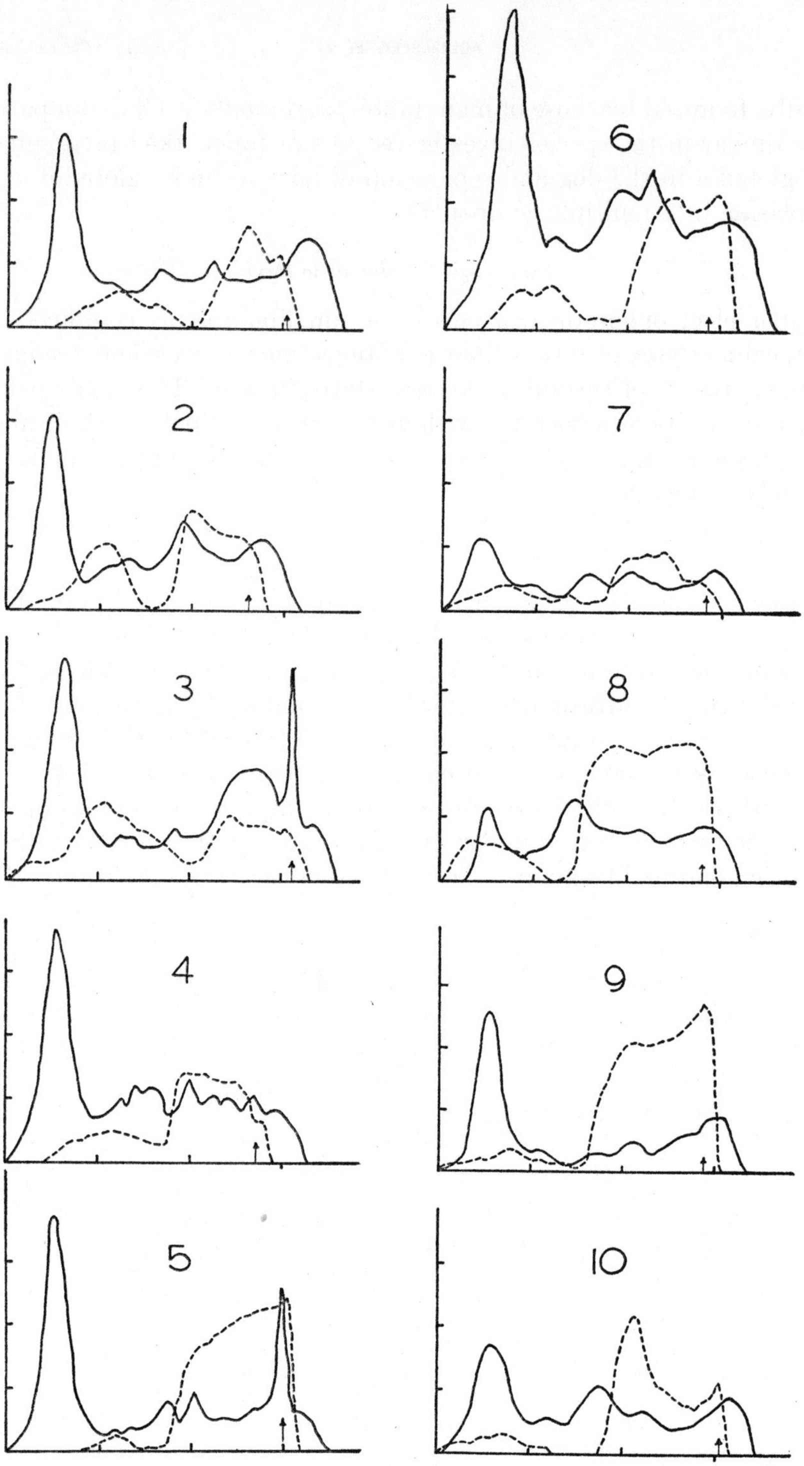

Figs. 1–10

rapidly, followed by those of man, rabbit, and monkey. Globulin patterns were similar in the species investigated except for marked predominance of β-globulin in the dog and separation of both α- and β-globulin in rabbit plasma into multiple components.

Pathologic Conditions in Man

Paper electrophoretic analyses of serum lipoproteins combined with chemical analyses of serum lipid partitions offer an excellent technic for detailed studies of certain pathologic states in man. This holds particularly for conditions associated with disturbances of lipid metabolism such as myxedema, the nephrotic syndrome, idiopathic hyperlipemia, and hypercholesteremia.

Myxedema

Table 2 shows the result in two cases of myxedema before and after treatment with thyroid extract. In Case 1 all serum lipids are increased including the zero fraction, while the α-fraction is reduced. Thyroid therapy resulted in restitution of normal values and profile along with a clinical response (Figs. 6 and 7). Case 2 is less typical, possibly because of complicating cardiovascular disease; the patient later died following a myocardial infarction. Although the concentration of serum phosphatides and cholesterol decreased under thyroid treatment the persistent electrophoretic abnormality might reflect the atherosclerotic condition.

Nephrosis

The considerable elevation of all the lipid fractions in nephrosis is associated with visible lipemia in the first three cases of Table 3 (Fig. 8). The electropherograms show a reduction of the α-fraction and increase of

Table 2. Lipid Partition and Lipoprotein Patterns in Myxedema Patients

before (A) and after (B) thyroid treatment

Case No.	*Total lipids* (mg./100 ml. serum)	*Neutral fat* (mg./100 ml. serum)	*Phosphatides* (mg./100 ml. serum)	*Cholesterol* (mg./100 ml. serum)		*Percentage of sudanophilic lipids*		
				Total	*Est.*	α	β	"0"
1-A	1745	280	620	570	400	20	51	29
1-B	970	280	280	275	200	29	59	12
2-A	900	90	380	290	205	32	54	14
2-B	780	320	210	170	115	16*	57*	27
Normal	860	275	260	215	160	35	52	13

* Decreased mobility.

Table 3. Lipid Partition and Lipoprotein Patterns in Nephrosis

Patient No.	Diagnosis	Total lipids (mg./100 ml. serum)	Neutral fat (mg./100 ml. serum)	Phosphatides (mg./100 ml. serum)	Cholesterol (mg./100 ml. serum)		Percentage of sudanophilic lipids		
					Total	Est.	α	β	"0"
11	Nephrotic stage of nephritis	2920	1205	575	765	545	13[a]	42	45
12	Nephrotic stage of nephritis	4080	1970	850	865	575	6	61	33
13	Nephrosis in lupus erythematosus	2340	1430	370	380	235	8[a]	55	37
14	Kimmelstiel-Wilson syndrome (clear)	1335	425	335	385	280	23	53[a]	24
15	Kimmelstiel-Wilson syndrome (clear)	1445	540	340	390	260	22	49 + 21	8
Normal		860	275	260	215	160	35	52	13

[a] Accelerated mobility.

the "0"-fraction. There is considerable increase of the β-fraction in Cases 12 and 15. A similar behavior may be seen in Patient 13, whose nephrotic syndrome is associated with disseminated lupus erythematosus. In these cases β_1- and β_2-globulin fractions separated.

Patients 14 and 15 illustrate the abnormalities seen in Kimmelstiel-Wilson syndrome, a nephrotic syndrome associated with diabetes. The elevation of the lipids is less striking, but the shifts in the profile occur in the same direction: both cases showed hypoalbuminemia. The fact that the cholesterol rather than the neutral fat is increased in these cases may be responsible for the clearness of their sera. The lactescence of the serum appears to be caused by very high neutral fat concentrations rather than by high cholesterol.

Idiopathic Hyperlipemia and Hypercholesteremia

Idiopathic hyperlipemia is characterized by milky appearance of the serum, caused by the marked increase of neutral fat fraction which is associated to a lesser extent with elevation of other serum lipids. The severe alteration of serum lipids in these patients is not caused by any disease known to produce such changes. This disorder of lipid metabolism is, according to our observations (4, 5), often familial and represents in its severe form a predisposition for advanced premature atherosclerosis.

Table 4. Lipid Partition and Lipoprotein Patterns in Idiopathic Hyperlipemia and Hypercholesteremia

Patient No.	*Total lipids* (mg./100 ml. serum)	*Neutral fat* (mg./100 ml. serum)	*Phosphatides* (mg./100 ml. serum)	*Cholest.* (mg./100 ml. serum) *Total*	*Est.*	*Percentage of sudanophilic lipids* α	β	"0"
Idio. Hyperlip.								
21	3580	1735	695	795	515	5	61	34
22	2150	810	490	575	400	13	40 + 10	37
23	2400	1295	500	410	285	15	41 + 14	30
24	3260	1945	590	500	330	9	51	40
25 (diab.)	2885	1900	385	410	295	5	39 + 17	39
Idio. Hypercholest.								
31 (clear)	1375	335	370	450	320	10	71	19
32 (clear)	975	280	285	275	200	6	72	22
Normal	860	275	260	215	160	35	52	13

Milder forms of idiopathic hyperlipemia may remain asymptomatic for many years. The lipoprotein patterns of this entire group invariably show an abnormally low α-fraction and very high concentrations (30–40 per cent) of the "0"-fraction (Table 4, Fig. 9).

Patients 31 and 32 are cases of idiopathic hypercholesteremia. In this condition the serum is clear and shows elevation of the cholesterol and of the phosphatides. The lipoprotein profiles resemble those seen in the previous group in the decrease of the α-fraction; in contrast there is a marked increase in the β-fraction rather than in the "0"-fraction. (Fig. 10)

It may be noted that in the serum of Patient 24 the β-globulin fraction is split and that in Patient 31 α_2-globulin is increased. Elevated γ-globulin was noted in Patient 22, who had a markedly enlarged, probably cirrhotic liver.

Animal Experiments

No. 41 exemplifies the serum of pyridoxine-deficient monkeys.* The lowering of the phosphatides and cholesterol, without changes of the lipoprotein, are atypical and reflect the poor nutritional state of the animals.

Dogs, when rendered myxedematous by large doses of radioactive iodine, show considerable elevation of cholesterol and phosphatides and a corresponding increase of the β-fraction at the expense of α-fraction. Similar changes may be brought about by continued feeding of cholesterol. Administration of cortisone in daily doses of 200 mg. per animal to

* Provided through the courtesy of Dr. Gladys Emerson of Merck Research Institute.

Table 5. LIPID PARTITION AND LIPOPROTEIN PATTERNS IN INDUCED ABNORMAL STATES

	Species	*Total lipids* (mg./ 100 ml. serum)	*Neutral fat* (mg./ 100 ml. serum)	*Phosphatides* (mg./ 100 ml. serum)	*Cholest.* (mg./100 ml. serum)		Percentage of sudanophilic lipids		
					Total	*Est.*	α	β	"0"
40	Monkey normal	780	290	280	140	105	41	41	18
41	Monkey B_6 def.	650	455	165	90	55	39	50	11
50	Dog normal	910	315	315	190	135	70	22	8
51	Myxedema	1310	285	500	345	260	52	34	14
52	Cholesterol fed	1010	0	505	335	245	61	31	8
53	Chol. fed and cortisone	2470	610	805	735	465	49	44	7
60	Rabbit normal	440	230	120	60	45	32	50	18
61	Cholesterol fed	2400	250	380	1210	965	2	53	45
62	Chol. fed and cortisone	7020	270	2970	2580	1750	3	97	

cholesterol-fed dogs resulted in additional enormous enhancement of all plasma lipids. The plasma became milky and the α-fraction was reduced to below 50 per cent, a low value for the dog. The changes brought about by cortisone administration confirm our previous observations on the important role played by the adrenal cortex in lipid metabolism (4). (Table 5).

The most striking lipid changes were brought about in the rabbit. One gram of cholesterol was fed to normal rabbits by a technic previously described by Wang, Schaefer, and Adlersberg without the use of a fat vehicle or stomach tube (7). Plasma cholesterol rose to a value twenty times the normal, and the phosphatides and the total lipid to three and five times their normal values. The plasma had the appearance of cream. This was accompanied by extreme changes in the lipid electropherogram: α-lipoprotein was almost absent, while the "0"-fraction rose to 45 per cent. Marked atherosclerosis, as well as cholesterol deposition in skin, joints, and other tissues, was observed. The combination of cortisone injection of 1.25 mg./Kg./day with cholesterol feeding resulted in further elevation of all the lipid levels and in a complete distortion of the lipoprotein profile. As the total lipid content of the plasma in this instance reached or even surpassed the total protein content, it becomes impossible to interpret the electropherogram in the customary terms (Table 5, Fig. 5).

Lipoalbumin

A protein-lipid system which lends itself much better than the above complex mixtures to in vitro studies and model experiments is the system serum albumin-fatty acids (18). As the latter lend themselves particularly well to the building up technic of Blodgett and Langmuir, we have studied the reaction of such monomolecular layers of stearic acid and its homologs with serum albumin preparations. Since one partner of the reaction, the fatty acid, is present in extremely small quantities, one can get along with very small amounts of albumin, on the average 5 mg. in 30 ml.

An 0.016% albumin solution is placed in a square glass cell; against one of its walls we place the metal slide with a known number of layers of stearic acid. The solution is rapidly stirred and kept at a given temperature. After short intervals of 10 or 20 minutes, the stearic acid plate is removed and its thickness reexamined by monochromatic interferometry or by the ellipsometer. It will invariably be found that a number of layers have been ripped off during exposure to the albumin solution (19). It should be noted that the ripping-off phenomenon is greatly accelerated by phosphate buffer, possibly because of the solubilizing influence of the phosphate upon the albumin-fatty acid complex.

From the physicochemical point of view, it is of interest to observe that the stearic acid film, which consists of a mixture of stearic acid and barium stearate, is not dissolved completely, layer by layer, from the plate. The action of the albumin is rather selective, as it takes off stearic acid and leaves a skeleton of barium stearate behind. This circumstance can not be detected by the optical method which only indicates the overall loss on the plate, but it may be demonstrated by filling out holes, left by the stearic acid, with a suitable substance, whereupon optical methods will show the original thickness to be restored.

Another peculiarity of monolayers is their penetrability to other molecules, due to a lowering of their cohesion, and even their melting point, as compared to the same compound in the three-dimensional state. Thus, the stearic acid film may be covered with as many as ten monolayers of cholesterol, ca. 200 Å thick, which are not attacked by albumin themselves, but which permit the reaction to go on between the stearic acid below and the albumin solution above. Moreover, water molecules will penetrate without difficulty through the cholesterol layers and refill the skeletonized film.

The ripping-off effect is highly specific for both components. Serum globulin, ovalbumin, synthetic polypeptides, etc., leave the stearic acid plate unchanged. On the other hand, built-up plates of cholesterol remain undisturbed by the albumin treatment. Amongst homologous fatty acids, the effect is of the same order of magnitude for palmitic acid. Monolayers of shorter chain fatty acids are difficult or impossible to handle at room temperature. Surprisingly enough, acids with more than 18 carbon atoms, such as arachidic, behenic, and lignoceric acid, also the terminally branched isoarachidic acid and the unsaturated elaidic and brassidic acids do not react with serum albumin.

One may calculate the molar ratio of stearic acid to albumin when the reaction has reached equilibrium. The values vary for different albumin preparations from 2.3 to 2.7 moles of fatty acids per mole of albumin. This corresponds to about 1.5 per cent by weight of the albumin, figures much smaller than the percentage of mixed lipoids combined with globulin fractions. We have to keep in mind that the original albumin may contain, before the experiment, some fatty acids or related aliphatics. Crystalline Bovine Serum Albumin (Armour) contains approximately one molecule dodecyl alcohol, which has been added to enhance crystallization.

There is a great number of anionic and neutral substances whose reaction with serum albumin has been studied. We should like to mention amongst them a number of carboxylic acids, primarily the lower fatty acids, studied by Murray Luck and his coworkers (20–23). Their combination with serum albumin seems to stabilize the protein against heat coagulation. The adsorption of anionic dyes of varying molecular dimensions has been investigated by Klotz *et al.* (24, 25, 26, 27) who found molecular ratios from about 2:1 to 4:1 in methyl orange:albumin by a diffusion technic. Westphal *et al.* (28, 29) have developed this technic for the study of serum albumin in pathologic and experimental conditions. They report that the dye affinity of the albumin is reduced by the addition of various fatty acids and that this competitive effect is maximal for myristic acid with 14-C-atoms and falls off sharply to reach zero for the homologs above stearic acid. This observation seems to dovetail with ours. Also our findings that the adsorption of azorubin on albumin reduces its affinity for stearic acid, indicates that we are dealing with the same site on the albumin molecule.

We have compared various fractions of human and horse serum albumin, obtained by a variety of methods. Their ability to rip off and dissolve stearic acid parallels their affinity for the dyestuffs. If one extracts the original lipid contained in the albumin and estimates it colorimetrically by Swahn's technic (30), one finds that affinity for stearic acid decreases as the actual lipid content increases.

Whether the lipid content determines the physicochemical behavior of individual albumin fractions or whether inherent differences in chemical constitution of the albumin fractions govern their lipid content, remains to be seen. The heat coagulability of various albumin fractions is undoubtedly a function of their lipid content. On the other hand, deviations from the normal coagulation point have been correlated with various groups of diseases such as rheumatic and infectious conditions and, in particular, cancer. We are at present studying the individual albumin fractions in patients' sera in respect to their lipid affinity and coagulation temperature.

One of the primary problems in serum lipoprotein research is the correlation of the individual types of lipids with the protein-bound lipid. While we have advanced some ideas as to which lipids are bound to which protein fractions, an accurate quantitative assignment is necessary as basis for the understanding of the reactions and properties of the serum lipoproteins, the nature of the linkages which hold them together, and the character of the agents which break them up—like *Clostridium welchii* toxin—or which act as clearing factors, like heparin.

SUMMARY

The chemical analysis of the lipids in serum or plasma yields data for total lipids, phosphatides, total and esterified cholesterol, and by subtraction, for neutral fat. Zone electrophoresis, for which experimental details are given, shows the distribution of the serum lipids between α-globulin, β-globulin, and a fraction which does not move in the electric field. Values are given for normal man, monkey, dog, and rabbit. Their distinctive patterns are correlated with differences in the propensity of these species to develop atherosclerosis.

Combined studies of the lipid partition and the electrophoretic profile were carried out on patients with disturbed lipid metabolism, particularly myxedema, nephrosis of various etiology, and idiopathic hyperlipemia and hypercholesteremia. The lactescence of lipemic sera is ascribed primarily to increases of the neutral fat and corresponding increases of the electroneutral fraction of the lipoprotein electropherogram. In the Kimmelstiel-Wilson syndrome, the nephrotic syndrome in diabetes, and in idiopathic hypercholesteremia, where the cholesterol level is increased but the neutral fat level normal, the sera usually remain clear.

In animal experiments the destruction of thyroid tissue and, in particular, the feeding of cholesterol induces hypercholesteremia and hyperphosphatidemia in dog and rabbit. The signs of lipemia are further enhanced by the simultaneous administration of cortisone, when the total lipids in the rabbit run sometimes above 7 per cent of the serum. This experimental condition is associated with severe atherosclerotic lesions.

A model for lipoproteins is provided by the reaction between serum albumin and fatty acids, the latter in the form of monomolecular layers.

The technic is described. The specificity of the ripping-off reaction and its parallelism with the dyestuff affinity of serum albumin are illustrated and discussed. The application of the reaction to the study of the "albumin defect" in infectious, rheumatic, and malignant disease is suggested.

REFERENCES

1. Chargaff, E., *Advances in Protein Chem.*, New York, Academic, Vol. 1, p. 1 (1944).
2. Sperry, W. M., *Ind. Eng. Chem., Anal. Ed.*, **14**, 88 (1942).
3. Schoenheimer, R., and Sperry, W. M., *J. Biol. Chem.*, **106**, 745 (1934).
4. Adlersberg, D., Schaefer, L. E., and Dritch, R., *Proc. Soc. Exp. Biol. Med.*, **74**, 877 (1950).
5. Adlersberg, D., Schaefer, L. E., and Wang, C., *Science*, **120**, 319 (1954); cf. Adlersberg, D., and Wang, C., *Ann. Meet. Am. Diab. Ass.*, San Francisco (to be published).
6. Bossak, E. T., Adlersberg, D., and Wang, C., *Circulation*, **10**, 602 (1954).
7. Wang, C., Schaefer, L. E., and Adlersberg, D., *J. Mt. Sinai Hosp.*, **21**, 19 (1954).
8. Durrum, E. L., *J. Am. Chem. Soc.*, **72**, 2943 (1950).
9. MacDonald, H. J., Lapper, R. J., Marbach, E. P., Spitzer, R. H., and Urbin, M. C., *The Clin. Chem.*, **5**, 17, 35, 51 (1953).
10. Kunkel, H. G., *Methods of Biochemistry*, New York, Interscience Anal. **1**, 141 (1954).
11. Sobotka, H., and Carr, J. J., *Ann. Rev. Med.*, in press (1955).
12. Crook, E. M., Harris, H., Hassan, F., and Warren, F. L., *Biochem. J.*, **56**, 434 (1954).
13. Durrum, E. L., Paul, M. H., and Smith, E. R. B., *Science*, **116**, 428 (1952).
14. Rosenberg, I. N., *Proc. Soc. Exp. Biol. Med.*, **80**, 751 (1952).
15. Kunkel, H. G., and Slater, R. J., *Proc. Soc. Exp. Biol. Med.*, **80**, 42 (1952).
16. Smith, E. R. B., Crawford, T. M., Jetton, E. R., and Durrum, E. L., *Fed. Proc.*, **12**, 269 (1953).
17. Carlson, L. A., *Acta Chem. Scand.*, **8**, 510 (1954).
18. Sher, I. H., and Sobotka, H., *J. Coll. Sci.*, **10**, in press (1955).
19. Trurnit, H. J., *Arch. Biochem. Biophys.* **47**, 251 (1953).
20. Ballou, G. A., Boyer, P. D., Luck, J. M., and Lum, G. F., *J. Biol. Chem.*, **153**, 589 (1944).
21. Ballou, G. A., Boyer, P. D., and Luck, J. M., *J. Biol. Chem.*, **159**, 111 (1945).
22. Boyer, P. D., *J. Biol. Chem.*, **158**, 715 (1945).
23. Teresi, J. D., and Luck, J. M., *J. Biol. Chem.*, **194**, 823 (1952).
24. Klotz, I. M., Walker, F. M., and Pivan, R. B., *J. Am. Chem. Soc.*, **68**, 1486 (1946).
25. Klotz, I. M., and Ayers, J., *J. Am. Chem. Soc.*, **74**, 6178 (1952).
26. Klotz, I. M., Burkhard, R. K., and Urquhart, J. M., *J. Am. Chem. Soc.*, **74**, 202 (1952).
27. Klotz, I. M., *The Proteins.* (H. Neurath and K. Bailey, eds.) New York, Academic, Vol. I, part B, p. 727 (1953).
28. Westphal, U., and Gedigk, P., *Proc. Soc. Exp. Biol. Med.*, **76**, 838 (1951).
29. Westphal, U., Stets, J. F., and Priest, St. G., *Arch. Biochem. Biophys.*, **43**, 463 (1953).
30. Swahn, B., *Scand. J. Clin. Lab. Inv.*, **5**, Suppl. 9, 7 (1953)

Effects of Diet on Blood Lipids In Man

Particularly Cholesterol and Lipoproteins

Ancel Keys, Joseph T. Anderson, Flaminio Fidanza, Margaret Haney Keys, and Bengt Swahn†*

THERE ARE GOOD REASONS for the current great interest in the effects of the diet on the blood lipids. It is now generally agreed that there is an important relationship between the concentration of certain lipid fractions in the blood and the development of atherosclerosis and the coronary heart disease it produces. The outstanding characteristic of atherosclerosis is the presence of lipid deposits, mainly cholesterol, in the walls of the arteries. And both in man and animals the most obvious factor that affects the blood lipids is the diet.

Broadly speaking, as indicated in Table 1, the lipids in the blood are carried in two forms, as emulsions or "chylomicrons," and in the form of complexes with proteins. The present discussion is concerned primarily with the latter, the lipoproteins. These may be separated analytically by fractional precipitation, as in Cohn's alcoholic system; by ultracentrifugation in a medium of known density; by paper electrophoresis; or, with less success so far, by chromatography. Both alcoholic

---

From the Laboratory of Physiological Hygiene, University of Minnesota, Minneapolis, Minnesota.

Some of the data cited here were obtained in research supported in part by grants from the National Dairy Council, Chicago, and the American Heart Association.

We are grateful for generous aid in providing facilities and subjects to Professors Gino Bergami and F. Di Lorenzo and Dr. M. Mattioli in Naples, to Professors G. Sotgiu, A. Poppi and T. Postelli in Bologna, and to Dr. R. Rossen in Hastings, Minnesota. Important help in Naples was given by Drs. R. Buzina of Zagreb, B. Bronte Stewart of Cape Town, and Robert Dale of London, and by Drs. V. Scardi, Dr. Di Giulio, Mr. A. Orengo and Miss N. Corrao, all of Naples. Dr. A. R. P. Walker of Johannesburg kindly supplied a copy of the paper by him and Arvidsson (31) on the Bantu in advance of publication.

Presented at the Symposium on Lipids and Lipoproteins at the 126th National Meeting of the American Chemical Society, Division of Biological Chemistry, in participation with the American Association of Clinical Chemists, September 16, 1954. New York, N. Y.

* Present address: Istituto di Chimica Biologica, University of Naples, Italy.

† Present address: Department of Medicine, University of Lund, Sweden.

Table 1. Primary Forms of Serum Lipids and Approximate Distribution, in Healthy Persons, of Lipoprotein Lipid (LPL), and Total Serum Cholesterol (Chol.) in These Forms

Class	Distribution	
	LPL (%)	*Chol.* (%)
A. Emulsions ("chylomicrons")	0	0
B. Solutions (lipoproteins)	100	100
1. α lipoproteins	20–30	20–30
2. β lipoproteins[a]	70–80	70–80

[a] Includes Gofman's "giant molecules."

precipitation and paper electrophoresis reveal two distinct fractions, the alpha lipoproteins and the larger beta lipoproteins which are more readily precipitated and move more sluggishly in an electrical field. Subfractions of these two classes are less sharply differentiated and their significance is more obscure. But all of the lipoproteins are notable in that they contain cholesterol and phospholipids, apparently as essential ingredients, as well as proteins and other lipids. The main interest in regard to lipids in atherogenesis is centered on the cholesterol and on the beta lipoproteins which contain most of this cholesterol.

Quantitative analysis of the lipoprotein system in the blood is technically not simple but progress in methods has been rapid recently. It has become increasingly easy to carry out controlled dietary experiments on animals so as to study the effects on the various items of the lipoprotein system. Unfortunately, different animal species differ markedly and in none of the species studied is there a close quantitative resemblance to man, either in regard to the effects of the diet on the blood or in regard to the tendency to deposit cholesterol in the coronary arteries.

This is most easily shown, as in Table 2, by the results of cholesterol-feeding experiments. The rabbit and the chick are at one end of the scale of sensitivity to exogenous cholesterol while man is far removed at the other. The addition to the diet of an amount of cholesterol that produces a rise in the serum cholesterol in the rabbit of 1000 per cent or more, produces in man either no change or perhaps a 10 per cent rise when the cholesterol load is consumed for months on end.

Accordingly, if it is desired to discover quantitative relationships in man, it is necessary to study man himself. But controlled human dietary experiments are difficult and costly. Many individuals must be studied in prolonged experiments because the significant time scale is long and individual variability is large. Finally, there is always the question as to what may be the influence of the previous lifetime of dietary habitus.

Table 2. Effect, in Various Species, on the Concentration of Total Cholesterol in the Blood Serum of Addition of Cholesterol to the Diet

Species	*References*	*Cholesterol*		
		Diet (mg./Cal.)	*Weeks*	*Serum* (% increase)[a]
Rabbit	37–43	0.4–5.0	5–16	200–3000
Chick	44–46	0.8–6.0	5–25	50–600
Rat	37, 47–49	3–30	4–22	50–200
Guinea pig	37	5	5	180
Dog	50, 51	2	1–2	100
Monkey	52, 53	3	29	22
Child	54	0.4–1.0	1–3	0
Woman	55, 56	1.0	16	0
Woman	57	1.4[b]	4	8
Man	58	1.5	6	"Slight"
Man	59	2[b]	6–7	11–18
Man	59	16[c]	4	3
Man	59	16[c]	9	5

[a] As a percentage of the initial (control) level.
[b] As egg yolks.
[c] As egg yolk powder.

Nevertheless, there is a growing accumulation of knowledge from controlled dietary experiments on man. Some of this will be presented here but the main emphasis will be on data obtained from samples of human populations habitually subsisting on different diets.

METHODS

The serum cholesterol values cited here were obtained by the method of Abell *et al.* (1) ("Kendall method") which involves saponification prior to the eventual estimation with the Liebermann-Burchard reagent. This method has checked repeatedly, with fully satisfactory agreement, with the method involving precipitation with digitonin (2, 3). A systematic comparison of 134 serum samples, in quadruplicate, analyzed by the Kendall method and by the ordinary application of the Liebermann-Burchard reagent to the Bloor extract, as previously used by us (4, 5–8), gave the prediction equation: $Y = 0.836X$, where Y is the Kendall method result and X is the result with the Bloor extract method. The standard error of estimate in this prediction proved to be ± 10.23 mg. per 100 ml.

Ultracentrifugal analysis was made in two stages by the flotation method of Gofman (9), with modifications as recommended by Dr. Gofman and other experts in the U.S.P.H.S. Cooperative Study.

Cholesterol in the alpha and beta lipoprotein fraction of the serum was analyzed in the fractions separated by a modification of Cohn's Method X which uses low-temperature precipitation in alcoholic solution.

The amount of lipid in the alpha and beta lipoproteins and in the chylomicrons was estimated by Swahn's (10) paper electrophoresis method; the lipid is measured by the amount of Bismarck or Sudan Black adsorbed on the paper after electrophoresis.

Relative obesity was estimated in terms of relative body weight and of the thickness of the skinfolds. Relative body weights are expressed as percentages of the average weight for given height and age as given in the tables of the Medico-Actuarial Investigations on Mortality of 1912; these are sometimes referred to as Davenport's Height-Weight Tables. Skinfold thickness, comprising a double layer of skin and subcutaneous fat, was measured with skinfold calipers at constant tension (11).

SUBJECTS

Most of the data to be cited here were obtained from the groups indicated in Table 3, all of whom were physically healthy men between the ages of 18 and 65. The experimental subjects were schizophrenic patients found to be metabolically "normal" on careful study. During the experiments on them they were separately housed and fed in a special diet kitchen and were under rigid 24-hour control, both as to diet and

Table 3. Principal Groups of Men Represented in Diet and Blood Lipid Studies Considered in This Paper

1. Minnesotans	(Business and professional men)
2. Experimental subjects	(Hastings State Hospital Patients)
3. U. S. Army	(Enlisted men in the United States)
4. Neapolitan clerks	(Naples Tax Offices)
5. Neapolitan firemen	(Naples Fire Department)
6. Neapolitan heavy workers	(ILVA Steel Works)
7. Neapolitan "bankers"	(Naples Rotary Club)
8. Bologna policemen	(Bologna Police Department)
9. Swedish clerks	(Kochums Shipyard, Malmö)
10. Swedish firemen	(Malmö Fire Department)
11. Swedish heavy workers	(Kochums Shipyard, Malmö)
12. South African Bantu	(Johannesburg)
13. South African Europeans	(Johannesburg)
14. Spanish lower class	(Madrid)
15. Spanish professional men	(Madrid)
16. Englishmen	(London, light industry)

as to physical activity. Finally, measurements were made on ambulatory patients who had definite coronary disease as indicated by previous myocardial infarction and/or angina pectoris and electrocardiographic changes.

INTERRELATIONS BETWEEN LIPID FRACTIONS

Cholesterol and Phospholipid

There is a general tendency for some of the lipid fractions to be interrelated so it might be expected that the measurement of the response of one fraction to the diet would allow the prediction of changes in other fractions. This assumption is not tenable, however, even in clinically healthy men and with such closely related items as cholesterol and phospholipid. For example, in blood serum samples from 59 healthy young men we found a correlation coefficient of $r = 0.847$ between total cholesterol and phospholipid. This is very impressive but even so it does not allow accurate prediction of one from the measurement of the other item. Incidentally, the ratio of cholesterol to phospholipid in the serum has been advocated frequently as a useful device to detect men who have or may be threatened with coronary heart disease.

Alpha Lipoprotein and Chylomicron Lipids

As shown in Table 4, the amount of lipid in the lipoproteins is very largely independent of the amount of lipid in the emulsion or "chylomicron" form in the serum. In healthy men there was no correlation at all between alpha lipoprotein lipid and chylomicron lipid concentrations. The small correlation indicated between beta lipoprotein lipid and chylomicrons could be an artifact owing to the uncertainty of separation of a portion of these fractions in paper electrophoresis. Finally, the concentration of total cholesterol in the serum shows only a trivial relationship with the concentration of chylomicron lipid in the same serum.

Table 4. Correlation Coefficients between the Concentration of Chylomicron Lipid and the Lipid in Alpha and Beta Lipoproteins the Total Cholesterol Concentration in Blood Serum from 247 Clinically Healthy Men in Naples, Italy

No.	*Age*	*Lipoprotein lipid*		*Cholesterol*
		α	*β*	
104	18–34	−0.12	0.28	0.15
143	35–50	0.00	0.41	0.20

Table 5. CORRELATION COEFFICIENTS OF TOTAL CHOLESTEROL WITH ALPHA LIPOPROTEIN LIPID ($r_{c,\alpha}$) AND WITH BETA LIPOPROTEIN LIPID ($r_{c,\beta}$) IN CLINICALLY HEALTHY MEN IN NAPLES, ITALY

No.	*Category*	*Correlation coefficient*	
		$r_{c,\alpha}$	$r_{c,\beta}$
119	Heavy workers	0.04	0.69
150	Firemen	0.03	0.63
26	Clerks	≅0	0.69
26	Bankers	≅0	0.60

Beta Lipoprotein and Chylomicron Lipids

The total cholesterol concentration in the serum shows no correlation with the amount of lipid in the alpha lipoprotein fraction but it is highly correlated with the amount of lipid in the beta fraction. Table 5 shows the results of serum analyses for 321 men in Naples. It will be observed that the correlations are substantially identical in all four categories of men, in spite of their differences in physical activity and the marked difference of the diet of the "Bankers" from the diets of the other men. Since only single analyses for lipoprotein lipids were available and there are appreciable method errors involved in the cholesterol method and particularly in the paper electrophoresis method, the true correlation between total cholesterol and beta lipoprotein lipid in these men is higher and is estimated to be of the order of $r = 0.7\text{–}0.8$.

Gofman (12) has insisted that there is very little correlation between the total serum cholesterol concentration and that of his S_f 12–20 fraction separated in the ultracentrifuge. Actually, the correlation is always significant and in many series is of the order of $r = 0.6$ (13, 14).

Alpha and Beta Lipoprotein Lipids

Among the cholesterol fractions in the serum it is obvious that there must be a very high correlation between the total cholesterol and the cholesterol in the beta lipoprotein since the latter contains some three quarters of the former. In a series of 54 healthy men aged 50–60 years, we found four fifths of the total cholesterol was in the beta lipoprotein fraction and in a series of 54 men of the same age with coronary disease, the beta lipoprotein fraction accounted for an average of 87.5 per cent of the total cholesterol. However, there is almost complete independence between the amounts of cholesterol in the alpha and in the beta lipoproteins. In the two series noted above the correlation coefficients between total cholesterol and alpha lipoprotein cholesterol were, respectively, $r = 0.063$ and $r = 0.195$.

All of the foregoing indicates that the effects of the diet on each of the several blood lipids should be separately considered though, as will appear, there are important common trends in the responses.

DIETARY CHOLESTEROL

The lack of effect on the blood cholesterol of man of adding large amounts of cholesterol to the diet has already been mentioned (cf. Table 2). Population surveys (4, 15, 16) have confirmed the lack of response in man to the cholesterol level of the diet so this point requires no further consideration. Where serum cholesterol differences have been found to be associated with differences in dietary cholesterol intake, other dietary differences have been involved (17, 18).

EFFECTS OF CALORIES AND RELATIVE OBESITY

The "calorie habitus" of a man may be inferred from its result as seen in his relative emaciation or obesity. And, in turn, the relationship between the calorie habitus and the serum lipids may be inferred by comparing the serum lipids of men of differing relative obesity, provided other factors, such as age and occupation, are constant. Five years ago we reported (4) that among sedentary businessmen aged 48–55 in Minnesota, the fatter men tended to have very slightly higher serum total cholesterol concentrations than their thinner counterparts. A similar slight tendency is observed among Danes when they are classed into "leptosomatic" and "pyknic" types (19). A more significant relationship in 46 young Englishmen, with a correlation coefficient of $r = 0.43$, between total serum cholesterol and subcutaneous fat thickness, was reported by Tanner (20). Among both men and women of the lower class of Madrid, Spain, and among men of the working class of Naples, Italy, we found significantly higher serum total cholesterol concentrations in the fatter persons than in their thinner counterparts (5, 8, 16, 21, 22). On the other hand, among men of the professional class in Madrid and among employees in light industry at Slough, near London, the tendency for a relationship between relative obesity and serum total cholesterol was slight, like that seen in Minnesota, and proved to be statistically not significant (6). These studies indicated that there is no general obligatory relationship between relative obesity and the serum total cholesterol concentration.

In the past six months it has been possible to collect more extensive data on the relationship between obesity and serum lipids. Table 6 summarizes data from heavy workers, firemen, and clerks in Naples, Italy. The concentration of lipid in the serum alpha lipoprotein fraction was

Table 6. Coefficients of Correlation for Relative Body Weight with the Concentrations in the Blood Serum of Total Cholesterol, of Alpha Lipoprotein Lipid and with Beta Lipoprotein Lipid in Healthy Men in Naples

No.	*Age*	*Occupation*	*Mean rel. body wt.* (%)	*Correlation with:*		
				Chol.	*α*	*β*
55	19–34	Heavy labor	98.7	0.35	−0.07	0.39
49	19–34	Firemen	103.8	−0.13	−0.07	0.15
22	19–34	Clerks	96.9	0.44	..	..
64	35–54	Heavy labor	97.7	0.41	0.12	0.38
101	35–54	Firemen	101.7	0.33	0.09	0.32
37	35–54	Clerks	97.4	0.46	..	..

Table 7. Fatness and Serum Cholesterol

Healthy Men of the Working Class in Naples, Segregated for Fatness by Skinfold Thickness (Arm + Scapula)

	No.	*Skinfold* (mm.)		*Cholesterol* (mg./100 ml.)	
		Range	*Mean*	*Mean*	*S. E.*
	64	8–23	15.8	151.7	±3.4
	64	23–83	36.6	180.8	±4.0
Difference				29.1	±5.2

completely independent of relative body weight both in younger (19–34 years) and older (35–54 years) men. But significant correlations with relative body weight were found for both total serum cholesterol and for the lipid in the beta lipoprotein fraction.

Relative body weight is not an exact measure of true obesity or fatness, and skinfold thickness, which is a direct measure of subcutaneous fat, may be more satisfactory. As shown in Table 7, skinfold thickness and serum total cholesterol are also correlated in these Neapolitans of the working class so there is no doubt about the effect of obesity in this population.

In contrast to the Neapolitans, Table 8 summarizes a simultaneous study on 134 clinically healthy Minnesotans. In these men relative obesity is not related to the serum cholesterol concentration. Only one point of consistency seems to emerge so far. In populations where the general level of cholesterol in the blood is low, as in Naples (5) or in poor men in Madrid (8), the cholesterol concentration tends to be correlated with relative obesity. And in populations characterized by high serum cholesterol, as in England (6), Minnesota, and among rich people in Madrid (8), there is little relationship to obesity.

Table 8. Relative Body Weight vs. Serum Total Cholesterol Concentration, in 134 Clinically Healthy Men, Aged 50–62, in Minnesota

No.	*Relative body weight* (Kg.)		*Cholesterol* (mg./100 ml.)	
	Range	*Mean*	*Mean*	*S. E.*
51	<95	86.9	222.7	±4.7
44	95–104.9	100.4	228.0	±5.9
39	>105	112.7	225.1	±6.6

Table 9. Serum Cholesterol Concentration and Weight Gain from Simple Overeating
Means and Standard Errors for 20 Men

Period	*Weight* (Kg.)	*Cholesterol* (mg./100 ml.)
Control	68.4 ± 2.2	228.5 ± 7.4
5 weeks	71.1 ± 2.3	248.8 ± 9.1
20 weeks	78.9 ± 3.1	252.2 ± 12.7

This is the situation when we study men who are constantly thin or fat in a stable situation. Among men who are losing weight and are actively underfed, the serum cholesterol is almost always low (22, 23, 24). And, as shown in Table 9, among men who are actively gaining weight from overeating, the serum cholesterol tends to rise when weight gain starts but to increase little thereafter as weight gain continues.

This is observed in controlled experiments where the diet is not changed in kind but is merely eaten in excess so that from a few to over 20 Kg. weight is gained in six months. A similar serum cholesterol response is seen in populations who gain weight after the privations of war (23, 24). And it may be remarked that in such populations there is also a parallel change in the incidence and mortality from arteriosclerotic heart disease.

CHARACTER OF THE DIET: HUMAN EXPERIMENTS

It is now well known that when patients are put on extremely low fat diets, such as Kempner's rice-fruit diet, there usually is a prompt and substantial fall in the blood cholesterol (7, 25–28). Some years ago we showed that the absence of cholesterol in the diet is not responsible but that any diet low in fat tends to have this effect (7, 13). During the past four years we have studied this question systematically and Table 10 summarizes some of the results.

Table 10. Change in Serum Lipid Concentrations in Physically Healthy Men, as Percentages of the Control Values, after 3 to 4 Weeks on Experimental Diets

Mean Values, and Standard Errors, for Total Cholesterol, S_f 12–20 Lipoprotein, α and β Lipoprotein Cholesterol, and Phospholipids

Item	*% calories from fats*		
	24	*18*	*9*
Cholesterol	-7.6 ± 2.0	-8.7 ± 2.4	-9.8 ± 2.2
S_f 12–20	-8.4 ± 5.4	$+12.2 \pm 17.5$	-0.3 ± 5.2
α Cholesterol	-8.2 ± 2.0	..	-5.3 ± 2.7
β Cholesterol	-6.0 ± 3.0	..	-10.8 ± 3.4
Phospholipid	$+1.8 \pm 3.4$	..	-6.7 ± 4.2

The control diet provided 38 to 39 per cent of calories from fats. Thirty-five to 48 men in each experiment except on the 18 per cent fat diet where there were 23 men.

Table 11. Change in Serum Cholesterol from Control Level after Change to a Moderately Low-fat Diet Rigidly Constant for 32 Weeks

Means for 9 Men

Weeks	*Serum cholesterol change* (mg./100 ml.)	*Weeks*	*Serum cholesterol change* (mg./100 ml.)
1	−17	16	−31
2	−16	28	−28
4	−24	32	−26

In these experiments each subject was stabilized for at least a month on the control diet and the intake of calories, proteins, vitamins, and cholesterol was constant throughout. The only alteration was the substitution of carbohydrate calories for fat calories. This dietary manipulation clearly resulted in a change in the serum concentration of total cholesterol and of the cholesterol in both the alpha and beta lipoprotein fractions. The changes in the S_f 12–20 ultracentrifugal fraction and in the phospholipids, however, were not statistically significant.

Such experiments are difficult to continue for long but, as shown in Table 11, it was possible to carry out one experiment for 36 weeks, including 32 weeks on the reduced fat diet. The serum lipid responses to such dietary changes persisted as long as we were able to maintain the changed diet.

This is borne out also by the data summarized in Table 12, from the experiment of Groen *et al.* (18) on 60 normal human volunteers. During twelve weeks on each controlled diet there was a major change in serum cholesterol in the first month and subsequently a slight tendency for the change to increase as the diet was continued for the next

Table 12. Mean Serum Total Cholesterol Values for 60 Healthy Volunteers Before and at Intervals during Subsistence on a Luxurious Diet and on a Vegetarian Diet

Diet	*Mean serum total cholesterol values*		
	Control	*During diets* (weeks from start)	
		3, 4, 5	*10, 11, 12*
Luxurious	216	242	248
Vegetarian	224	202	199

Data from Groen *et al.* (18).

two months. It is not possible to identify the responsible dietary factor or factors in this Dutch experiment because there were simultaneous changes in fats, calories, proteins, and cholesterol in the diet, but it is clear that a more luxurious high-fat diet caused the cholesterol to rise and a vegetarian diet caused it to fall. On the luxurious diet 45 per cent of the calories were supplied as fats while the corresponding figure for the vegetarian diet was 37 per cent.

POPULATIONS ON DIFFERENT DIETS

We have repeatedly stressed the value of the study of properly selected populations for comparisons of dietary effects as they actually occur in nature (13, 16, 21, 22, 29). If the interest is on diets differing in fat content, then there is a wide range of choice, as indicated in Table 13. Fats provide from less than 10 per cent of the calories, as in Japan, among the South African Bantu, and in many parts of Asia and Africa, to our own level of over 40 per cent in the United States. Most Eskimos have much lower fat diets (30). Swedes and Canadians eat relatively

Table 13. Approximate Percentage of Dietary Calories Supplied from Total Fats in the Period 1951–1953

Country	*Calories from fat (%)*	*Country*	*Calories from fat (%)*
Japan	8	Greece	24
S. A. (Bantu)	10	France	30
India	13	Holland	34
Turkey	14	England	35
Brazil	18	Australia	38
Portugal	20	Sweden	38
Italy	20	Canada	38
Spain	22	U. S. A.	41

Compiled from data of F. A. O. and other sources.

high fat diets, while Spaniards and Italians, on the average, have diets low in fat. It is interesting that in the Western countries, where racial, cultural, and climatic differences are minimal, the range of fat consumption is great but the proportion of calories supplied by proteins is remarkably constant, being consistently from 11 to 14 per cent, usually between 12 and 13 per cent.

From our dietary experiments in Minnesota we expected that differences in fat consumption of populations should be reflected in the serum concentrations of cholesterol and perhaps other components of the lipid system. Explorations in 1951–1952 demonstrated both the feasibility of field work on these questions and the general soundness of the approach (5, 6, 8). In 1954 more extensive studies were possible in Italy and in Sweden. Some of the most recent results are summarized here.

In Naples, where the general diet averages about 20 per cent of calories from fats, we studied 356 heavy workers, firemen, and clerks and 46 men of the wealthy class who eat a diet higher in fats than the general population. As a sample of Italians on a diet much higher in fats than that of Naples or Italy as a whole, we studied 54 policemen of Bologna. The average diet in Bologna is estimated to provide 28 to 30 per cent of the calories from fats. Finally, we studied, simultaneously, 205 men in the Twin Cities of Minnesota in whose diets fats provided slightly over 40 per cent of the calories. The men in the various groups were suitably distributed from age 18 to age 60 and all were clinically healthy. The cholesterol findings are summarized in Fig. 1.

Clearly, the men of the general Naples population have much lower serum cholesterol values than the Minnesotans, the difference of some 40 mg. in the twenties rising to a difference of nearly 60 mg. per cent in the fifties. All of the groups of men show an age trend but this is trivial among the Neapolitan working men after the early thirties. The Naples "bankers" and the Bolognese policemen are intermediate, about as would be predicted on the theory of the controlling effect of the proportion of fat in the diet.

It should be observed that the cholesterol differences summarized in Fig. 1 are considerably greater than we have found in controlled experiments on man with similar diets. This suggests, as is reasonable, that lifelong subsistence on these diets produces more effect than results in a few weeks or months. However, consideration should be given to other factors in the diet or in the mode of life of possible relevance. There are several obvious questions.

First, are there differences in calorie habitus and relative obesity which might be involved? The answer to this is no. The average relative body

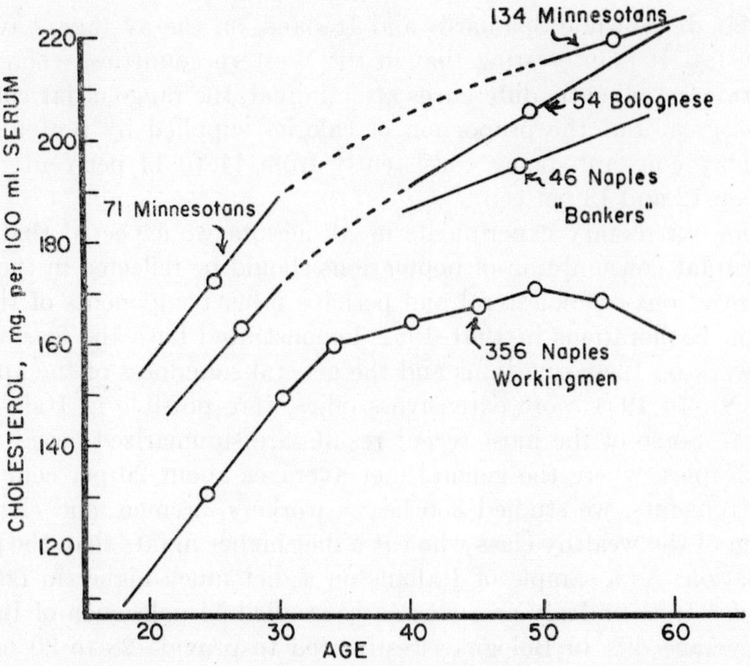

Fig. 1. Serum cholesterol data obtained in 1954 in Minnesota and in Italy. Mean values.

weights of the Neapolitans and of the Minnesotans are both in the range of 98 to 102 per cent of U. S. standards and matching the groups exactly in regard to relative body weight does not affect the observed cholesterol differences. The Bolognese policemen tended to be overweight, averaging 108 per cent for their height and age but, as shown in Table 14, this does not explain the large difference between them and the Neapolitans. A difference of 31.8 mg. per 100 ml., or 18 per cent of the Naples average, remains.

Considerations of differences in physical activity is not helpful either. The physical activity of the Naples firemen is much like that of the Bologna policemen and the physical activity of our Minnesota subjects resembles that of the Naples clerks. And among the Neapolitans, there were no significant cholesterol or other lipid differences related to physical activity; heavy workers, moderate workers, and sedentary clerks were substantially the same.

The factor of race does not seem to be significant; at least it does not explain the serum lipid differences observed between groups of Spaniards (8) or between the various groups of Italians.

It is conceivable that other dietary differences besides those in total fat consumption may affect the serum lipids. In all of the various popu-

Table 14. Serum Cholesterol Concentrations in Bolognese and in Neapolitans Matched for Age and Relative Body Weight

No.	*City*	*Mean age*	*Mean rel. wt.* (Kg.)	*Cholesterol* (mg./100 ml.) *Mean*	*S.E.*
34	Bologna	49.3	108.4	209.3	
34	Naples	49.1	107.9	177.5	
Difference, 34 pairs				31.8	±7.3

lations studied here the proportion of the total calories supplied from proteins is substantially constant and in none of the subjects were there evidences of vitamin or mineral deficiencies. Further and more detailed studies on the diets are desirable but only the factor of fat intake appears important so far.

Studies on Bantu

As a follow-up of our first (1952) report on studies in Italy, Walker and Arvidsson (31) made a study on populations in the Johannesburg area of South Africa. A part of their findings, with the cholesterol values converted to equivalence of the method used here, is summarized in Table 15. The South African Europeans, whose diet follows the North European and American pattern of high fat, are similar in cholesterol concentration to Minnesotans, but the Bantu, whose diet provides only some 10 to 20 per cent of calories from fats, have much lower values. Europeanized Bantu, whose diets are slightly more luxurious than that of their fellows, tend to have slightly higher cholesterol values.

Table 15. Mean Serum Cholesterol Values of Bantu and of Minnesotans (1953–1954), with Equivalent Methods and at Equal Age, Expressed as Percentage of the Mean for South African Europeans (S. A. E.) at Age 28

Group	*Mean age 28*		*Mean age 46*	
	No.	*Chol.* (mg./100 ml.)	*No.*	*Chol.* (mg./100 ml.)
S. A. E.	55	100	46	116
Minnesota	70	106	46	125
Bantu	85	81	54	87
Bantu, Eur.[a]	69	86	..	..

Computed from data of Walker and Arvidsson (31) on ordinary Bantu, Europeanized Bantu (Eur.), and S. A. E., and new data on Minnesotans.

[a] Mean age 31 years.

The findings in South Africa fit nicely into the picture of a dominating influence of dietary fats on the serum cholesterol.

Studies in Sweden

Immediately after the end of the work in Italy last spring, parallel studies on men in Malmö, Sweden, were undertaken by Professor H. Malmros and Drs. Gunnar Biörck and Bengt Swahn (32), who had participated in some of the work in Italy. A comparison of some of the findings in Sweden with those obtained in Naples is shown in Fig. 2. There were 459 men in the Swedish series, equally divided among heavy workers, firemen, and clerks.

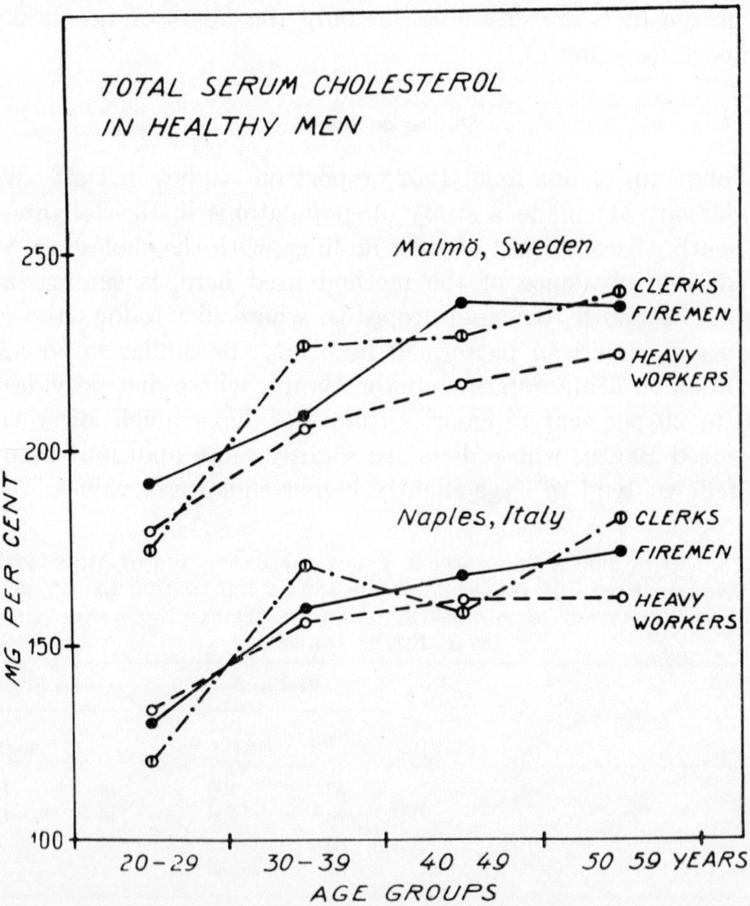

Fig. 2. Comparison of 1954 cholesterol findings in Naples, Italy, and in Malmö, Sweden, the latter being obtained by Prof. H. Malmros and Drs. Gunnar Biörck and Bengt Swahn.

As in Naples, there was little difference between the men according to their physical activity, though there may be a slight tendency for the heavy workers to have lower cholesterol values, especially at the older ages. But the difference between these Swedes and the Neapolitans is very impressive, averaging 50 to 60 mg. per 100 ml. There was a similar but not quite so striking difference between the concentrations of lipid in the beta lipoproteins when the Swedes and the Neapolitans were compared.

There are no reliable figures on the local diet in Malmö but there is no doubt that the fat content there is at least as high, and probably is higher, than the average for the whole of Sweden. For 1953 the average Swedish diet was estimated from official figures to provide 37.5 per cent of the calories from fats and 11.5 per cent from proteins.

Figure 2 compares the approximate average cholesterol concentrations in the serum in several populations of healthy men of age 25 and at age 50. At age 25, the highest averages, in Minnesota and in Southern Sweden, are some 50 mg. of cholesterol per 100 ml. above the averages for Naples and for the Bantu; at age 50 the maximum difference between averages is about 75 mg. per 100 ml. The regularity of the relationship is notable.

Other Studies

The conclusions reached here about the important effect of the level of total fat metabolism on the blood cholesterol in man are supported by other observations. The cholesterol and the beta lipoprotein concentration is low in the serum of Guatemala Indians, who live on a low-fat diet (33, 34). After the war the Germans, who were forced to live on a low-fat diet, had low serum cholesterol values and these rose as the dietary fat was increased (23, 24). Patients put on low-fat, low-cholesterol diets show declines in serum cholesterol and in the beta lipoprotein S_f 12–20 fractions (12).

There are also some questions that need further investigation. It has been reported that heavy drinkers have low serum cholesterol values (35). And it has been reported that artificial diets extremely high in fats, with fats contributing 70 per cent or more of the calories, may actually lower the blood cholesterol (36). What may be involved in these situations is obscure.

Neither space nor presently available knowledge allow a detailed discussion of the mechanisms involved in this dietary fat control of the blood lipids. They are unquestionably very complex.

SUMMARY

1. Lipids exist in the blood serum as emulsions ("chylomicrons") and as solutions of lipoproteins containing proteins, cholesterol, and other lipids. Interest in relation to atherosclerosis is centered on the cholesterol and the beta lipoproteins which contain most of the cholesterol.

2. The diet influences the blood lipids in man and animals but great quantitative differences between species makes it essential to study man himself to discover the effects of the diet on the blood lipids in man.

3. The amount of lipid in the chylomicron form in the serum is practically independent of the concentration of cholesterol and lipoproteins in the serum. The correlation between the concentrations of alpha and beta lipoproteins is very low.

4. Experiments on man show that dietary cholesterol per se, even in large amount, has no important influence on the serum cholesterol concentration but that the latter is markedly affected by the total fat content of the diet.

5. Calorie intake per se has little influence on the blood lipids. Such effect as it has may be secondary to fat metabolism differences commonly associated with differences in calorie intakes.

6. Studies on population samples of healthy men show a marked direct relationship between the content or proportion of fat in the diet on the one hand and the concentration of total cholesterol and of beta lipoproteins in the serum on the other. The effect of the diet tends to be greater in middle-aged men than in younger men.

7. The average concentration of cholesterol in the serum of men in areas where the diets are very high in fats (of the order of 40 per cent of calories), is 25 to 50 per cent greater than the average in areas where the diets are low in fats (of the order of 20 per cent, or less, of calories).

8. A significant effect of dietary fat level on the serum cholesterol concentration is evident in man in a few weeks on a changed diet. The effect tends to increase very slowly with time thereafter and it is most pronounced when comparison is made between populations habitually subsisting on different diets.

9. It is not known how the dietary fat intake exerts its controlling influence on the blood lipids of man but the mechanisms must be complex.

REFERENCES

1. Abell, L. L., Levy, B. B., Brodie, B. B., and Kendall, F. E., *J. Biol. Chem.* **195**, 357 (1952).

2. Schoenheimer, R., and Sperry, W. M., *J. Biol. Chem.* **106,** 745 (1934).
3. Sperry, W. M., and Webb, M., *J. Biol. Chem.* **187,** 97 (1950).
4. Keys, A., *Fed. Proc.* **8,** 523 (1949).
5. Keys, A., Fidanza, F., Scardi, V., Bergami, G., Keys, M. H., and di Lorenzo, F., *Arch. Internal Med.* **93,** 328 (1954).
6. Keys, A., and Keys, M. H., *Brit. J. Nutrition* **8,** 138 (1954).
7. Keys, A., Mickelsen, O., Miller, E. v. O., and Chapman, C. B., *Science* **112,** 79 (1950).
8. Keys, A., Vivanco, F., Miñon, J. L. R., Keys, M. H., and Mendoza, H. C., *Metabolism* **3,** 195 (1954).
9. Lindgren, F. T., Elliott, H. A., and Gofman, J. W., *J. Physical Colloid Chem.* **55,** 80, (1951).
10. Swahn, B., *Scan. J. Clin. Lab. Invest.* **5,** Supplement 9 (1953).
11. Keys, A., and Brozek, J., *Physiol. Rev.* **33,** 245 (1953).
12. Gofman, J. W., *Bull. New York Acad. Med.* **28,** 279 (1952).
13. Keys, A., *Circulation* **5,** 115 (1952).
14. Kinsell, L. W., Michaels, G., de Wind, G., Partridge, J., and Boling, L., *California Med.* **78,** 5 (1953).
15. Gertler, M. M., Garn, S. M., and White, P. D., *Circulation* **2,** 696 (1950).
16. Keys, A., and Anderson, J. T., *Nat. Res. Council Symposium on Atherosclerosis,* March, 1954, in press.
17. Groen, J., Kamminga, C. E., and Reisel, J. H., *Ned. Tijds. v. Geneesk.* **94,** 728 (1950).
18. Groen, J., Tjiong, B. K., and Kamminga, C. E., *Voeding* (Amsterdam) **13,** 556 (1952).
19. Kornerup, V., *Arch. Internal Med.* **86,** 212 (1950).
20. Tanner, J. M., *J. Physiol.* **115,** 371 (1951).
21. Keys, A., *Voeding* (Amsterdam) **13,** 539 (1952).
22. Keys, A., *J. Mt. Sinai Hosp.* **20,** 118 (1953).
23. Schettler, G., Verh. Deut. Geselis. inn. Med., **59,** 194 (1953).
24. Schettler, G., *Deut. med. Wschr.* **78,** 989 (1953).
25. Chapman, C. B., Gibbons, T., and Henschel, A., *New Eng. J. Med.* **243,** 899 (1950).
26. Kempner, W., *Amer. J. Med.* **4,** 545 (1948).
27. Nelson, A. M., *Northwest Med.* **51,** 860 (1952).
28. Schwartz, W. B., and Merlis, J. K., *J. Clin. Invest.* **27,** 406 (1948).
29. Keys, A., *Assoc. Life Insur. Med. Directors Amer.* **38,** (1954) in press.
30. Sinclair, H. M., *Proc. Nutr. Soc.* **12,** 69 (1953).
31. Walker, A. R. P., *J. Clin. Invest.* (1954), in press.
32. Malmros, H., Biörck, G., and Swahn, B., *Proc. Third Internat. Congress Internal Med.,* Stockholm, Sept. 1954.
33. Mann, G. V., Munos, J. A., and Scrimshaw, N. S., *Fed. Proc.* **13,** 467 (1954).
34. Mann, G. V., and Stare, F. J., *Nat. Res. Council Symposium on Atherosclerosis,* March 1954, in press.
35. Hobson, W., Jordan, A., and Roseman, C., *Lancet* 961 (Nov. 1953).
36. Kinsell, L. W., Partridge, J., Boling, L., Margen, S., and Michaels, G., *J. Clin. Endocrin. Metab.* **12,** 909 (1952).
37. Cook, R. P., and Thomson, R. O., *Quart. J. Exp. Physiol.* **36,** 61 (1951).
38. Forbes, J. C., and Petterson, O. M., *Proc. Soc. Exp. Biol. Med.* **83,** 665 (1953).
39. Kesten, H. D., and Silbowitz, R., *Proc. Soc. Exp. Biol. Med.* **49,** 71 (1942).
40. Kritchevsky, D., Moyer, A. W., Tesar, W. C., Logan, J. B., Brown R. A., Davies, M. C., and Cox, H. R., *Amer. J. Physiol.* **178,** 30 (1954).
41. Nichols, C. W., Siperstein, M. D., and Chaikoff, I. L., *Proc. Soc. Exp. Biol. Med.* **83,** 756 (1953).
42. Seifter, J., Baeder, D. H., Beckfield, W. J., Sharma, G. P., and Ehrich, W. E., *Proc. Soc. Exp. Biol. Med.* **83,** 468 (1953).

43. Strumpf, H. H., and Wilens, S. L., *Proc. Soc. Exp. Biol. Med.* **86,** 219 (1954).
44. Katz, L. N., and Stamler, J., *Experimental Atherosclerosis*, Thomas, Springfield, Ill., 1953.
45. Rodbard, S., Bolene, C., and Katz, L. N., *Circulation* **4,** 43 (1951).
46. Stamler, J., and Katz, L. N., *Circulation* **2,** 705 (1950).
47. Horlick, L., and Havel, L., *J. Lab. Clin. Med.* **33,** 1029 (1948).
48. Sperry, W. M., and Stoyanoff, V. A., *J. Nutrition* **9,** 131 (1935).
49. Swell, L., and Flick, D. F., *Amer. J. Physiol.* **174,** 51 (1953).
50. Gould, R. G., *Amer. J. Med.* **12,** 209 (1951).
51. Gould, R. G., Taylor, C. B., Hagerman, J. S., Warner, I., and Campbell, D. J., *J. Biol. Chem.* **201,** 519 (1953).
52. Greenberg, L. D., and Rinehart, J. F., *Proc. Soc. Exp. Biol. Med.* **76,** 580 (1951).
53. Mann, G. V., Andrus, S. B., McNally, A., and Stare, F. J., *J. Exp. Med.* **98,** 195 (1953).
54. Heymann, W., and Rack, F., *Amer. J. Dis. Child.* **65,** 235 (1943).
55. Moses, C., *Amer. J. Med. Sci.* **224,** 212 (1952).
56. Moses, C., Rhodes, G. L., Leathem, E., and George, R. S., *Circulation*, **6,** 103 (1952).
57. Okey, R., and Stewart, D., *J. Biol. Chem.* **99,** 717 (1933).
58. Steiner, A., *Amer. J. Med.* **6,** 117 (1949).
59. Messinger, W. J., Porosawska, Y., and Steele, J. M., *Arch. Int. Med.* **86,** 189 (1950).

Oxidation and Synthesis of Fatty Acids in Soluble Enzyme Systems of Animal Tissues

David E. Green

During the past two years the complete reconstruction of fatty acid oxidation with combinations of highly purified enzymes has been successfully accomplished. Now that the excitement of the participating groups has died down it may be desirable to review the general field of fatty acid oxidation and synthesis according to a logical plan without stressing unduly the chronology of developments.

To the best of our knowledge fatty acids are oxidized exclusively within one site in animal cells, the mitochondrion (1, 2). When we say that the process of fatty acid oxidation is localized within the mitochondrion just what do we mean? Do we infer that the mitochondrion is like a red blood corpuscle—a structure with a membrane separating the internal fluid content from the outside medium—and that within the internal fluid all the enzymes and coenzymes of the fatty acid oxidation system are in solution reacting with one another by a process of random collision? Or are we to think of the mitochondrion in terms of the concept of the cyclophorase complex of enzymes (3)—a giant macromolecule arising from the complexing and association of hundreds of separate enzymes—arranged in a very precise and intricate pattern of organization? According to this concept juxtaposition of the enzymes which follow one another serially in a particular metabolic sequence is the principle which makes random diffusion and collision unnecessary, and which makes possible interactions that are difficult to duplicate with combinations of separate, unassociated enzymes. In the closing part of the present review I intend to mention some recent work in our laboratory on one of the enzymes of the fatty acid oxidation system

---

From the Institute for Enzyme Research, University of Wisconsin, Madison, Wisconsin.
Presented at the Symposium on Lipids and Lipoproteins, 126th National Meeting of The American Chemical Society. In participation with the American Association of Clinical Chemists; September 16, 1954, New York City, N. Y.

Table 1. PRODUCTS OF OXIDATION OF FATTY ACIDS

Source of mitochondria	*Even-numbered acids* (C_4 *to* C_{18})	*Odd-numbered acids* (C_5 *to* C_{17})
Heart	CO_2, H_2O	Propionate, CO_2, H_2O
Kidney	CO_2, H_2O	Propionate, CO_2, H_2O
Liver	Acetoacetate, CO_2, H_2O	Acetoacetate, CO_2, H_2O

that may have considerable bearing on the questions which I have just raised.

Let us begin by examining some of the characteristics of fatty acid oxidation as it is catalyzed by suspensions of mitochondria. In presence of kidney or heart mitochondria and with appropriate additions even numbered fatty acids from C_4 to C_{18} (Table 1) are oxidized completely to CO_2 and H_2O (4). The corresponding β-hydroxy acids, α-β unsaturated acids, and β-ketoacids are also oxidized to completion and at about the same rate. The odd numbered fatty acids are oxidized as rapidly as the even numbered fatty acids but with the difference that propionic acid accumulates as an end product in addition to CO_2 and water. When liver mitochondria are used instead of kidney or heart mitochondria, two important differences emerge in the pattern of fatty acid oxidation. In the first place, acetoacetate also accumulates as one of the end products of the oxidation of even numbered fatty acids (4–6). Second, propionic acid does not accumulate as the end product of the oxidation of odd numbered fatty acids since propionic acid is readily oxidized, at least by rabbit liver mitochondria, to CO_2 and water (7).[1]

THE CITRIC ACID CYCLE

Fatty acids as such are not oxidized by mitochondria (8). Unless some member of the citric acid cycle is undergoing oxidation simultaneously fatty acid oxidation does not start (Table 2). Members of the citric acid cycle or substances which give rise to members of the cycle are referred to as sparkers since their oxidation sparks the oxidation of fatty acids. There are two functions served by the sparker which we will consider separately.

First, when any member of the citric acid cycle undergoes oxidation by molecular oxygen, inorganic phosphate in the suspending medium becomes esterified and ultimately converted to adenosine triphosphate (ATP) (9). It is the generation of ATP by oxidative phosphorylation which is one of the two functions of the sparker. ATP triggers the first

[1] Rat liver mitochondria do not show this capacity for oxidizing propionate (5).

Table 2. Sparking of Fatty Acid Oxidation by Fumarate Kidney Cyclophorase System

Additions	*Oxygen uptake*
Butyrate (30 μm)	10
Butyrate + fumarate (0.5 μm)	200
Butyrate + fumarate (3.0 μm)	287
Octanoate (5 μm)	0
Octanoate + fumarate (0.5 μm)	140

The values for the sparked oxidations have been corrected for the oxygen uptake due to the oxidation of fumarate (8).

step of fatty acid oxidation, the conversion of the fatty acid to the corresponding coenzyme A derivative (10–12). Coenzyme A (CoA) is a complex nucleotide whose structure (shown in Fig. 1) has recently been established by Lipmann and his group (13, 14). For present purposes it can be conceived of as merely a vehicle for an SH group which can readily become acylated to form an acyl thiol ester.

Now we come to the second function of the sparker. These thioesters —the fatty acyl derivatives of CoA—are oxidized by repetitions of a cyclical process which has been called the β-oxidation cycle (15) (Fig. 2). At each turn of the cycle, acetyl CoA is liberated. For reasons which will become clear later, acetyl CoA cannot accumulate as such without bringing the process to a quick stop. The sparker in the course of oxidation gives rise to oxalacetate which condenses with acetyl CoA to form citrate, CoA being liberated in the process. This condensation reaction, discovered and documented so brilliantly by Ochoa and his group (16), may be considered as a device not only for regenerating coenzyme A needed in the initial activation of fatty acids but also for perpetuating

Structural Units of Coenzyme A

Adenine—ribose (-3 phosphate)-phosphate
|
HS-CH_2-CH_2-NH-β-alanine-pantoic-phosphate

CoASH—thiol form of CoA

CoASCOR—acyl thiolester of CoA

Fig. 1. Structural units of coenzyme A.

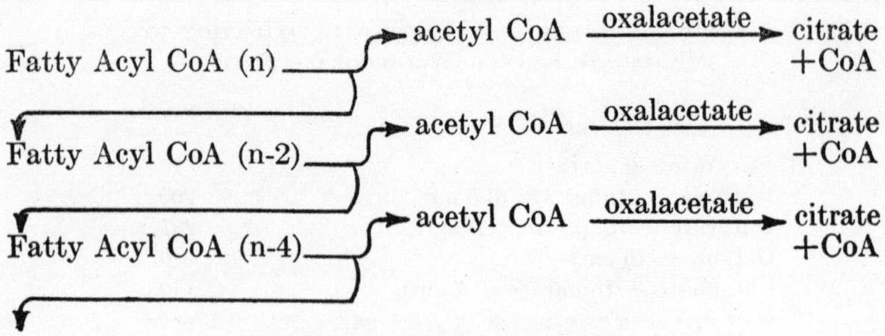

Fig. 2. Scheme for β-oxidation.

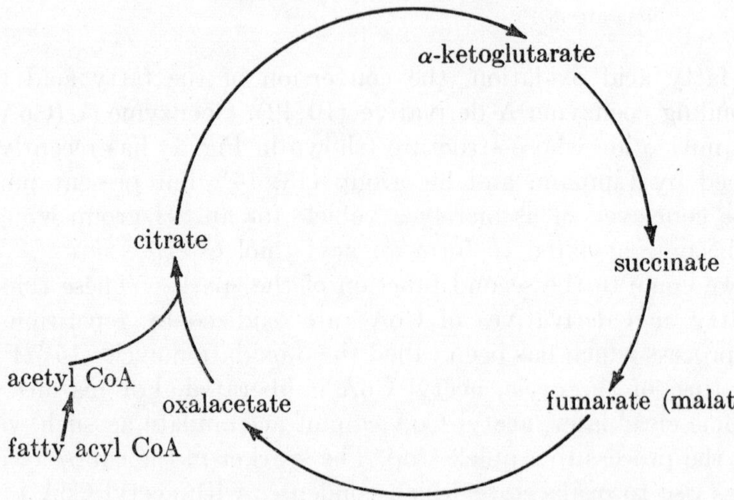

Fig. 3. Citric and fatty acid oxidation cycles.

sparker (Fig. 3). Citrate formed as the product of the condensation can now undergo oxidation back to oxalacetate through α-ketoglutarate, succinate, and malate as intermediates. This is in fact the pathway of the citric acid cycle. In addition each one of these intermediary oxidative steps generates ATP needed for the initial activation of the fatty acid. Thus the conversion of one mole of citrate to oxalacetate is attended by the formation of some 12 moles of ATP.

In theory, at any rate, a catalytic amount of sparker should spark the oxidation of an unlimited amount of fatty acid. Once initiated the process should be self-perpetuating. In practice that is not entirely true. Some fraction of the total number of molecules of oxalacetate formed undergoes decarboxylation to pyruvate or transamination with glutamate or other amino acids. There is, in other words, a constant loss of sparker in side reactions. Thus, to keep the fatty acid oxidation pot always on the boil, a not inconsiderable amount of sparker must be present at all times.

Acetyl CoA cannot accumulate as the end product of fatty acid oxidation in mitochondria since CoA is present only in catalytic amounts. Thus, unless CoA can go through a cycle of esterification and deesterification, the oxidation would grind to a halt as soon as all the CoA became esterified. The citrate condensation step is one device for release of coenzyme A (16). We shall discuss later the formation of acetoacetate as another device evolved by liver for accomplishing the same purpose. But we will forego consideration of acetoacetate formation until the individual enzymes of fatty acid oxidation have been discussed in more detail.

THE STEPS OF FATTY ACID OXIDATION

It is essentially impossible to recognize the individual steps of fatty acid oxidation in the mitochondrial system. This system is designed for the initial fatty acids to go directly to CO_2 and water without accumulating more than catalytic amounts of intermediary products. Two preliminary steps were necessary for the study of intermediates and of the enzymes which accomplish these transformations: ways and means had to be found of releasing the individual enzymes of the fatty acid oxidation system from mitochondria, and at the same time, methods and technics had to be devised for studying one-step reactions. In point of fact until appropriate methods became available there was no way of recognizing the individual enzymes involved in one-step reactions.

Availability of Coenzyme A

Fatty acid oxidation as it proceeds in mitochondria involves catalytic amounts of CoA and an elaborate cycle to regenerate CoA. If one had to reproduce such an arrangement for regeneration of CoA it would be virtually impossible to study in a test tube any one enzyme process in simple fashion. Clearly the proper substrate of each of the enzymes has to be provided in excess, and that means preparing the various acyl derivatives of CoA in substrate amounts. There are two different ways of accomplishing this preparative task. The first involves the use of the very enzymes which carry out the task in the mitochondrion—in other words, the activation enzymes which carry out the ATP-catalyzed esterification of CoA by fatty acids or by fatty acid derivatives as shown in Equation 1:

1. ATP + CoASH + fatty acid $\rightleftharpoons$ S-fatty acyl CoA + AMP + inorganic pyrophosphate (11, 12)

The second is that of chemical synthesis of which there are now three variations shown in Equations 2–4:

2. Fatty anhydride + CoASH → S-fatty acyl CoA + fatty acid (17)
3. Fatty acyl thiophenol + CoASH → S-fatty acyl CoA + thiophenol (18)
4. Fatty thioacid + CoASH → S-fatty acyl CoA + H_2S, (19)

One of the simplest involves the condensation of fatty anhydrides with SHCoA in bicarbonate solution. Other methods make use of thioacids or acylthiophenols as the acylating agents for coenzyme A.

I should add parenthetically that none of these preparative methods would be practical unless coenzyme A were available in relatively large amounts. It is perhaps no coincidence that the solution of the problem of reconstructing fatty acid oxidation followed almost immediately on the publication of a method for large-scale isolation of coenzyme A which made possible commercial production of this hitherto rare coenzyme on an almost unlimited scale (20).

Isolation of Mitochondria

When aqueous mitochondrial suspensions are treated with some 10 volumes of acetone the resulting acetone powder contains dried, damaged mitochondria which when extracted with dilute salt solutions readily release the enzymes of the fatty acid oxidation cycle (21, 22). These enzymes after solubilization can now be separated one from another by the conventional methods of protein purification.

Since the enzymes in question are localized in mitochondria it is obvious that great initial purification can be obtained by first separating particles generally from the soluble constituents of the cell and then separating mitochondria by differential centrifugation from other cell particulates. While the isolation of mitochondria by this type of procedure had been accomplished some years previously through the efforts of Hogeboom and Schneider (23) the technic had been applied exclusively to tissues of laboratory animals. In our own laboratory it has been found possible to prepare mitochondrial suspensions suitable for isolation of enzymes on a very large scale from slaughter-house material (11, 24). This development has simplified enormously the task of purifying the enzymes of fatty acid oxidation.

The Four Basic Reactions

Even Numbered Fatty Acids

Now let us make an over-all survey of the four basic reactions in the fatty acid oxidation cycle as summarized in Equations 5–8:

5. $RCH_2CH_2COS\overline{CoA} \xrightarrow{-2H} RCH{=}CHCOS\overline{CoA}$ (25, 27)

6. $RCH{=}CHCOS\overline{CoA} + H_2O \rightarrow RCHOHCH_2COS\overline{CoA}$ (28, 29)

7. $RCHOHCH_2COS\overline{CoA} \xrightarrow{-2H} RCOCH_2COS\overline{CoA}$ (15, 30)

8. $RCOCH_2COS\overline{CoA} + CoASH \rightarrow RCOS\overline{CoA} + CH_3COS\overline{CoA}$ (15, 31)

The fatty acyl CoA is oxidized by a flavoprotein enzyme to the corresponding α-β unsaturated acyl CoA derivative (25). In turn this unsaturated derivative is hydrated to form the L configurational β-hydroxyacyl CoA (32). Then a second oxidation takes place at the β-carbon atom leading to the formation of the β-ketoacyl CoA (33, 34). Finally the β-ketoacyl CoA is cleaved in the presence of a molecule of free CoA, resulting in two products of cleavage, acetyl CoA and a fatty acyl CoA with two carbon atoms less than the parent fatty acyl CoA (15, 31).

This new acyl CoA now undergoes a repeat of the four above mentioned reactions while acetyl CoA is condensed with oxalacetate to form citrate. These four reactions constitute one turn of the β-oxidation cycle which continues until eventually all the fatty acid molecule has been transformed into acetyl CoA (Fig. 4). This point is reached when the β-ketoacyl CoA has only four carbon atoms. The cleavage of this derivative leads to two molecules of acetyl CoA and no residue is left.

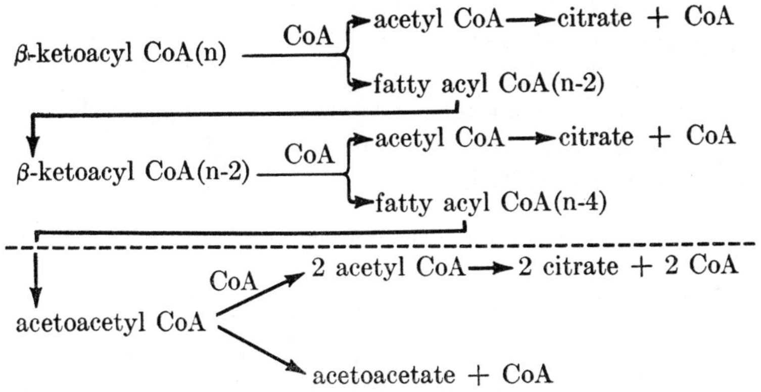

Fig. 4. Alternative pathways of fatty acid degradation.

Odd Numbered Fatty Acids

Let us consider what happens when a fatty acid with an odd number of carbon atoms is subjected to the β-oxidation sequence. Successive degradation eventually leads to a five carbon β-ketoacyl CoA which on cleavage yields acetyl CoA and propionyl CoA. There is no possibility of further reaction for propionyl CoA in the case of mitochondria other than from liver. Deacylation of propionyl CoA by enzymes present in kidney and heart mitochondria yields propionic acid which accumulates as such.

Action of Liver Mitochondria

In the case of liver mitochondria an alternative pathway is provided at the stage of acetoacetyl CoA (Fig. 4). In addition to the possibility of cleavage to two molecules of acetyl CoA, acetoacetyl CoA can be deacylated to form acetoacetate and free CoA (35). When any reagent which interferes with the citric acid cycle, such as malonate, is added to liver mitochondria (5, 6) or when a physiologic situation exists—as in diabetes mellitus—where generation of members of the citric acid cycle is interfered with or suppressed, then the deacylation mechanism becomes the exclusive mechanism for disposal of acetoacetyl CoA. The accumulation of the so-called acetone bodies (derived from acetoacetic acid) is a token that the level of sparker in liver has been reduced well below normal.

There is a very simple explanation for the fact that acetoacetate accumulates only in liver. Liver is by no means the only tissue which contains an enzyme capable of deacylating acetoacetyl CoA. However, liver is the only known tissue which lacks an enzyme capable of converting acetoacetate to acetoacetyl CoA in presence of ATP and CoA. Thus while other tissues can form acetoacetate, no accumulation of acetoacetate can be observed since it is pushed back into the metabolic hopper as fast as it is pushed out.

Thus far we have skirted around the edges of the individual enzymes of the β-oxidation cycle and I propose now to consider in more detail each of the pertinent enzymes.

THE KNOWN INDIVIDUAL ENZYMES

Acylation

There are four known enzymes which catalyze the acylation of CoA by fatty acids or by substituted fatty acids in presence of ATP (Table 3). One is specific for acetic and propionic acids (24, 35, 36); a second acts upon fatty acids from C_4 to C_{12} and upon a wide variety of substituted,

Table 3. Fatty Acid Activation Enzymes

Designation	*Chain-length range*	*Specificity*
Acetate (heart)	C_2, C_3	Fatty acids
Mahler-Wakil enzyme (liver)	C_4–C_{12}	Fatty acids + branched, phenyl, β-hydroxy, α-β
Kornberg-Pricer (liver)	C_{10}–C_{18}	Fatty acids + . . .
β-Ketoacid (kidney)	C_4–C_{12}	β-ketoacids

branched, and phenyl fatty acids (11); a third acts upon fatty acids in the range of chain length from C_{10} to C_{18} (12); while a fourth acts generally upon β-ketoacids—a species of substituted acid which is left severely alone by the other enzymes in the group (37). ATP is the only nucleotide which can initiate the acylation and even adenosine diphosphate (ADP) is inactive in this regard. The precise mechanism by which the acylation of CoA is initiated by ATP is still undetermined. In a general way it may be assumed that ATP reacts with the activating enzyme to form pyrophosphoryl enzyme with liberation of adenosine monophosphate (AMP). A series of replacements then take place: fatty acid for the pyrophosphoryl group, and then CoASH for the enzyme. The net reaction is then the conversion of ATP to AMP and P-P, coupled to the acylation of CoA by the fatty acid (cf. Equations 9–11):

9. ATP + enzyme → pyrophosphoryl enzyme + AMP
10. Pyrophosphoryl enzyme + fatty acid + fatty acyl enzyme + pyrophosphate
11. Fatty acyl enzyme + CoASH + S-fatty acyl CoA + enzyme

Jones *et al.* (38, 39) have proposed another mechanism in which the interaction of ATP with enzyme leads to the formation of adenosine-monophosphoryl enzyme with liberation of inorganic pyrophosphate.

The acylation reaction is readily followed by measuring the SH function of CoA. As acylation proceeds the SH group of CoA disappears. The delicate nitroprusside reaction for free SH groups serves as the basis of a very simple and convenient method of assay of the activation enzymes (11).

It should be mentioned that the activation reaction is a reversible one and that the equilibrium constant for the reaction at 30° is about 1 (11).

Dehydrogenation of Fatty Acyl CoA's

There are two known enzymes which catalyze the dehydrogenation of fatty acyl CoA's: a green copper-containing flavoprotein which acts in the C_4 to C_8 chain length range (25, 40), and a yellow, iron-containing flavoprotein which acts on all acyl CoA's from C_4 to C_{18} (26, 35). It can readily be demonstrated that the flavoproteins are reduced coincident with the oxidation of the substrate. The metal plays no role in the primary oxidation of the substrate, as shown by the fact that preparation of these flavoproteins which have been freed of metal are still readily reducible by substrate. The metal is concerned with interaction of the reduced flavoprotein enzyme with one-electron acceptors (40, 41).

The interaction of the two flavoproteins with electron acceptors is a complex process which will be discussed in detail later on. For present purposes it is sufficient to stress that there are two important problems which remain unsolved with respect to the mode of action of the fatty acyl CoA dehydrogenases: first, which oxidant oxidizes their reduced forms physiologically, and second, which reductant reduces them in their oxidized form when the reaction is reversed as in synthesis of long-chain fatty acids from acetyl CoA. The enzymatic oxidation of the fatty acyl CoA's is a reversible process. The oxidation-reduction potential at *p*H 7 is about +0.2V which is the most positive E'_o known for a substrate system (40).

There is no one simple method of following the action of the fatty acyl CoA dehydrogenases which is free from complication or possible sources of error. To make matters worse the interaction of the primary dehydrogenase with electron acceptors is not a direct process and thus does not lend itself to a simple assay. But in a general way the direct reduction of the enzyme by the substrate is the least ambiguous way of demonstrating the dehydrogenase and this can be made the basis of a method for evaluating purity levels (26).

The unsaturated acyl CoA hydrase acts on α,β- and β,γ-unsaturated acyl CoA's regardless of chain length (28). The hydration reaction is reversible. At equilibrium three species are present—the α,β-unsaturated acyl CoA, the β,γ-counterpart, and the β-hydroxyacyl CoA.

The oxidation of L(+),β-hydroxyacyl CoA's by diphosphopyridine nucleotide (DPN) is catalyzed by an enzyme which acts upon derivatives covering the entire gamut of chain length according to Equation 12 (30):

12. β-Hydroxyacyl CoA + $DPN^+ \rightarrow$ β-ketoacyl CoA + DPNH + H^+

The reaction is readily followed kinetically by observing the change in absorption at 340 mμ which accompanies reduction of DPN (15, 30).

At neutral *p*H the equilibrium of the reaction lies almost completely to the left while above *p*H 9 the equilibrium is shifted almost completely to the right. This fact is taken advantage of as the basis of a method for preparing β-ketoacyl CoA's.

The estimation of hydrase is based on the coupling of the hydrase reaction with the subsequent dehydrogenation reaction at *p*H 9 (28). The rate of reduction of DPN can be used as a measure of the rate of hydration of the unsaturated acyl CoA providing the β-hydroxyacyl CoA dehydrogenase is present in excess.

The β-ketoacyl CoA cleavage enzyme acts upon derivatives from C_4 to at least C_{12} (31). The reaction probably proceeds through the sequence shown in Equations 13–14 below:

13. $RCOCH_2COSCoA + Enzyme \rightarrow RCO\ Enzyme + CH_3COSCoA,$
14. $RCO\ Enzyme + CoASH \rightarrow RCOSCoA + Enzyme.$

The enzyme breaks the carbon-to-carbon bond between the α and β carbon atoms of the β-ketoacyl CoA—the acyl group becoming attached to the enzyme while the two-carbon fragment is liberated as acetyl CoA. The acyl enzyme complex is then dissociated by coenzyme A with formation of acyl CoA and liberation of the free enzyme. This process has been aptly called thiolysis by Lynen (33).

The cleavage of acetoacetyl CoA to two molecules of acetyl CoA has been shown to be reversible. The equilibrium point lies almost completely to the side of acetyl CoA (42).

Reductive Synthesis of Fatty Acids

It is of great importance to know whether physiologically the same group of enzymes which catalyze the oxidative breakdown of fatty acids can also bring about the reductive synthesis of long-chain acids from acetyl CoA. Since all the reactions of the fatty acid cycle have been shown to be reversible it should in principle be possible to accomplish synthesis by reversal of the reactions of the β-oxidation cycle.

A partial synthesis has already been reported by Beinert and Stansly (43) who were able to demonstrate the formation of butyryl CoA from acetyl CoA in presence of the four enzymes of the cycle under conditions suitable for synthesis. The key to synthesis lies in the maintenance of reducing conditions. The two oxidative steps can be reversed only when appropriate reducing agents are present.

The problem of the second oxidative step is a simple one since the physiologic electron acceptor is known to be DPN^+. To reverse this oxidation step it is merely sufficient to introduce a dehydrogenase system which can generate DPNH and there are many systems known which can serve in that capacity.

The reversal of the first oxidative step is a somewhat more sticky problem. Cytochrome *c* is the only natural acceptor which is reducible by the acyl CoA dehydrogenase. While there are dehydrogenase systems available which can maintain cytochrome *c* in the reduced state it has been assumed on the basis of oxidation-reduction potential consideration that the head of potential between reduced cytochrome *c* and the acyl CoA dehydrogenase system would not be sufficient to drive the reduction efficiently. In consequence Beinert and Stansly used reduced benzyl viologen as the driving force for the reduction of the unsaturated acyl CoA to the fatty acyl CoA. Benzyl viologen is an artificial acceptor of very negative oxidation-reduction potential which is readily reduced by any of several dehydrogenase systems such as milk xanthine oxidase.

The fact that butyryl CoA was synthesized from acetyl CoA in the Beinert-Stansly system rules out the possibility of inadequate reducing conditions. The failure to synthesize fatty acyl CoA's higher than butyryl CoA must be ascribed to another cause. There is reason to believe that the fault lies with the cleavage enzyme. The equations describing the synthesis of β-ketoacyl CoA's by reversal of the cleavage reaction are shown in Equations 15–17 below:

15. Acetyl CoA + acetyl CoA → β-ketobutyryl CoA + CoA
16. Acetyl CoA + butyryl CoA → β-ketocaproyl CoA + CoA
17. Acetyl CoA + fatty $acyl_n$CoA → β-$ketoacyl_{n+2}$CoA + CoA

If the cleavage enzyme is presented with a mixture of acetyl CoA and butyryl CoA three possibilities of reaction exist. Either Reaction 15 or 16 or both can take place. The particular cleavage enzyme which Beinert and Stansly worked with carried on only Reaction 15 when presented with a mixture of acetyl CoA and butyryl CoA. The explanation for this selectivity is probably as follows. The cleavage enzyme carries out a condensation between acetyl CoA and a fatty acyl CoA. If the affinity of the cleavage enzyme for the fatty acyl CoA increases sharply with decreasing chain length then the condensation of acetyl CoA with the shortest fatty acyl CoA—another molecule of acetyl CoA—will take complete precedence over the condensation of acetyl CoA with a higher fatty acyl CoA such as butyryl CoA.

Popjak and Tietz in England (44) and Gurin *et al.* (45, 46) in this country have been able to show synthesis of long-chain fatty acids from acetate in homogenates and extracts of mammary tissue and liver respectively. It is possible that there are two types of cleavage enzyme.

The first type which is important in oxidation has the characteristics noted by Beinert and Stansly. The second which is important in reductive synthesis may show highest affinity for the long-chain fatty acyl CoA's. That would mean that such a cleavage enzyme would preferentially form long-chain β-ketoacyl CoA's rather than acetoacetyl CoA.

ISOLATION OF DEHYDROGENASES OF ACYL CoA's

The two enzymes which catalyze the dehydrogenation of acyl CoA's to their unsaturated derivatives can be isolated in the form of a complex in which these two flavoproteins are linked to still another flavoprotein which Beinert and Crane have called the electron-transferring flavoprotein (47). The functional interrelationships of these three flavoproteins may be represented diagrammatically, as in Fig. 5. The interaction of the two dehydrogenases with electron acceptors is not direct but has to go through the electron-transferring flavoprotein as an intermediary. Electrophoresis is essentially the only effective procedure for separating the two dehydrogenases from one another and from the electron-transferring flavoprotein. However, the three enzymes form a very tightly associated complex which is not resolved by any of a large number of preparative procedures.

First, let us consider the significance of there being two separate enzymes in the same complex with the same catalytic function which differ only in the range of substrate chain length over which they are effective. The yellow dehydrogenase is active on acyl CoA's from C_4 to C_{18}, but the affinity of the enzyme for the substrate increases with increasing chain length (26). The properties of the yellow dehydrogenase are such that when presented with a mixture of acyl CoA's it will prefer to oxidize the derivatives of longer chain length at the expense of the shorter chain derivatives. This would lead to an undesirable situation under physiologic conditions, namely the accumulation of shorter-chain acyl CoA's and the consequent tying up in enforced idleness of valuable coenzyme A. The green dehydrogenase solves this particular dilemma. At the point in chain length where a fatty acyl CoA cannot compete favorably with the C_{18} derivative (about C_8), it can be acted upon by the green dehydrogenase without interference by the long-chain acyl CoA's since the affinity of the green dehydrogenase for acyl CoA's decreases as the chain length of the acyl CoA's increases.

It is entirely possible that the device of a complex of two enzymes with similar catalytic activities but with different affinities with respect to substrate chain length is not confined to the acyl CoA dehydrogenases but may have its counterpart in all the other enzymes of the β-oxidation sequence. This possibility has yet to be tested experimentally.

Fatty acyl CoA's

short chain → ↓ → green dehyd. ↘

long chain → ↓ → yellow dehyd. ↙

Electron transfer flavo.

↙ ↓ ↘

O_2 cytochrome c dyes

Fig. 5. Electron transfer scheme. According to H. Beinert and F. Crane.

Finally may I call attention to the fact that in the complex of the three flavoproteins which are concerned with the oxidation of fatty acyl CoA's we have a model in miniature of the kind of forces which hold the mitochondrion together and of the remarkable way in which juxtaposition of enzymes with serial function minimizes the random diffusion of substrate molecule from one enzyme to another.

REFERENCES

(1) Schneider, W. C., and Potter, V. R., *J. Biol. Chem.* **177,** 893 (1949).
(2) Lehninger, A. L., and Kennedy, E. P., *J. Biol. Chem.* **179,** 957 (1949).
(3) Green, D. E., *Biol. Rev.* **26,** 410 (1951).
(4) Grafflin, A. L., and Green, D. E., *J. Biol. Chem.* **176,** 95 (1948).
(5) Cheldelin, V. H., and Beinert, H., *Biochim. Biophys. Acta* **9,** 661 (1952).
(6) Lehninger, A. L., *J. Biol. Chem.* **164,** 291 (1946).
(7) Huennekens, F. M., Mahler, H. R., and Nordmann, J., *Arch. Biochem.* **30,** 66 (1951).
(8) Knox, W. E., Noyce, B. N., and Auerbach, V. H., *J. Biol. Chem.* **176,** 117 (1948).
(9) Cross, R. J., Taggart, J. V., Covo, G. A., and Green, D. E., *J. Biol. Chem.* **177,** 655 (1948).
(10) Drysdale, G. R., and Lardy, H. A., *J. Biol. Chem.* **202,** 119 (1953).
(11) Mahler, H. R., Wakil, S. J., and Bock, R. M., *J. Biol. Chem.* **204,** 453 (1953).
(12) Kornberg, A., and Pricer, W. E., Jr., *J. Biol. Chem.* **204,** 329 (1953).
(13) Lipmann, F., Kaplan, N. O., Novelli, G. D., Tuttle, L. C., and Guirard, B. M., *J. Biol. Chem.* **186,** 235 (1950).
(14) Lipmann, F., *Harvey Lect.* **44,** 99 (1948–9).
(15) Lynen, F., and Ochoa, S., *Biochim. Biophys. Acta* **12,** 299 (1953).
(16) Stern, J. R., and Ochoa, S., *J. Biol. Chem.* **191,** 161 (1951).
(17) Simon, E. J., and Shemin, D., *J. Am. Chem. Soc.* **75,** 2520 (1953).
(18) Wieland, T., and Koppe, H., *Ann.* **581,** 1 (1953).
(19) Wilson, I. B., *J. Am. Chem. Soc.* **74,** 3205 (1952).
(20) Beinert, H., Von Korff, R. W., Green, D. E., Buyske, D. A., Handschumacher, R. E., Higgins, H., and Strong, F. M., *J. Biol. Chem.* **200,** 385 (1953).
(21) Drysdale, G., and Lardy, H. A., *in* McElroy, W. D. and Glass, B. (eds.): *Symposium of Phosphorus Metabolism* **2,** 281 (1952).
(22) Beinert, H., Bock, R. M., Goldman, D. S., Green, D. E., Mahler, H. R., Mii, S., Stansly, P. G., and Wakil, S. J., *J. Am. Chem. Soc.* **75,** 4111 (1953).
(23) Schneider, W. C., and Hogeboom, G. H., *Cancer Research* **11,** 1 (1951).
(24) Hele, P., *J. Biol. Chem.* **206,** 671 (1954).
(25) Green, D. E., Mii, S., Mahler, H. R., and Bock, R. M., *J. Biol. Chem.* **206,** 1 (1954).
(26) Crane, F., Beinert, H., Mii, S., and Green, D. E., *J. Biol. Chem.*, to be published.

(27) Lynen, F., Wessely, L., Wielland, O., and Rueff, L., *Z. angew. Chem.* **64,** 687 (1952).
(28) Wakil, S. J., and Mahler, H. R., *J. Biol. Chem.* **207,** 125 (1954).
(29) Stern, J. R., Coon, M. J., and Del Campillo, A., *J. Am. Chem. Soc.* **75,** 2277 (1953).
(30) Green, D. E., Dewan, J. G., and Leloir, L. F., *Biochem. J.* **31,** 934 (1937).
(31) Goldman, D. S., *J. Biol. Chem.* **208,** 345 (1954).
(32) Lehninger, A. L., and Greville, G. D., *J. Am. Chem. Soc.* **75,** 1515 (1953).
(33) Lynen, F., *Fed. Proc.* **12,** 683 (1953).
(34) Beinert, H., *J. Biol. Chem.* **205,** 575 (1953).
(35) Beinert, H., Green, D. E., Hele, P., Hift, H., Von Korff, R. W., and Ramakrishnan, C. V., *J. Biol. Chem.* **203,** 35 (1953).
(36) Lipmann, F., Jones, M. E., Black, S., and Flynn, R. M., *J. Am. Chem. Soc.* **74,** 2384 (1952).
(37) Mahler, H. R., unpublished observations.
(38) Jones, M. E., Black, S., Flynn, R. M., and Lipmann, F., *Biochim. Biophys. Acta* **12,** 141 (1953).
(39) Jones, M. E., Lipmann, F., Hilz, A., and Lynen, F., *J. Am. Chem. Soc.* **75,** 3285 (1953).
(40) Mahler, H. R., *J. Biol. Chem.* **206,** 13 (1954).
(41) Mahler, H. R., and Green, D. E., *Science* **120,** 7 (1954).
(42) Beinert, H., and Stansly, P. G., *J. Biol. Chem.* **204,** 67 (1953).
(43) Stansly, P. G., and Beinert, H., *Biochim. Biophys. Acta* **11,** 600 (1953).
(44) Popjak, G., and Tietz, A., *Biochem. J.* **56,** 46 (1954).
(45) Dituri, F., and Gurin, S., *Arch. Biochem. and Biophys.* **43,** 231 (1953).
(46) Van Baalen, J., and Gurin, S., *J. Biol. Chem.* **205,** 303 (1953).
(47) Beinert, H., and Crane, F., *J. Am. Chem. Soc.* **76,** 4491 (1954).

American Association of Clinical Chemists

President's Address

Monroe E. Freeman

Over the past few years The American Association of Clinical Chemists has established an outstanding record of progress and achievement. Today, the state of the Association is excellent. For the future, there are ambitious plans and favorable prospects. The past history, the objectives, and accomplishments of the Association are familiar to the readers of the Clinical Chemist and detailed review would add little. However, it is interesting to note, in passing, that Dr. Max M. Friedman's address[1] to the Association in 1949 forecast the many important tasks to be done and the subsequent record of accomplishment is convincing evidence of the rapidly growing strength of the Association.

Rather than detail the record of accomplishment, it seemed more appropriate to examine the fundamental elements of purpose that seem to have contributed the most to the success of this enterprise. It is these simple fundamentals that should be the soundest guidance for future efforts.

First, there should be a real need for an organization of clinical chemistry. Second, there must be a comprehensive program to fill that need. Third, there must be individuals who are willing and able to effectively implement the program.

At first glance, it might seem unnecessary to debate the need for such an organization in the field of modern medical science. Certainly the members of this association as well as a large segment of the medical profession would not dissent, but at the same time there has been a body of contrary opinion. Opinion, pro or con, however, counts for little in the face of such facts as the rapid growth of the American Association, the

---

Lt. Col., Medical Service Corps.
Delivered at the Annual Meeting, New York, September 17, 1954.
[1] *Chem. & Eng. News* 27, 3116 (1949).

rise of similar organizations throughout Western Europe, recognition by other scientific societies, and the assembly of 300 clinical chemists from 23 nations and five continents at the First European Congress of Clinical Chemistry.

From this positive assertion of the need for an organization of clinical chemistry, we can derive two specifications. First, in the public interest, there is a need for an organized effort to advance the science and practice. It is obvious that the increasing complexity of chemical theory and technic involved in modern medical practice requires a comprehensive organization of the pertinent and applicable chemical knowledge. Second, in the interests of the individual chemist, there is a need for a strong organization to protect and improve his professional identity, and to facilitate his professional improvement through educational guidance and the free exchange of technical information. This requirement is particularly significant in the newly developing field of clinical chemistry because the individual should not carelessly nor inadvertently trespass in the field of medical practice and medical responsibility, nor should he retreat into the circumscribed area of mere technical analysis. Authoritative guidance is needed to help the clinical chemist clearly define his position in the field of medical science.

The second element of purpose was a comprehensive program, and a program has been derived from Article II of the Constitution. Since few people read Constitutions, quotation will not be superfluous:

> In the interest of the public welfare, it is the aim and object of this association to raise the level at which chemistry is practiced in the clinical laboratories to stimulate the development of new methods for use in the clinical laboratories; to encourage highly trained chemists to enter the field of clinical chemistry; to encourage those engaged in this field to pursue advanced studies so as to more effectively render service to the public; and to create and maintain a forum where chemists engaged in applying the science of clinical chemistry may exchange ideas and information concerning their scientific, technical, and professional problems.

These are fine words but they mean little unless effectively implemented by positive action. In short, what have we done? What are we doing? and What do we intend? This deserves special emphasis because there is some reason to believe that scientific societies may be approaching a "buyer's market." There are many worthwhile scientific organizations, so many that few young scientists can afford membership in all. They will become more critical in their selections and it is only logical to assume that the best of the younger generation will be attracted by real accomplishment and by prospects of progressive action.

Illustrations of accomplishment and current activities include; the first volume of *Standard Methods*, substantial progress on volumes two and three, and the new CLINICAL CHEMISTRY, important steps for a society as young as ours. Another most important accomplishment was the formalization of a Code of Ethics. The latter is a most significant step in defining the position of the clinical chemist, a position that has long been confused by controversy, prejudice, and legal restrictions that were, in themselves, capable of compounding confusion in forty-eight different ways. As the lines become more finely drawn in the next few years, it is most important that this Code of Ethics be maintained in a form that is acceptable and applicable to new conditions and situations. This is as much the responsibility of individuals and of the local sections as it is of the national officers and committees. It is essential that local sections maintain continued interest and surveillance over the Code of Ethics and critically review and recommend changes and improvements necessary or advisable.

By the same token, local sections and individuals must assume primary responsibility for the legislative problems that appear in their localities. The Association does not have the resources to support a central secretariat that could monitor the legislative proposals throughout the country. However, the national legislation committee under Dr. John G. Reinhold will provide competent advice and experienced counsel upon request. This committee will be most effective if it is kept fully informed regarding legislative matters in your locality so that the position and actions of the Association may be properly coordinated.

Other activities that are beginning to assume more significance are the employment exchange services and the personnel and laboratory standards. Some thought has been given to the problem of technical surveys. Standard samples have been circulated by different groups for different purposes, some for the evaluation of technician or laboratory proficiency, some for the evaluation of methods and primary standards. Surveys of this sort have been conducted by public health laboratories, by local sections of the association, by large laboratory systems such as the Army, and on an international scale under the sponsorship of the International Federation of Clinical Chemists. For the most part these have been independent and uncoordinated operations that could conceivably lead to as many different primary definitions and standards. Sooner or later, these efforts should be coordinated and reduced to a national or international definition of standards for materials, methods, and performance. This will be large task and a difficult one but there is no doubt that this

Association should be prepared to assume an appropriate share of the responsibility for such an effort.

The third element of success was the willingness of capable individuals to carry out the program. Special tribute must be paid to the leaders and officers of the past few years, to the committee members and to the individuals who have done the most in forwarding this enterprise. Most of them have done more than their share and continued responsibility would be an imposition. Their successors should represent the nation-wide scope of this Association, and their selection will result almost automatically from the interest and activity of the local sections in carrying on the program that has been so successfully begun.

the Clinical Chemist

Nominations for the 1955 Ernst Bischoff Award

The National Executive Committee of the American Association of Clinical Chemists has announced that the Association Award Committee will consider nominations for the 1955 Ernst Bischoff Award in Clinical Chemistry.

The Ernst Bischoff Award is presented annually to an outstanding clinical chemist selected by the Association. The Award consists of a scroll, a bronze medal, and an honorarium of $500.00. It was first presented in 1952, to Jos Kahn (posthumous). The other recipients have been Michael Somogyi (1953) and John G. Reinhold (1954).

Candidates for this award are proposed by the membership of the A.A.C.C. A member may place in nomination the name of any individual by submitting in triplicate a letter of recommendation and any other pertinent data relative to the nomination to the Chairman of the Award Committee. Nominations must be received on or before March 30, 1955, to be considered for the 1955 Award.

Nominations should be sent to Dr. Joseph H. Roe, 1335 H. St., N. W., Washington, D. C.

Executive Committee Meeting

The National Executive Committee of the American Association of Clinical Chemists met at the Mount Sinai Hospital, New York, on September 15, 1954. Present were Monroe E. Freeman, *President*; Max M. Friedman, *National Secretary*; Louis B. Dotti, *National Treasurer*; Robert M. Hill, Hugh J. McDonald, Marschelle H. Power, Miriam Reiner, Albert B. Sample, Harold D. Appleton (by invitation), John G. Reinhold (by invitation), Joseph I. Routh (by invitation), and Harry Sobotka (by invitation).

The Treasurer's report was given for the fiscal year July 1, 1953–June 30, 1954.

Income	
Membership dues	$3736.30
Clinical Chemist	1136.25
Membership list	50.00
Certificates	20.00
Bank interest	32.48
TOTAL INCOME	$4975.03
Expenses	
Clinical Chemist	$3754.22
Treasurer	88.41
Secretary	321.24
Executive Committee	100.40
Membership Committee	56.00
Section allotments	50.10
Membership fee refunds	8.20
TOTAL EXPENSES	$4378.57
Balance for year	$596.46
Bank balance, as of June 30, 1953	1911.67
Unaccounted credit	10.00
Bank balance, July 1, 1953	$2518.13

John G. Reinhold reported for the Nominating Committee and recommended the following slate of officers for 1955–56:

President: Otto Schales

Vice-President: Robert M. Hill

National Secretary: Max M. Friedman

National Treasurer: Louis B. Dotti

Executive Committee: Monroe E. Freeman, Joseph H. Gast, William H. Goldwater, Icie M. Hoobler, and Samuel Natelson.

REPORTS AND ACTIVITIES

The Committee on Membership reported a total of 624 members in the Association as of September 15, 1954.

Nelson F. Young reported for the editorial board working on Volume II of *Standard Methods* that the manuscript for this volume is nearly complete. Kurt M. Dubowski reported that work has already been started on Volume III of *Standard Methods* and will include toxicologic technics for use in hospital laboratories as emergency procedures.

Albert E. Sobel reported that a collaborative program has been started with the American Association for the Advancement of Science and approval has been received for a symposium as well as a series of contributed papers to be presented at the Atlanta meetings on December 26–31, 1955.

Oliver H. Gaebler reported that the Intersociety Committee met in Atlantic City on April 11, 1954, and has tentatively scheduled the next meeting for Buffalo, N. Y.

Otto Schales reported that John G. Reinhold was voted the recipient of the third Ernst Bischoff Award for his outstanding contributions to clinical chemistry.

Max M. Friedman reported that the committee appointed to recommend revision of the constitution is now progressing in its study.

Joseph I. Routh reported that the activity of the Employment Clearing House had increased considerably and various openings for clinical chemists are now being handled.

Emmett B. Carmichael reported that the Committee on Education was now organized and a program will soon be under way.

Robert L. Dryer reported for the Committee on Laboratory Standards and Personnel. A questionnaire had been distributed and the returns are now being evaluated.

NEW COMMITTEES

The following committees were appointed: *Program Committee:* Marschelle H. Power, chairman; *Ernst Bischoff Award:* Joseph H. Roe, chairman; Ferrin B. Moreland and Arnold G. Ware; *Committee on Ethics:* Hugh J. McDonald, chairman; Albert L. Chaney and Harry Sobotka. *Legislative Committee:* John G. Reinhold, chairman.

George T. Lewis was invited to join the Board of Editors of CLINICAL CHEMISTRY.

RESOLUTIONS PASSED

It was moved, seconded, and passed that only five issues of *The Clinical Chemist* shall be published during 1954 so as to save expenses and conserve scientific material for the new journal, CLINICAL CHEMISTRY.

It was moved, seconded, and passed that the bylaws of the Chicago, Midwest and Washington-Baltimore-Richmond sections be approved, with the recommendation to the sections that their local officers be designated as chairman and vice-chairman rather than president and vice-president, respectively, in order to avoid confusion between national and local offices.

It was moved, seconded and passed that membership shall be terminated for those who have not paid their annual dues by March 15 of any calendar year and their subscriptions to CLINICAL CHEMISTRY withdrawn.

It was unanimously agreed that an invitation from the American Society of Biological Chemists for a joint symposium at the Federation meetings shall be accepted.

The Executive Committee agreed to propose to the membership that the dues for 1955 include the assessment for the journal.

It was moved, seconded, and passed that the seventh annual meetings of the A.A.C.C. shall be held in conjunction with the American Chemical Society in Minneapolis, Minnesota, from September 11–16, 1955.

ABSTRACTS

Editor: Ellenmae Viergiver. *Contributors:* Joseph A. Annino, Clyde A. Dubbs, Alex Kaplan, Margaret M. Kaser, Miriam Reiner, Herbert Thompson

Studies of the thymol turbidity, cephalin flocculation, and thymol flocculation tests. E. J. Katz, R. J. Hasterlik, and F. E. Snapp (*Health Services Division and the Division of Biological and Medical Research, Argonne National Laboratory, Lamont, Ill.*)

Four thymol reagents were studied: (I) Maclagen reagent, *p*H 7.72; (II) thymol reagent modified by Huerga and Popper, *p*H 7.72; (III) Maclagen reagent modified by Mateer *et al.*, *p*H 7.55; and (IV) thymol reagent modified by Huerga and Popper, *p*H 7.55.

Calculation of thymol turbidity measurements was based on the precalibrated colloidal glass standard of Reinhold. Results indicated that Reagent II was best for screening both normal individuals and patients with liver disease. The thymol flocculation test, regardless of the reagent used, was unsatisfactory as a screening test. Two cephalin cholesterol antigens, Difco and Wilson, were compared, and it was found that the latter gave fewer positive results in normal individuals and patients ill with diseases other than liver disease. Results in patients with liver disease were approximately the same with both antigens.—*J. Lab. & Clin. Med.* **44,** 353 (1954).

E.V

Clinical value of the plasma butanol-extractable (thyroxin) I^{131} in the diagnosis of hyperthyroidism and myxedema. A. L. Schultz, S. Sandhaus, H. L. Demorest, and L. Zieve (*Veterans Admin. Hosp., Minneapolis, Minn.*)

Butanol-extractable I^{131}: A 5 ml. aliquot of plasma is extracted twice with 20 ml. of *n*-butanol and three times with one half volume of 4N NaOH which contains 5 per cent Na_2CO_3 to remove the nonthyroxine I^{131} carried into the butanol phase. The butanol extract is concentrated over a waterbath and adjusted to a volume of 6 ml. Radioactivity is counted in a well-type scintillation counter.

Plasma protein-bound I^{131}: A 5 ml. aliquot of plasma is placed in a flat-bottom 20 ml. counting tube. Proteins are precipitated with 10 ml. of 20 per cent trichloroacetic acid. After centrifugation, the proteins are washed four times with trichloroacetic acid, care being taken not to pour off or remove protein particles. The solidly packed protein is then counted in a well-type scintillation counter.

Butanol-extractable I^{131} and protein-bound I^{131} levels in plasma 24 hours after administration of a tracer dose of I^{131} were studied in 50 euthyroid, 12 hyperthyroid, and 5 myxedematous subjects. The two measures are closely correlated, the butanol-extractable fraction comprising four fifths of the protein-bound iodine, but has no diagnostic significance. Euthyroid individuals can be separated from hyperthyroid cases, but the test is not useful in distinguishing myxedematous patients.—*J. Clin. Endocrinol. & Metab.* **14,** 1062 (1954).

M. R.

Comparison of incineration and chloric acid methods for determination of chemical protein-bound iodine. L. Zieve, M. Dahle, and A. L. Schultz (*Dept. of Medicine, and the Radioisotope Unit, Veterans Administration Hospital and the Univ. of Minnesota, Minneapolis, Minn.*)

A comparison was made between the values obtained with an incineration method and a chloric acid method. Although there was no significant difference between the two methods in hypothyroid and hyperthyroid groups, it was found that euthyroid values obtained by the chloric acid method were shifted upward approximately 1–1.5 μg. per 100 ml. Since the hyperthyroid levels were not shifted correspondingly, there was a loss in discriminative effectiveness of the test. The chloric acid procedure did not prove to be significantly more rapid to perform in terms of actual technician-time spent on the procedures.—*J. Lab. & Clin. Med.* **44,** 374 (1954).

E.V.

An improved method for multiple rapid determinations of arterial blood *p*H. D. A. Holaday (*Dept. of Anesthesiology, Columbia University, College of Physicians & Surgeons, and the Anesthesiology Service, Presbyterian Hospital, New York*)

Details of construction are presented for an instrument which permits direct transfer of blood from the patient into a glass electrode for serial determinations of *p*H at body temperature. The volume of blood required for each determination is approximately 2 ml. The apparatus is designed for use in the presence of explosive gas mixtures in the operating room.—*J. Lab. & Clin. Med.* **44,** 149 (1954).

A.K.

Conductometric titration method for determination of serum chloride. H. A. Teloh (*Evanston Hospital Association, Evanston, Ill., and Northwestern University Medical School, Chicago, Ill.*).

Proteins are precipitated from 0.5 ml. of serum by the addition in drops of 5 ml. of absolute alcohol. After vigorous shaking, the tube is centrifuged at 1500–2000 r.p.m. for 2 minutes. The supernatant liquid is decanted into a 45 ml. Pyrex glass-stoppered Freas conductance cell. Five milliliters of absolute alcohol is added to the precipitate and the contents are thoroughly mixed by shaking and stirring. After centrifuging, the supernatant is also added to the Freas cell, followed by approximately 40 ml. of double-distilled chloride-free water. The contents of the cell are mixed by shaking and brought to room temperature. The cell is connected to the conductance measuring apparatus (H. G. Davis, *to be published*) and the conductance measured after consecutive additions of

0.1 ml. of 100 mEq./l. $AgNO_3$ solution. Contents of the cell should be mixed after each addition. The end point, graphically calculated, is associated with an abrupt and marked increase in conductance. Sulfates, monohydrogen phosphates, and bicarbonates in concentrations up to 20–30 mEq./l. exerted no effect on the endpoint. Normal serum chloride levels by this method range from 97.4 to 106 mEq./l., with a mean of 101.0 mEq./l. Accuracy of this procedure was established in control experiments. Advantages of this method are not stated.—*Am. J. Clin. Pathol.* **24,** 1095 (1954).

H.E.T.

The control of variable influences on the electrolyte content of sweat and their application to clinical study of adrenal function. C. R. Kleeman, M. Quinn, and D. E. Bass (*Yale Univ. Med. School, New Haven, Conn.*)

Nonhormonal or local factors such as skin and air temperature, method of collection, rate and duration of sweating, and interval between the onset of sweating and its collection, play a fundamental role in determining the electrolyte composition of thermal sweat, irrespective of the level of adrenocortical activity. There is no reciprocal relationship between the concentrations of sodium (or chloride) and potassium in thermal sweat collected under controlled conditions from young, healthy males. When the nonhormonal or local influences on sweat are controlled, electrolyte concentrations in random samples of thermal sweat may serve as indices of adrenocortical activity.—*J. Clin. Endocrinol. & Metab.* **14,** 1126 (1954).

M. R.

Simultaneous determination of sucrose and inulin in biologic fluids. M. K. Young and J. F. Prudden (*Surgical Research Unit, Brooke Army Medical Center, Fort Sam Houston, Tex.*)

An anthrone procedure is presented for the determination of sucrose and the simultaneous determination of sucrose and inulin. The latter is accomplished by the measurement of the optical densities of samples before and after inversion and subsequent digestion with sodium hydroxide.—*J. Lab. & Clin. Med.* **44,** 160 (1954).

E.V.

Simplified sensitive test for thyroid function, using protein-bound I^{131}. L. Van Middlesworth, C. E. Nurnberger, and A. Lipscomb. (*Univ. Tennessee, Knoxville*)

Twenty-four hours after a 50 μc tracer dose of I^{131} is given, 5–10 ml. of venous blood is obtained. A 3–5 ml. plasma sample is placed in the 3 mm. annulus of a special plastic cup and the radiation is counted. Four to five drops of 3 per cent NaI carrier are delivered into the plasma, and 8–12 ml. of 20 per cent trichloroacetic acid is added. After centrifugation and washing twice with 10 ml. of 10 per cent trichloroacetic acid, the precipitate remaining in the plastic cup is counted. The conversion ratio equals $\frac{\text{count/min. of ppt.}}{\text{count/min. of plasma}}$ times 100. Conversion ratios of over 50 per cent are considered indicative of hyperthyroidism, ratios of normal subjects are less than 50 per cent, ranging from 10 per cent to 30 per cent.—*J. Clin. Endocrinol. & Metab.* **14,** 1056 (1954).

M. R.

The use of substances depressing antithrombin activity in the assay of prothrombin. P. Fantl. (*Alfred Hospital, Melbourne, Australia*).

For the assay of prothrombin, a reaction mixture was prepared which consisted of 0.5 ml. of thromboplastin preparation (a 6% suspension of acetone-dried human or rabbit brain powder); 0.6 ml. of 0.025M $CaCl_2$; 0.45 ml. of 0.15M NaCl and 0.3 ml. of 0.18M pyrocatechol in Veronal buffer, *p*H 7.4. To this mixture was added 0.3 ml. of the material to be tested. At periods of 1 minute after the last addition, 0.2 ml. was blown into a mixture of 0.2 ml. of prothrombin-free human plasma (oxalated plasma stirred with 10–20 mg. $BaSO_4$ or $BaCO_3$ per ml. at 0° for 30 min.) and 0.05 ml. of 0.18M pyrocatechol and the clotting time determined. Reactions were carried out at 28° ± 1°. Values of 470–720 prothrombin units per ml. were found in an examination of 126 normal subjects.—*Biochem. J.* **57,** 416 (1954).

A.K.

The interaction of dyes with proteins on paper with special reference to paper electrophoresis. G. T. Franglen and N. H. Martin (*St. George's Medical School, London*)

The spectral absorption characteristics of bromophenol blue, bromocresol green, azocarmine B, and naphthalein black 12B have been examined. Azocarmine B is heterogeneous in chromatography on filter paper. Bromophenol blue slowly fades in 0.01N NaOH. The dye-binding characteristics of human albumin and human gamma globulin with bromocresol green have been studied individually and in mixtures of known composition. The results suggest that existing quantitative methods of analysis by paper-strip electrophoresis require reassessment. —*Biochem. J.* **57,** 626 (1954).

A.K.

Influence of hyperglycemic factor (Glucagon) on 17-hydroxysteroids in plasma and urine of man. P. P. Van Arsdel, Jr., H. H. Romizawa, and R. H. Williams (*University of Washington School of Medicine and King County Hospital, Seattle, Wash.*).

The subjects were 8 fasting hospital patients with normal renal and hepatic function and no signs of congestive heart failure. Four were given purified hyperglycemic factor in a dose of 10 μg./kg. body weight by intravenous infusion during a 30-minute period. Blood glucose and plasma 17-hydroxysteroids in samples taken just before and at the end of the infusion, and plasma steroids 1 hour after the start of the infusion, were determined. A 3-hour control urine specimen was collected prior to the infusion and a 2-hour specimen was collected during and after administration of the hyperglycemic factor. Seventeen-hydroxysteroids in plasma were estimated by the method of Nelson and Samuels [*J. Clin. Endocrinol. and Metabolism* **12,** 519 (1952)] and in urine by the method of Glenn and Nelson [*J. Clin. Endocrinol. and Metabolism* **13,** 911 (1953)].

In the remaining 4 patients similar doses of hyperglycemic factor were injected intravenously during a 30-second period. Blood sugar was determined and the plasma hydroxysteroids were estimated before, at 20 minutes, and at 40 minutes after injection, and, in 2 patients, 80 minutes after injection. Urinary steroids were determined in 3-hour specimens. No significant changes in plasma steroid values occurred, and the results for urinary steroids were variable. No direct action of hyperglycemic factor on the adrenal cortex was demonstrated by these methods.—*Proc. Soc. Exp. Biol. Med.* **86,** 844 (1954).

M.K.

Diminished plasma 17-ketosteroid concentration in pregnancy. L. I. Gardner, R. L. Walton, W. Ellis, and E. C. Hughes (*State University of New York, Syracuse, N. Y.*).

Neutral 17-ketosteroids in plasma were determined by a method previously reported [Gardner, *J. Clin. Endocrinol. and Metabolism* **13,** 941 (1953)]. A control group of 17 men and 16 women showed a mean value of 61 μg. per 100 ml. of plasma with no significant sex difference. The mean for 30 pregnant women was 18 μg. per 100 ml., which was significantly lower than the controls ($p < .001$).—*Proc. Soc. Exp. Biol. Med.* **86,** 804 (1954).

M.K.

The light sensitivity of the Liebermann-Burchard reaction during spectrophotometric determination of cholesterol. J. K. Kabara (*Argonne Research Hospital, University of Chicago, Chicago, Ill.*)

The whole absorption curve of the color developed in the dark and in the light was investigated using cholesterol standards in a polar solvent (glacial acetic acid) and in a nonpolar solvent (toluene). The optical density of the two solutions, measured from 580 to 740 mμ, was the same in either solvent. The difference in shade that is seen is explained by the light sensitivity of the solution in the region of 450 mμ. Unless the range 340–450 mμ is used for the determination, no special precautions concerning light are necessary.—*J. Lab. & Clin. Med.* **44,** 246 (1954).

E.V.

Flame photometric determination of electrolytes in tissue and of calcium in serum. J. R. Denson (*Biochemistry Dept., Army Medical Research Laboratory, Fort Knox, Ky.*)

Flame photometric methods are presented for the simultaneous determination of calcium, magnesium, sodium, and potassium in tissue, and for the determination of calcium in blood serum. The instrument used was the Beckman Model DU with No. 9200 flame attachment.—*J. Biol. Chem.* **209,** 233 (1954).

E.V.

BOOK REVIEWS

Clinical Chemistry in Practical Medicine (ed. 4)

C. P. Stewart and D. M. Dunlop. Baltimore, Md., The Williams and Wilkins Company, 1954, 320 pp., $5.00

The authors have set as their goal a discussion of the application of clinical chemistry to the everyday practice of clinical medicine. The book is intended to give the clinician and the senior medical student the knowledge of biochemical backgrounds where a chemical examination may be helpful, and the interpretation and significance to be placed on the laboratory results.

The reviewer has been impressed with the authors' awareness of the problems of the laboratory in their everyday dealings with the practicing physician. Throughout the book the reader is reminded of this; for example: "[though] chemical methods have established their right to be considered among the major aids of diagnostic medicine . . . [laboratory tests] supplement, but do not replace examination of the patient"; and ". . . if analysts are relieved of the necessity of doing useless work, the quality and therefore the value of the remainder is more likely to be maintained at a high level."

The chapters are well organized and the discussions are clearly presented. It must be remembered that the authors have always kept in mind their intended audience, and therefore the practicing biochemist and research worker may find the subject-matter presentation shallow.

Good discussions are found in the chapters "Water and Electrolyte Metabolism," "Neutrality Regulation," "Carbohydrate Metabolism," "Renal Function," "Plasma Proteins," "Tests of Gastric, Pancreatic and Hepatic Functions," "Cerebrospinal Fluid," and "Calcium and Phosphorus."

In the chapter "Thyroid Function," the basal metabolism determination is given preference. Under this heading there is also an adequate presentation of the use of radioactive iodine. The protein bound iodine determination is not mentioned.

The appendices contain a selection of simple methods which the practicing physician can perform as part of the office routine and a description of the clinical chemical procedures and laboratory methodology which are in use in the authors' laboratories.

Though references for further reading are not given, this book would make a good basic text for instruction of residents, interns, and technicians assigned to the clinical chemistry laboratory.

Chemotherapy of Infections

H. O. J. Collier. New York, John Wiley and Sons, Inc., 1954, 248 pp., $4.00

This small volume describes the general aspects of chemotherapy and the various groups of chemotherapeutic agents. Dr. Collier discusses the application of chemical substances used against microbes infecting the body, and though he admits that his book ignores many interesting substances, the chemical agents which are included are those in which important results have recently been achieved, and those compounds and experiments which clearly show the basic principles of chemotherapy and the historic development of these principles.

Dr. Collier adequately illustrates the newer approach to therapy which may be called "chemical pharmacology." The subject matter makes very interesting reading and does not demand a great background in either chemistry or microbiology. This book will prove interesting and instructive to those who have the authority to prescribe these drugs as well as those who wish to keep informed on the progress of a neighboring science.

A Practical Manual of Medical and Biological Staining Techniques

E. Gurr. New York, Interscience Publishers, Inc., 1954, 320 pp. $4.00

This is an excellent manual dealing with preparation of material and staining procedures in all phases of microbiology. It is well written, giving the maximum information and directions in concise terminology.

The appendix contains formulas for stain preparation, tables of stain solubilities, and tables of refractive indices of the solvents and oils used in microbiological work.

This book is highly recommended as the laboratory supplement to the standard texts on microbiology and cytology.

Statistical Analysis in Chemistry and the Chemical Industry

C. A. Bennett and N. L. Franklin. New York, John Wiley and Sons, Inc., 1954, 724 pp. $8.00

This book has been sponsored by the Committee on Applied Mathematical Statistics, National Research Council of the National Academy of Sciences. The authors present those aspects of applied mathematical statistics which will be continually useful to both the chemist and chemical engineer. The subject matter is developed very completely with the theoretical basis, derivation of the methods, and the computational procedures. The reader is given a good background of mathematical theory so that he has a firm basis for judging application. The selection of methods is aimed specifically at the chemist and the examples given are taken from many branches of chemistry and chemical industry. The more recent developments in applied mathematical statistics have been included, with illustrations of their application to chemistry.

Human Biochemistry (ed. 4)

I. S. Kleiner. St. Louis, Mo., The C. V. Mosby Co., 1954, 746 pp., $7.50

This well-known text has been revised in many aspects in keeping with the recent rapid advances in biochemistry.

The discussions of blood coagulation, enzymes and coenzymes, biologic oxidations, cholesterol metabolism, urea formation, and action of insulin have been completely rewritten. There also has been extensive revision of other sections and the recent knowledge gained through the use of isotopes is found almost throughout.

The author has kept his original purpose of creating a useful, understandable, and compact volume for use as a text in the standard courses in biochemistry. The subject matter is presented clearly. For the more inquisitive student, each chapter contains a well-rounded reference list of pertinent papers.

Laboratory Instructions in Biochemistry (ed. 4)

I. S. Kleiner and L. B. Dotti. St. Louis, Mo., The C. V. Mosby Co., 1954, 285 pp., $3.50

This excellent laboratory manual is the laboratory partner of Kleiner's *Human Biochemistry*. The directions are set forth clearly and concisely and the experiments for illustrating the points in the subject matter will give the student clear-cut results, which in turn emphasize the reaction under study.

The fourth edition has been revised to include experiments with ion exchange resins, paper chromatography, the phosphatase test for pasteurization, and the Somogyi-Nelson true blood sugar procedure.

The practicing clinical chemist will find this manual useful as a ready reference for rapid toxicologic determinations and for procedures not "routine." The Appendix contains a rather complete list of formulas for the preparation of the reagents and solutions. It is the reviewer's opinion that the formulas could have been made part of the specific procedures in order to acquaint the student with the contents of the reagent used, the time required in its preparation, and any necessary precautions, even though in course work these reagents are provided on the shelf.

The soft cover, with printed matter on the left hand page and the right side blank for notes, makes for ease of handling in a laboratory with many students and a minimum of laboratory table space.

Serum Lipoproteins

Chemical and Enzymatic Studies

Ray K. Brown, Louis S. DeLalla, and Dorothy L. Kauffman

ALTERATION IN BLOOD LIPIDS is associated with a wide variety of diseases, among them xanthomatosis and atherosclerosis. Excessive loss of carbohydrate or protein from the body, as in diabetes, nephroses, multiple myeloma, or chronic hemorrhage, is frequently accompanied by blood-lipid derangement. Studies of the structure and linkages which bind lipids to protein molecules and of the mechanisms controlling their concentration may give clues to the varied diseases associated with deranged lipid metabolism.

The unusual solubility properties of the serum lipids have been attributed to lipid protein complexes for over half a century.[1] Macheboeuf was among the early workers to isolate a lipoprotein and determine its composition.[2] Serum lipoproteins are usually divided in those of high density, α_1, and α_2 lipoproteins; those of low density, the β lipoprotein described by Oncley, Gurd, and Melin;[3] and larger lipoproteins of Sf 10 and greater as described by Lindgren, Elliott, and Gofman.[4] There is considerable evidence that several of these lipoproteins consist of more than one macromolecular entity. The fractionation experiments of Batchelor[5] and ultracentrifuge studies of Boyle *et al.*[6] indicate the heterogeneity of α_1 lipoproteins, the immunochemical investigations of Gitlin[7] suggest the heterogeneity of the β lipoproteins,* and the electron microscope studies of Beischer[8] on Sf 30 lipoproteins indicate that these substances are not homogeneous. Although chylomicrons are probably heterogeneous aggregates of lipids, it is possible that subfractions of

From the Division of Laboratories and Research, New York State Department of Health, Albany, N. Y.

Presented at the Symposium on Lipides and Lipoproteins, at the 126th National Meeting of the American Chemical Society—In participation with the American Association of Clinical Chemists, September 16, 1954, New York City.

* Recent gradient tube experiments of Oncley and Mannick also support this view.

smaller lipoproteins are homogeneous molecular entities. It is only by attempting to further purify these lipoproteins that an answer to these questions can be found.

PREPARATION OF LIPOPROTEINS

Preparation of α_2 Lipoproteins

When plasma is fractionated by Cohn's method,[9] most of the low-density lipoproteins and considerable amounts of α_2 lipoprotein fall into fraction III-O. This fraction can be further purified by dialyzing the freshly prepared paste twice at $-5°$ C. for twenty-four hours against 30 volumes of a 1.65 M solution in sodium chloride. The alcohol is thus removed and the paste brought into solution at a solvent density of 1.06. This solution is ultracentrifuged for eighteen hours at 97,720 G and the floating low-density lipoprotein concentrate is sliced from the top of the tube by means of a sharp blade in a rigid holder. This material is saved for further purification. The solution immediately below the low-density lipoproteins is discarded and the proteins in the bottom of the tube are decanted from the pellicle. These proteins are fractionated with neutral ammonium sulfate at 0°. The fraction precipitating between 33- and 42-per-cent saturation is dissolved in a minimal amount of H_2O, brought to a solvent density of 1.20, and ultracentrifuged as before. The α_2 lipoproteins sliced from the top are ultracentrifugally homogeneous at a density of 1.20 and the solution has a single electrophoretic peak with a mobility of -2.56×10^{-5} in barbital buffer, pH 8.6, $\Gamma/2 = .1$. Their minimum solubility lies near pH 4.9 (Fig. 1). However, when these lipoproteins are tested immunochemically on an agar plate, they still give faint lines with anticrystalline albumin, antigamma globulin, and anticrystalline glycoprotein sera.[10]

Preparation of β Lipoproteins

The low-density lipoprotein concentrate from fraction III-O may be further purified by diluting it with 3.07 volumes of physiological saline to a density of 1.02 and ultracentrifuging as before. This separation is less sharp than that at density 1.06. The lipoproteins of Sf 10 and greater are sliced from the top of the tube. The β lipoproteins are more than 95 per cent homogeneous electrophoretically. They will not form a boundary in the descending limb due, presumably, to density differences. The hexose content of this material is typical of that of most proteins, about 0.4 per cent.

If the β lipoproteins are to be preserved for any appreciable time, the pH should be adjusted to 6.5 and Merthiolate, .01%, added. This pH range is similar to that of maximum stability for serum albumin and gamma globulin. Beta lipoproteins stored for a few weeks below *p*H 6.0 form very turbid solutions. The turbidity is not affected by ethylene diamine tetracetate or *p*H shift.

Beta lipoproteins prepared as described have remained stable without turbidity change for several months at 0° and have not, as yet, permitted any observations on the effects of esterase inhibitors, antioxidants, and chelating agents. Studies of other agents on the stability of beta lipoproteins have been made by Gurd.[11]

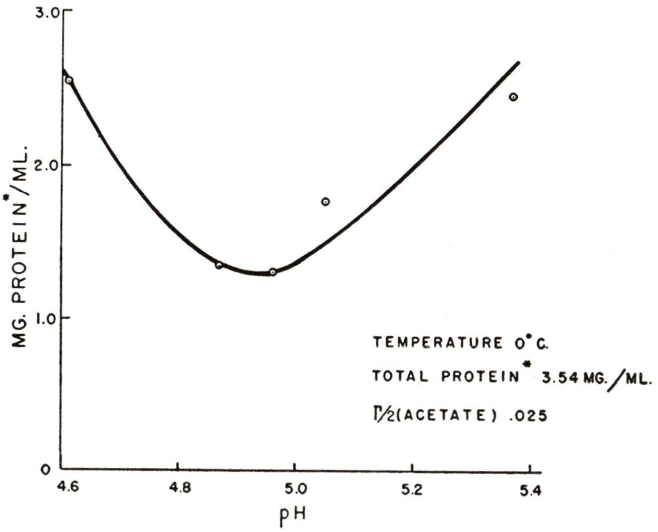

Fig. 1. Solubility of α_2 lipoprotein at various *p*H's.

Preparation of α Lipoproteins

A lipoprotein fraction of human plasma, which was 90 per cent homogeneous electrophoretically and ultracentrifugally, was isolated under conditions similar to those used by Cohn and coworkers[12] and by Kominz.[13]

The material used was fraction IV-I paste separated from plasma by Cohn's Method 6. A weighed amount of paste was dissolved in twice its weight of water containing sufficient sodium bicarbonate to raise the *p*H above 6. The addition of water was begun with the paste at −5° and completed at 0°. All subsequent manipulations were carried out at 0°. The solution containing fraction IV-I was dialyzed against distilled water for four or five days. The reddish brown precipitate which formed was removed by centrifugation. The supernatant was adjusted to an ionic strength of 0.1 with sodium chloride and to *p*H 5.1–5.2 with acetate buffer, *p*H 4.0, $\Gamma/2 = .01$, eighty times concentrated. The resulting suspension was separated by centrifugation and the precipitate was washed once with 0.1 M sodium chloride buffered to *p*H 5.2. The washed precipitate was dissolved in a suitable buffer at approximately neutral *p*H.

This lipoprotein fraction has been partially characterized chemically and its composition resembles closely that of fraction IV-I (1) reported by Rosenberg.[14] It has a protein:cholesterol ratio of 0.6 and a cholesterol:phospholipid ratio of 0.2. A 1% solution has an S_{20W} of 4.5 and an electrophoretic mobility of -4.8×10^{-5} at *p*H 8.6 in .1 M barbital buffer.

ALTERATION OF LIPOPROTEINS BY ENZYMES

Previous workers have shown that administration of heparin clears the turbidity of alimentary lipemia[15] and causes alterations in the serum lipoproteins[16] as determined ultracentrifugally. Lipoproteins of high Sf are broken into smaller lipoproteins. These alterations may be divided into two major steps, the formation of clearing factor and its action on lipoproteins.

Formation of Clearing Factor

In the intact animal, injection of many different substances may give rise to clearing activity. All are acidic substances of relatively large molecular weight or salts of these substances. Many are sulfates, although phosphotungstic acid, a substance very different from heparin, has been found by Bragdon and Havel[17] to produce clearing factor in rats.

The recent work of Korn[18] indicates that ammonia extracts of an acetone powder of normal rat heart contain clearing factor. Previous work with heart minces indicated that a component of plasma was necessary for formation of the clearing factor.[19] This action is probably solubilization, which would agree with the results of Nikkilä[20] who found some clearing activity in mortar-ground heart extracts in the absence of plasma, although plasma extracts were more effective. It is inadvisable to use the term precursor for this activity. If clearing factor must be solubilized before it can act under physiologic conditions, a plasma component may be involved. Some clearing activity in normal rat serum has been reported[19] and Jeffries[21] has extended these observations. Anfinsen[22] has suggested that clearing may occur in the tissues and that clearing factor may not normally be in solution. The stability of lipemic serum is in accord with this hypothesis.

Substrate Specificity

It has been shown that serum containing clearing factor has no greater activity toward β naphthyl laurate than preheparin serum from the same animal.[23] Similar results are obtained when β carbonaphthoxy choline iodide or β naphthyl chloracetate is used as substrate, which indicates that the esterase activity of clearing factor is not responsible for the histochemically demonstrable staining of mast cells with β naphthyl chloracetate as observed by Gomori.[24]

Emulsions of most triglycerides of short chain,[25] long chain, or unsaturated fatty acids are cleared by clearing factor. The rate of attack on triglyceride emulsions seems related more to the size of the emulsion than to the triglyceride used. The data in Table 1, which are typical of six experiments, indicate that monopalmitin is also attacked by clearing factor. Korn[18] has shown that lipoproteins are needed before clearing factor made in vitro can attack triglyceride emulsions. Since these experiments were done with clearing factor prepared in vivo, it is uncertain whether lipoprotein components are required for the substrates.

Table 1. Hydrolysis of Monopalmitin by Clearing Factor

	Fatty acid liberated (μ) m
Preheparin serum	0.15
Clearing factor serum	2.7

1 ml. of dog serum incubated for 3 hours with 1 ml. of an emulsion in 1.5% gelatin containing 1.5 mg. (45 μ m) of 1 monopalmitin. With smaller amounts of monopalmitin hydrolysis is complete, indicating that monopalmitin rather than impurities is being attacked.

Substrate Competition Experiments with Clearing Factor

Although monoglycerides and triglycerides compete with β naphthyl laurate for esterase, alimentary lipemic lipoproteins do not unless clearing factor is present. Nor do they compete for choline esterase either in the presence or absence of clearing factor when β carbonaphthoxy choline iodide is used as substrate. Since no data are available on the affinity of this enzyme for its substrate, one cannot rule out the possibility that choline esterase plays a part in esteratic breakdown, although the lack of inhibition of clearing by eserine and diisopropyl fluorophosphate (DFP),* 10^{-5} M, suggests that it does not. These findings indicate that plasma aliphatic esterase has little to do with the initial reaction of lipoprotein breakdown and that it does play an important part in glyceride hydrolysis.

* We are indebted to Dr. Robert F. Sterner of Merck and Company and to Dr. William H. Summerson of the United States Army Chemical Corps for a supply of DFP.

ACTION OF INHIBITORS ON THE CLEARING SYSTEM

Previous reports have indicated that clearing factor is inhibited by a high concentration of salt and of protamine. It is not inhibited by most other enzyme poisons.[25] Shore, Nichols, and Freeman[26] have reported that arsenite is an inhibitor. At the concentrations employed, the *p*H is quite alkaline to the *p*H optimum and attempts to titrate the material toward neutrality cause precipitation of arsenous oxide. Under these conditions, no inhibition occurs. DFP is a fairly general inhibitor of hydrolytic enzymes. It inhibits clearing factor at low concentrations

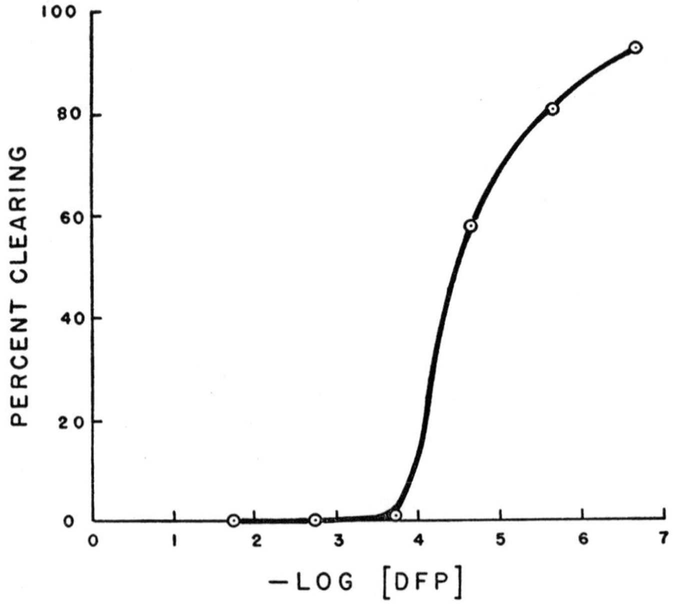

Fig. 2. Inhibition of clearing by DFP.*

(Fig. 2), which suggests that clearing factor may be a hydrolytic enzyme. In a crude way it gives an indication of its maximum concentration. If the concentration of clearing factor is assumed to be twice that of the DFP giving a 50 per cent inhibition, its concentration must be 3 × 10^{-5} M or less. However, it should be emphasized that the concentration

* Freshly opened DFP (.036 ml.) was emulsified in 2.0 ml. of *p*H 7.7 $\Gamma/2$ = .1 phosphate buffer. A series of 1:10 dilutions was made at once and .42 ml. of each was mixed immediately with 1.4 ml. of dog plasma containing clearing factor. They were allowed to stand, with occasional agitation, at room temperature for one hour and dialyzed against 4 L of saline, buffered with phosphate to *p*H 7,[34] in a rocking dialyzer for one hour. A control sample was treated similarly, except for DFP addition, and was dialyzed in a separate arm of the rocker. Clearing was observed in a tube containing 0.26 ml. of each sample, 0.2 ml. of dog alimentary lipemic serum, saline, phosphate buffer, and EDTA as described previously.

of clearing factor may be many times smaller since DFP may be lost from the system by spontaneous hydrolysis or by coupling to other proteins. There is no assurance that a 1:1 enzyme:inhibitor ratio will hold for clearing factor as it does for chymotrypsin.[27] In a typical experiment, corrected by these assumptions, 120 moles of fatty acid were liberated by one mole of clearing factor, a clear indication of the enzymatic nature of clearing factor.

Table 2 indicates that DFP inhibits clearing factor itself rather than any of the other components of the clearing mechanism. The addition of normal serum to a DFP-inhibited system does not remove the inhibition. Controls in which clearing factor containing serum was added show the expected amount of clearing which rules out the possibility that

Table 2. Effect of DFP on Clearing

	Decrease in optical density at 500 mμ in 1 hr.
1. Clearing factor	.194
2. DFP clearing factor	.010
3. DFP clearing factor + preheparin serum	.021
4. DFP clearing factor + clearing factor	.205

Dog serum heparinized *in vivo*, 0.2 ml. per determination, was used as clearing factor. DFP clearing factor was $2 \times 10^{-4}M$ in DFP. Ethylene diamine tetracetate (EDTA)-phosphate, 0.2 ml., was added to each tube, the volume was brought to 0.9 ml. with saline, and 0.1 ml. of lipemic dog serum was added. The tubes were incubated at 37°C.

free DFP remains and inhibits the added normal serum. Lipoproteins treated with DFP are cleared by clearing factor.

Surface active agents are another group of substances which inhibit clearing. The effect of Triton WR 1339 on lipoproteins had been described.[25] Lipoproteins treated with Triton and washed are not cleared. They do not inhibit the clearing of control lipoproteins which were treated similarly but with saline instead of Triton. This suggests that Triton inhibits clearing by altering the lipoprotein. Nikkilä's report[20] that Tween inhibits clearing has been confirmed. Cholate is also an inhibitor. It is probable, although not yet proved, that Tween and cholate act by the same mechanism as Triton.

Gordon *et al.*[28] have described another type of clearing inhibition in which fatty acid is added to the crude clearing factor in excess of the amount needed to saturate albumin. The addition of recrystallized serum albumin restores the activity. Robinson and French[29] have reported that serum albumin added to chyle and clearing factor brings about additional clearing.

Fatty acid or glycerol formation, ultracentrifugal alteration, and optical density change have been used frequently to assay clearing. In crude systems, where two methods have been used simultaneously, good agreement has usually been obtained. However, one should be cautious about interpreting the phenomenon in purified systems or in systems containing unusual substances. The clearing observed when chylomicrons are placed in 40% glycerol appears to be due merely to the approach of solvent and solute refractive index since glycine or sucrose solutions of the same refractive index cause similar clearing. Indeed, the experiment is like that of the magician who makes a glass ball disappear in a glass of so-called water, only repeated on a micro scale.

The determination of glycerol liberation in purified systems may not give reliable results unless care is taken to control carefully the concentration of aliphatic esterase since this substance plays a part in the breakdown of glycerides. Fatty acid determination is open to similar objections, although in properly controlled experiments most of the fatty acid is a result of clearing factor activity.

Action of Other Enzymes on Lipoproteins

Preparations containing pancreatic and gastric lipases attack lipoproteins and cause clearing, fatty acid formation, and often an increase in α lipoprotein concentration. Castor bean lipase has no effect. Although the clearing activity in plasma extracts of gastric lipase fractionates in a manner similar to clearing factor and is inhibited by salt and protamine, there is considerable evidence that they are not identical. Clearing factor made in vivo requires nonlipoprotein components during its course of activity, may be complexed onto coconut oil emulsions, and has no esterase activity with β naphthyl laurate as substrate. Extracts containing gastric lipase do not possess these properties. The course of clearing with gastric lipase often shows an initial lag period whose length is a function of the amount of lipase used.[30] Gastric and pancreatic lipase possess almost full activity at DFP levels one thousand times those that cause 50 per cent clearing factor inhibition. The substance causing clearing may be solubilized from mouse pyloric mucosa by α lipoproteins or by 0.025 M ammonium hydroxide. This suggests that α lipoprotein may merely serve as an extractant, perhaps by forming an enzyme–substrate analogue combination.

Rosenberg[31] has shown that proteolytic digestion of lipoproteins must proceed to a considerable extent before ultracentrifugal changes occur. Studies by Williams[32] on the action of *Clostridium welchii* lecithinase on lipoproteins indicate that the optical density of lipoprotein solutions, pretreated with lecithinase, is not affected by clearing factor.

Relationship of Clearing Factor to Plasma Esterases

It is apparent that clearing factor is neither of the enzymes that account for most of the esterase activity of plasma. Plasma choline esterase is inhibited by low concentrations of DFP, clearing factor is not. Grossman[33] has shown that clearing is not appreciably inhibited by physostigmine at levels that inhibit choline esterase, as confirmed here. Plasma aliphatic esterase is not inhibited by protamine in concentrations that inhibit clearing factor and is only about 50 per cent inhibited by DFP in concentrations that completely inhibit clearing factor. Both plasma aliphatic esterase and choline esterase attack β naphthyl laurate. Since no increase in β naphthyl laurate esterase activity occurs during formation of clearing factor, it cannot be either of the plasma esterases. As yet no inhibitor of plasma aliphatic esterase has been found which does not also inhibit clearing factor.

Whether appreciable amounts of specific lipase exist in plasma is uncertain. Both plasma choline esterase and plasma aliphatic esterase attack triglycerides. Thus far, attempts to use substances that partially inhibit or partially activate them have given equivocal results.

SUMMARY

The larger lipoproteins of Sf greater than 10 also contain triglycerides. The action of lipases on these lipoproteins, either heparin-induced clearing factor, pancreatic lipase, or gastric lipase, yields fatty acids, glycerol, and smaller lipoproteins. Crude clearing factor attacks monoglycerides and triglycerides and is inactive against several esters which plasma esterases attack. Albumin, plasma esterases, and probably other components are needed for optimal clearing factor activity. Low concentrations of diisopropyl fluorophosphate (DFP), a substance inhibiting most hydrolytic enzymes, inactivate crude clearing factor. Stoicheometric calculations made from this experiment indicate further the enzymatic nature of clearing factor. Evidence that clearing factor is different from other lipases and from esterases found in plasma is presented.

Studies with purified lipoproteins are needed to determine what alterations, if any, occur in smaller lipoproteins. The separation and purification of lipoproteins by chemical and ultracentrifugal means are described. Whole human plasma separated by Cohn's methods 6 and 9 serves as starting material for the preparation of α_1, α_2, β, and Sf 10 and greater lipoproteins.

Studies of lipoproteins may give clues to the varied diseases associated with deranged lipid metabolism, such as xanthomatosis and atherosclerosis.

REFERENCES

1. Nerking, J. Pflügers Arch. ges. Physiol., *85*, 330 (1901).
2. Macheboeuf, M. A. Bull. Soc. Chim. Biol., *11*, 268 (1929).
3. Oncley, J. L., Gurd, F. R. N., and Melin, M. J. Am. Chem. Soc., *72*, 458 (1950).
4. Lindgren, F. T., Elliott, H. A., and Gofman, J. W. J. Phys. and Colloid Chem., *55*, 80 (1951).
5. Batchelor, W. H. Personal communication, 1951.
6. Boyle, E., Bragdon, J. H., and Brown, R. K. Proc. Soc. Exper. Biol. and Med., *81*, 475 (1952).
7. Gitlin, D. Science, *117*, 591 (1953).
8. Beischer, D. E. Circulation Res., *2*, 164 (1954).
9. Oncley, J. L., Melin, M., Richert, D. A., Cameron, J. W., and Gross, P. M., Jr. J. Am. Chem. Soc., *71*, 541 (1949).
10. Brown, R. K., Baker, W. H., Peterkofsky, A., and Kauffman, D. L. J. Am. Chem. Soc., *76*, 4244 (1954).
11. Gurd, F. R. N. Ph.D. dissertation, Harvard University, Cambridge, Mass., 1949.
12. Cohn, E. J., Strong, L. E., Hughes, W. L., Jr., Mulford, D. J., Ashworth, J. N., Melin, M., and Taylor, H. L. J. Am. Chem. Soc., *68*, 459 (1946).
13. Kominz, D. Personal communication, 1953.
14. Tullis, J. L. (ed.) *Blood Cells and Plasma Proteins*. New York, Academic Press, 1953, p. 338.
15. Hahn, P. F. Science, *98*, 19 (1943).
16. Graham, D. M., Lyon, T. P., Gofman, J. W., Jones, H. B., Yankley, A., Simton, J., and White, S. Circulation, *4*, 666 (1951).
17. Bragdon, J. H., and Havel, R. J. Science, *120*, 113 (1954).
18. Korn, E. D. Science, *120*, 399 (1954).
19. Anfinsen, C. B., Boyle, E., and Brown, R. K. Science, *115*, 583 (1952).
20. Nikkilä, E. Scand. J. Clin. and Lab. Invest., *5*, Sup. 8, 101 (1953).
21. Jeffries, G. H. Quart. J. Exper. Phys., *39*, 77 (1954).
22. Anfinsen, C. B. Personal communication, 1954.
23. Brown, R. K., Boyle, E., and Anfinsen, C. B. J. Biol. Chem., *204*, 423 (1953).
24. Gomori,. G. J. Histochem. and Cytochem., *1*, 469 (1953).
25. Levy, S. W., and Swank, R. L. J. Physiol., *123*, 301 (1954).
26. Shore, B., Nichols, A. V., and Freeman, N. K. Proc. Soc. Exper. Biol. and Med., *83*, 216 (1953).
27. Jansen, E. F., Nutting, M. D. F., Jang, R., and Balls, A. K. J. Biol. Chem., *179*, 189 (1949).
28. Gordon, R. S., Jr., Boyle, E., Brown, R. K., Cherkes, A., and Anfinsen, C. B. Proc. Soc. Exper. Biol. and Med., *84*, 168 (1953).
29. Robinson, D. S., and French, J. E. Quart. J. Exper. Phys., *38*, 233 (1953).
30. Brown, R. K., Baker, W. H., and Kauffman, D. L. Fed. Proc., *13*, 563 (1954).
31. Rosenberg, R. Personal communication, 1953.
32. Williams, G. R. Biochim. Biophys. et Acta, *13*, 72 (1954).
33. Grossman, M. Personal communication, 1954.
34. Wadsworth, A. B. *Standard Methods of the Division of Laboratories and Research of the New York State Department of Health* ed. 3. Baltimore, Md., Williams and Wilkins, 1947.

Recent Studies of Fat Digestion and Absorption

Raymond Reiser

THE MECHANISM WHEREBY water-insoluble fat can pass through the intestinal epithelium and into the blood has been a very intriguing as well as a most refractory problem. Obviously, the fat must either pass as particles or it must be solubilized, and various theories have been devised based on both possibilities.

Most studies on the degree of hydrolysis of fat during digestion have been undertaken to obtain clues of the mechanism of the absorption of fat. If it could be demonstrated, for example, that fat is always completely hydrolyzed in the lumen of the intestine, it would be necessary to explain the absorption of fatty acid but not of glycerides. On the other hand, if it could be demonstrated that hydrolysis is not complete, then, *ipso facto*, glycerides must be absorbed and the mechanism of their absorption must be explained.

Up to the advent of the use of isotopes as tracers, no experiment was designed which could demonstrate unequivocally whether or not hydrolysis is complete or whether glycerides are absorbed.

IN VITRO DIGESTION

"Modern" studies on the mechanism of digestion of fat, and the action of lipases, may be said to have originated with the work of Artom and Reale in 1935 (1). These workers fractionated the products of in vitro pancreatic lipase digestion in alcohol–water and acetone–water solutions. They found that, contrary to opinion up to that time, lipase action produced little if any glycerol but mainly mono- and di-glycerides.

From the Department of Biochemistry and Nutrition, Texas Agricultural Experimental Station, College Station, Texas.

Presented at the Symposium on Lipids and Lipoproteins, 126th National Meeting of the American Chemical Society—In Participation with the American Association of Clinical Chemists; September 16, 1954, New York City, N. Y.

It was not until ten years later that Frazer and Sammons independently rediscovered this phenomenon and announced that during the first four hours of in vitro fat digestion little if any glycerol is produced and that considerable quantities of monoglycerides are produced (2).

Two years after Frazer's rediscovery of the limited hydrolytic capacity of pancreatic lipase on monoglycerides, Desnuelle and his coworkers (3, 4) verified the observation of these in vitro studies. These authors showed conclusively that pancreatic extracts produce diglycerides readily, that the production of monoglycerides requires more time and the presence of calcium ions, and that the digestion of monoglycerides requires "a large aqueous phase rich in bile salts" and much more time.

Schønheyder and Volqvartz have made confirmatory studies demonstrating the increasing difficulty of hydrolysis with increase in number of free hydroxyl groups (6). These workers found that the action of liver esterases on tripropionin produces the diglyceride easily, the monoglyceride with more difficulty, and free glycerol only after prolonged time. Under their conditions pancreatic lipase could hydrolyze the substrate only to the diglyceride.

In a study to determine the most susceptible glyceride ester linkages Desnuelle, Naudet, and Rouzier have reported (5) that the proportions of 1- and 2-monoglycerides formed are 2:1, an observation which, if confirmed, would indicate that there is no specificity for the 1- or the 2-positions.

In 1952 (7) and in 1954 (8) Borgström reported in vitro studies in which base exchange resins and silicic acid chromatography were utilized to separate the products of digestion, and C^{14} labeled fatty acids to trace the course of the reactions. Borgström reported that after one hour of digestion with pancreatic lipase the digestion mixture contained considerable quantities of tri- and mono-glycerides but that there was no free glycerol. In 24 hours digestion was complete (7).

In Borgström's studies (8) labeled fatty acids were added to digestion mixtures containing triglycerides. It was found that an equilibrium was reached between the free fatty acids and the glyceride fatty acids. At equilibrium the specific activity of the glyceride fatty acids, however, were less than that of the free fatty acids. Separation of the glycerides by silicic acid chromatography, and direct measurement of the specific activities of their constituent fatty acids showed that the triglycerides had about two thirds of the activity of the free acids, the diglycerides about one half, and the monoglycerides about one tenth.

Borgström explained these results according to the scheme shown in Fig. 1. If one assumes that only the 1- and 3-positions are in equilib-

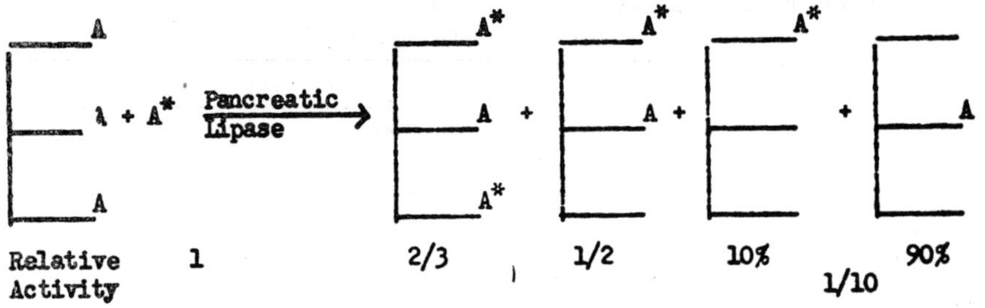

Fig. 1. The products of the digestion of triglycerides in the presence of labeled free fatty acid. From Borgstrom. (8)

rium with the free fatty acids the data are explainable. The fatty acid on the 1- and 3- positions would then have the same activity as the free fatty acids but those on the 2-position would remain inert. This hypothesis would require that 90 per cent of the monoglycerides are of the 2-isomer. To the contrary, Mattson, Benedict, and Beck have recently found by chemical analysis that only the 1- monoglyceride is formed in vitro but that 2- monoglycerides are the predominant monoglyceride formed in in vivo digestion (9).[1]

To sum up the results of in vitro studies beginning with the 1935 work of Artom and Reale, it has become increasingly evident that diglycerides are readily produced by in vitro lipase action, that monoglycerides are produced with more difficulty and require more time and more exacting conditions, and that the production of glycerol is slow and refractory.

The in vitro studies are conflicting with respect to the relative specificity of the 1-, 2-, and 3- positions. Desnuelle reported that twice as much 1- as 2- monoglycerides are formed, indicating equal specificity (5). Borgström adducted evidence to show that the 2-isomer is the predominant one formed (8), while Mattson, Benedict, and Beck found that in vitro pancreatic digestion produced mainly the 1-isomer (9).[1]

IN VIVO DIGESTION

The past two years have produced a number of important studies on in vivo lipolysis (Table 1). Desnuelle and Constantin (10) examined the intraluminary lipides three hours after olive oil ingestion and found that it consisted of approximately 50 per cent triglycerides, 21 per cent diglycerides, 5 per cent monoglycerides, and 16–24 per cent free fatty acids.

[1] In a recent communication, Dr. Mattson informed this author that in new studies by his group, the 2-monoglycerides have been identified in the products of in vitro digestion.

Table 1. Lipide Analyses of the Intestinal Contents after Triglyceride Digestion

	Glyceride species				
	Tri- (%)	Di- (%)	Mono- 1- (%)	Mono- 2- (%)	FFA (%)
Desnuelle *et al.* (10)	50	21	5		16–24
Mattson *et al.* (11)	41	36	3.2	4.3	15.5
Mattson *et al.* (9)	60–70	..	4–7	4–7	25
Kuhrt *et al.* (13)	..	..	37.6		..
			50.0		..
Harris *et al.* (14)	..	..	2.5	2.5	2–3 times the monoglycerides

Mattson, Benedict, Martin, and Beck (11) found that three hours after feeding triglyceride the lipides of the intestine consisted of 41 per cent triglyceride, 36 per cent diglyceride, 4.3 per cent 2-monoglyceride, 3.2 per cent 1-monoglyceride, and 15.5 per cent free fatty acid. These equal proportions of the 1- and 2- monoglycerides were in contrast to their in vitro findings (9)[1] but in confirmation of Desnuelle. That equal proportions do not mean equal susceptibility of the 1- and 2- positions to hydrolysis however, was demonstrated by an experiment with the use of 2-oleyl-dipalmitin (Fig. 2). After the ingestion of this compound by the rat, analyses of the intestinal lipides showed that there were about equal proportions of 1- and 2- monoglycerides. The iodine value of the mixed monoglycerides, however, was 64, and of the free fatty acids only 5. This indicates that the palmitic acid radicles must first have been hydrolyzed and half the resultant 2-monoolein rearranged to form 1-monoolein.

More recently Mattson, Benedict, and Beck (9) examined the lipides of the intestinal contents after the ingestion of cottonseed oil, of cottonseed oil with various proportions of 1-monoglyceride, cottonseed oil with varying amounts of 2-monoglyceride, and cottonseed oil with varying amounts of free fatty acids. Surprisingly, after 3 hours of digestion of the oil, alone or with any amount of either monoglyceride, the lipides of the digestion mixture had the same composition: 60–70 per cent triglycerides plus diglycerides, 4–7 per cent 1-monoglycerides, and about 25 per cent free fatty acids. When fed with free fatty acids, there was no 2-monoglyceride found, although there were 6–15 per cent 1-monoglycerides.

In an undetailed experiment, these authors reported that they fed 1-monoglyceride alone and found no 2-monoglyceride, diglyceride, or triglyceride.

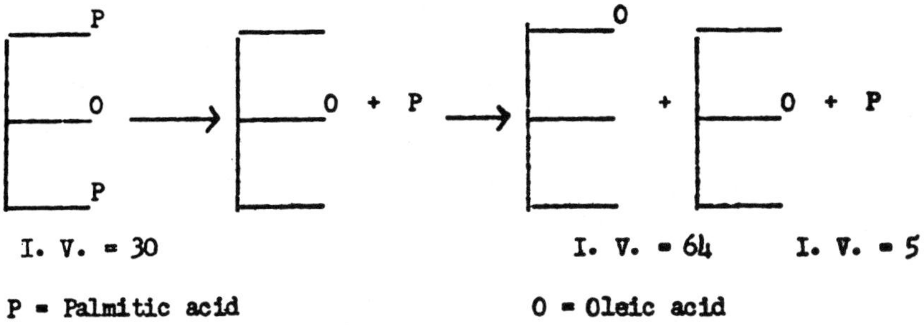

Fig. 2. Evidence that 2-monoglycerides are the product of in vivo fat digestion, followed by rearrangement to the 1-isomer from Mattson *et al.* (11)

The observations of Mattson, Benedict, and Beck, upon feeding monoglycerides alone, or triglycerides plus free fatty acids, are in strong contrast to a recent report by Borgström (12). Upon feeding olive oil with labeled palmitic acid, or monoolein with labeled oleic and palmitic acid, this worker found the label in mono-, di- and tri-glycerides, all apparently produced during digestion.

The resolution of these conflicting findings is not apparent at this time. Mattson's results indicating that the 2- position cannot be esterified during digestion is in support of older studies by Artom and Reale (13). Beginning with glycerol and fatty acids these workers found it much more difficult to esterify the 2- position than the 1- or 3-.

There have been two recent studies on in vivo lipolysis in humans. Kuhrt, Welch, Blum, Perry, Weber, and Nasset (14) examined the lipides of the intestinal contents of 2 humans after the ingestion of oil. They found the lipides to contain 37.6 per cent and 50 per cent monoglycerides in the 2 subjects. This figure is five to ten times as high as that found by others.

Recently Harris, Chamberlain, and Benedict (15) reported finding 4–11 per cent of monoglycerides, evenly divided between the 1- and 2-isomers, in the intestines of 11 human subjects after fat meals. The free fatty acid content was two to three times that of the monoglycerides. This is similar to the results obtained by Mattson *et al.* with rats (11).

Gidez and Karnovsky, in a private communication,[2] state that they have measured the degree of hydrolysis by comparing the rate of $C^{14}O_2$ excretion after the ingestion of free C^{14}-labeled glycerol and triolein, C^{14}-labeled in the glycerol. They found that about 12 per cent glycerol was hydrolyzed during the first hour, 14 per cent during the first two

[2] Private communication. L. I. Gidez, Brookhaven National Laboratory, Upton L. I., New York, M. L. Karnovsky, Department Biological Chemistry, Harvard Medical School, Boston, Mass.

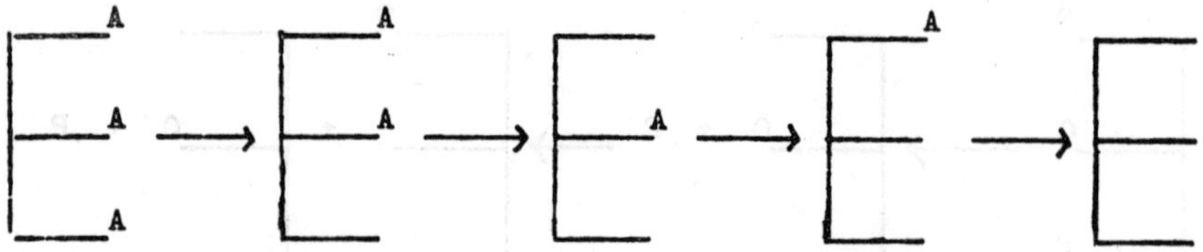

Fig. 3. Probable sequence of pancreatic lipolysis.

hours, 52 per cent at three hours and 97 per cent at eight hours. Although they have found some free labeled glycerol in the lumen of the intestine during fat digestion they believe intralumenary hydrolysis to glycerol to be slight and that the hydrolysis somehow takes place during transit of the ingested lipide from the mucosal cells to lymph.

In summary we can say that the bulk of both in vitro and in vivo experiments indicates that pancreatic lipolysis proceeds from triglycerides to glycerol stepwise with increasing difficulty, that the 1- and 3- positions are first split, that the 2- monoglycerides probably rearrange to the 1-isomer and that it is the 1-isomer that is finally hydrolyzed (Fig. 3).

ABSORPTION

Unfortunately our new knowledge of the steps in lipolysis allow us to draw no conclusions as to which species of glycerides are absorbed. The fact that pancreatic digestion is capable of hydrolyzing glycerides completely to fatty acids and glycerol does not mean that such happens and that no glycerides are absorbed. On the contrary, during the past two years unequivocal evidence has been obtained that the larger part of lipide glycerol is absorbed as glycerides. It remains to be determined whether all the lipide glycerol is so absorbed and whether it is in the form of only monoglycerides, or mixtures of monoglycerides with di- and triglycerides.

In 1951 Favarger, Collet, and Cherbuliez fed a mixture of triglycerides and deuterium-labeled glycerol to rats and examined the lymph glycerides for the labeled glycerol (16). They found that the glycerol was incorporated to the extent of only about 1.5–4.5 per cent into the resynthesized lipides and concluded that very little hydrolyses must take place and that 90 per cent of the fat must have been absorbed as mono-, di- and tri-glycerides (Fig. 4).

The rationale behind this experiment was that if hydrolysis were complete, the hydrolyzed glycerol would mix with the labeled free glycerol and the specific activity of the resynthesized fat, as it appears in the lymph, would reflect the degree of hydrolysis. Unfortunately their as-

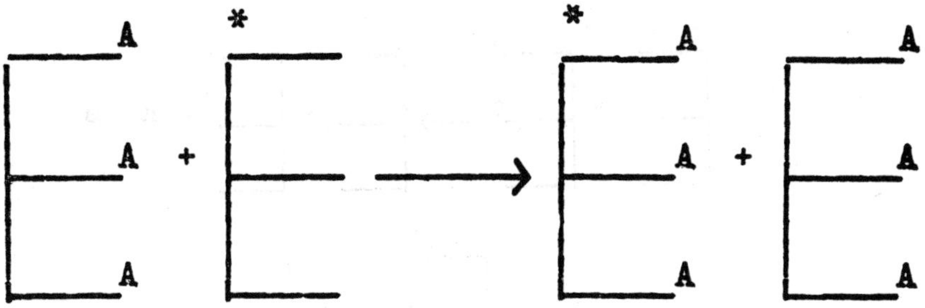

Fig. 4. Incorporation of ingested glycerol into lymph glycerides. From Favarger, Collet, and Cherbuliez. (16)

sumption was wrong. As it was later demonstrated, and several times confirmed, free glycerol in the intestinal lumen is not incorporated into resynthesized glycerides. Favarger's failure to incorporate labeled free glycerol into lymph glyceride need not then be due to lack of hydrolysis.

In 1952 we reported our first studies with glycerides labeled in both the glycerol and fatty acid moieties (17). In the first experiments rats were fed conjugated trilinolein in which the glycerol was labeled with C^{14}. Sixty per cent of the labeled glycerol was found in the lymph glycerides. (That is, after correcting for biological dilution, the lymph glycerol had a specific activity of 60 per cent as compared to that fed.)[3] It is possible either that the 60 per cent had been absorbed as glycerides or that the glycerides had been hydrolyzed and the labeled glycerol reutilized.

---

[3] In these calculations, in order to correct glycerol activity for biological dilution, it is assumed that ingested fatty acids undergo no metabolism before their appearance in the lymph and that the biological dilution of the glycerol is the same as that of the fatty acid. The following equation, therefore, may be used to determine the percentage of activity in the glycerol of the lymph or mucosa lipides as compared to the activity of the glycerol fed, corrected for biological dilution.

$$R = \frac{AF}{Ar} \times \frac{Gr}{Gf} \times 100$$

R = percentage of activity of recovered glycerol as compared to the glycerol fed;
Af = activity of fatty acid fed;
Ar = activity of fatty acid recovered;
Gf = activity of glycerol fed;
Ar = activity of glycerol recovered.

One may then calculate the percentage of glycerol activity lost (or, the percentage of labeled glycerol replaced with unlabeled glycerol) as "L" = 100 − R

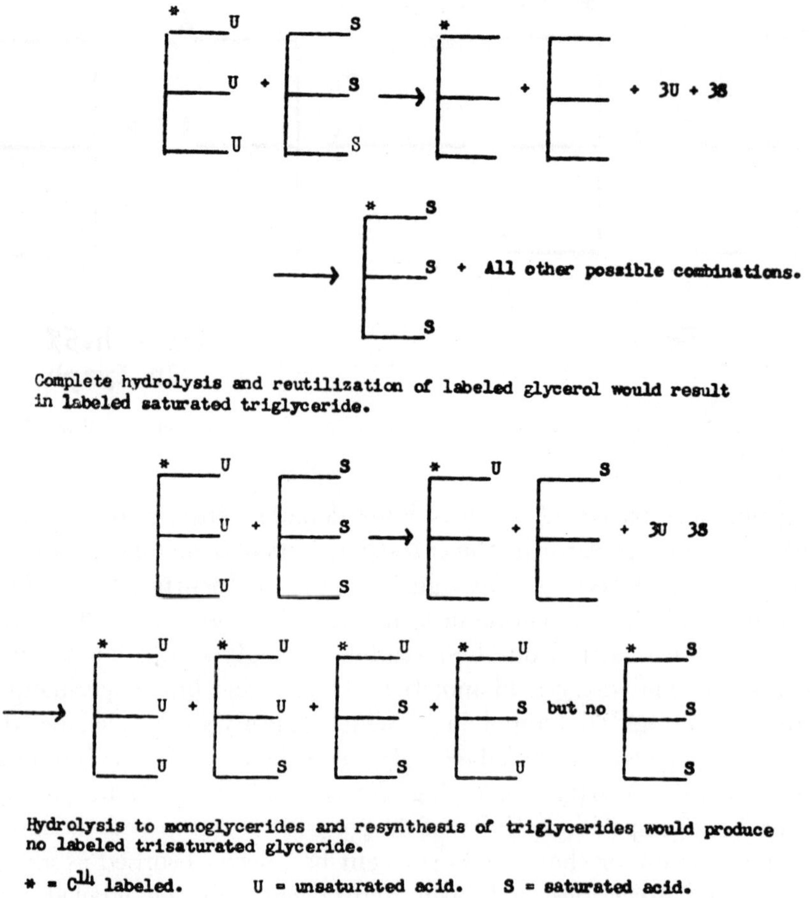

Fig. 5. Rational for determination of the degree of hydrolysis and of the glyceride species absorbed.

To test which possibility had occurred the labeled fat was mixed with saturated triglycerides and fed. The rationale for this study is diagramed in Fig. 5. In this example labeled unsaturated and unlabeled saturated triglycerides were administered in equal proportions: If all the triglycerides were completely hydrolyzed, and the labeled glycerol reutilized, some labeled trisaturated triglyceride would have been formed. If, however, the two compounds were hydrolyzed only as far as the monoglycerides, no labeled saturated triglyceride could be formed. Similarly, the theoretical relative specific activities of the various glyceride fractions can be calculated for any degree of hydrolysis. These calculations were made and compared to the experimental results (Table 2). It may be seen that the experimental results fit only the conditions that no

Table 2. Calculated Relative Specific Activities of the Glycerol of Hypothetically Possible Acetone-alcohol Soluble and Insoluble Lymph Glycerides after the Ingestion of Equal Parts of Glycerol-labeled Conjugated Trilinolein and Unlabeled Saturated Triglyceride

	Complete hydrolysis[a]	*No hydrolysis*	*Hydrolysis to diglycerides*	*Hydrolysis to monoglycerides*	*Found*
Acetone-soluble	40	80	75	60	60
Acetone-insoluble	100	0	0	60	59

[a] Reutilization of labeled glycerol.

completely hydrolyzed glycerol was reutilized and that only mono- but no di- or tri-glycerides were absorbed.

Confirmation that hydrolyzed glycerol is not reutilized has come from Wagner and Ritzel (18). These authors fed deuterium labeled glycerol, free and as triacetin, and found only traces in the lymph lipides. In the same report they presented data to show that triolein, deuterium labeled in the glycerol fraction, is only 24–53% hydrolyzed before its appearance in lymph fat, a figure close to that obtained in our laboratory.

That free glycerol, fed as such, or as glycerol phosphate, does not participate in glyceride resynthesis has been amply confirmed (18, 19). Furthermore, Borgström has been unable to incorporate glycerol and and fatty acids with pancreatic lipase in vitro under physiological conditions (11).

Since free glycerol or glycerol phosphate are not the precursor of glyceride glycerol, what is its precursor? The most logical compounds are glyceraldehyde or dihydroxyacetone. At the time this question arose, we had in our laboratory a few milligrams of 1-palmitoxy-3-hydroxyacetone labeled in the ketone and palmitic acid fractions. This compound was an intermediate in the synthesis of our labeled glycerol. (20) The material was fed to rats and appeared in the lymph as triglyceride, with the specific activity almost unchanged, acting very similar to labeled monopalmitin.

The appearance of labeled triglycerides in the lymph after the ingestion of either palmitoxy-hydroxyacetone or monopalmitin, with no loss of specific activity, indicates that just enough hydrolysis had occurred to permit the triglyceride synthesis. This suggested an enzymatically controlled reaction, such as would take place intracellularly, rather than digestion in the lumen of the intestine. That is, it seemed reasonable that monoglycerides are absorbed unchanged and converted to triglycerides in the intestinal mucosa.

A corollary of this hypothesis would be that phospholipides are not

Table 3. Relative Specific Activities of the Glycerol of Mucosa and Lymph Triglycerides and Phospholipides after the Ingestion of Glycerol-labeled Triglycerides

Mucosa		*Lymph*	
Triglycerides (%)	*Phospholipides (%)*	*Triglycerides (%)*	*Phospholipides (%)*
−154[a]	38–42	54–73	46 and 48

[a] This factor may be explained if the mucosa glycerides contained appreciable quantities of unlabeled fatty acids.

intermediate in the resynthesis of triglycerides. Studies have been made in our laboratory to test this hypothesis by comparing the specific activity of ingested triglyceride, mucosa triglyceride and phospholipide, and lymph triglyceride and phospholipide (Table 3). The relative specific activities R[3], of the lymph and mucosa phospholipide glycerol were between 38 per cent and 48 per cent, while those of the triglycerides were between 54 per cent and 73 per cent. It thus seems clear that phospholipide must be formed from triglycerides rather than the reverse.

Gidez and Karnovsky have just informed me that they have unpublished data also demonstrating that the mucosa phospholipide glycerol has a lower relative specific activity than the triglycerides. A surprising observation was the presence in the lumen of the intestine of phospholipide glycerol with a relative specific activity of 100.

The demonstrated limited capacity of lipase to hydrolyze monoglycerides, as well as their rapid absorption, the proven fact that hydrolyzed glycerol does not participate in glyceride resynthesis, and the relative specific activities of labeled glycerol in ingested and lymph triglycerides and in mucosa and lymph phospholipide, have tempted me to construct a modified hypothesis of fat absorption (Fig. 6). Considering, first, the changes when monoglycerides alone are fed, the hypothesis that these are absorbed into the mucosa and there converted to triglycerides with no loss of glyceride glycerol, fits the experimental data. Under these conditions there would be no loss in relative specific activity.

The hypothesis for the mechanism of the digestion and absorption of triglycerides is diagrammatically presented in Fig. 7.

Triglycerides are hydrolized in the intestine to monoglycerides. The absorbed fatty acids combine in the mucosa with the absorbed monoglycerides and with the glycerol precursor in the proper proportions to produce triglycerides with the observed relative specific activity of 60 per cent. This step requires the postulate that monoglycerides and endogenous glycerol (or its precursor) compete for the absorbed fatty acids in the ratio of 3:2. Two molecules of this triglyceride may then combine

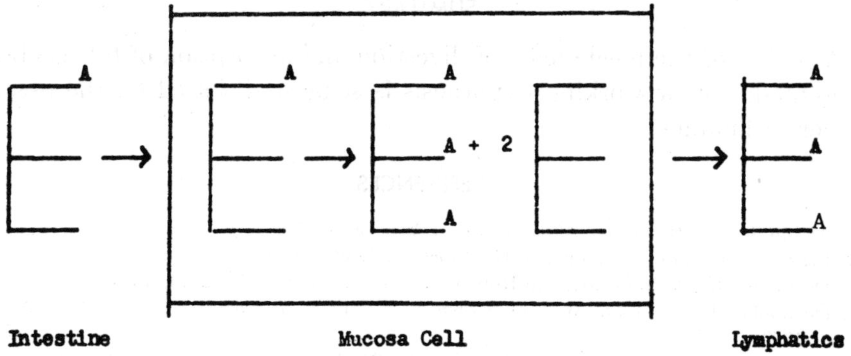

Fig. 6. Absorption of monoglycerides.

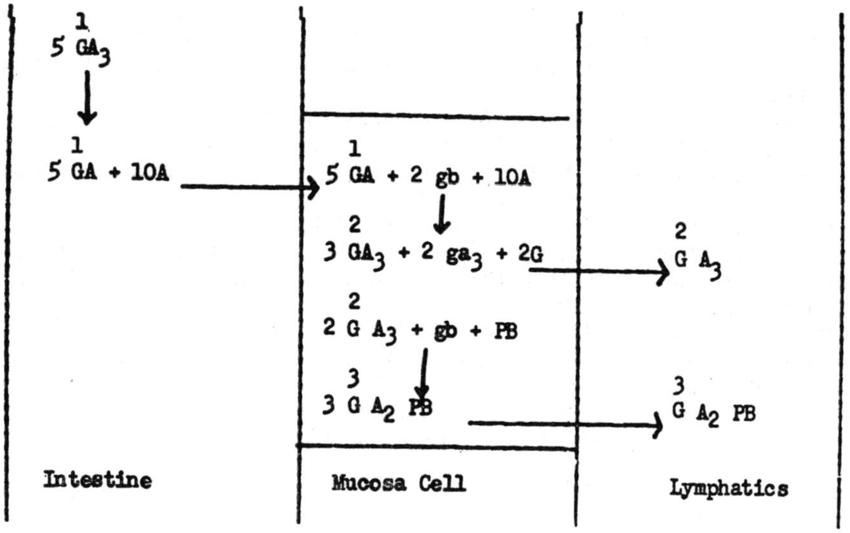

Fig. 7. Absorption of triglycerides. *G*, Labeled glycerol; *gb*, unlabeled glycerol precursor. *1*, Relative specific activity = 100; *2*, relative specific activity = 60; *3*, relative specific activity = 40.

with one molecule of glycerol precursor and one molecule of a phosphorylated base to produce phospholipide whose glycerol, therefore, has a relative specific activity of 40 per cent.

This scheme is presented as a working hypothesis only. Actually, there may be up to 10 per cent hydrolyses of monoglycerides in the intestine. Also, a number of alternative schemes could be designed which would fit the same data. However, this scheme seemed to be the simplest and most reasonable. I hope it may be of some help in clearing up the many mysteries which remain unanswered in this intriguing problem.

SUMMARY

A review of the mechanism of digestion and absorption of fat has been presented. A new working hypothesis is suggested, based on the uses of tracer techniques.

REFERENCES

1. Artom, C. and Reale, L., *Arch. Aci. Biol.* **21,** 368 (1935).
2. Frazer, A. C., and Sammons, H. G., *Biochem. J.* **39,** 122 (1954).
3. Desnuelle, R., Naudet, M., and Rouzier, J., *Arch. Sci. Physiol.* **2,** 71 (1948).
4. Desnuelle, P., Naudet, M., and Constantin, M. J., *Biochem. Biophys. Acta.* **5,** 561 (1950).
5. Desnuelle, P., Naudet, M., and Rouzier, J., *Biochem. Biophys. Acta.* **2,** 561 (1948).
6. Schønheyder, F., and Volqvantz, K., *Biochem. Biophys. Acta.* **8,** 407 (1952).
7. Borgström, Bengt, *Acta Physiol. Scand.* **25,** 328 (1952).
8. Borgström, Bengt, *Biophysica Acta.* **13,** 491 (1954).
9. Mattson, F. H., Benedict, J. H., and Beck, L. W., *J. Nutrition* **52,** 575 (1954).
10. Desnuelle, P., and Constantin, J. H., *Biochem. Biophys. Acta.* **9,** 531 (1952).
11. Mattson, F. H., Benedict, J. H., Martin, J. B., and Beck, L. W., *J. Nutrition* **48,** 335 (1952).
12. Borgström, Bengt, *Arch. Biochem. Biophys.* **49,** 268 (1954).
13. Artom, C., Reale, L., *Bull. Sci. Chem. Biol.* (Paris) **18,** 959 (1936).
14. Kuhrt, N. H., Welch, E. A., Blum, W. P., Perry, E. S., Weber, W. H., and Nasset, E. S., *J. Am. Oil Chemists. Soc.* **29,** 261 (1952).
15. Harris, R. S., Chamberlain, J. W., and Benedict, J. H., *Fed. Proc.* **13,** 525 (1954).
16. Favarger, P., Collet, R. A., and Cherbuliez, E., *Helv. Chim. Acta.* **34,** 1651 (1951).
17. Reiser, Raymond, Bryson, M. J., Carr, Mary J., and Kuiken, K. A., *J. Biol. Chem.* **194,** 131 (1952).
18. Bernhard, K., Wagner, H., and Ritzel, G., *Helv. Chim. Acta.* **35,** 1404 (1952).
19. Buensod, M., Favarger, P., and Collet, R. W., *Helv. Physiol. et Pharmacol. Acta.* **11,** 45 (1953).
20. Schlenk, H., and DeHaas, Bernice, W., *J. Am. Chem. Soc.* **73,** 3921 (1951).
21. Reiser, Raymond, and Williams, Mary C., *J. Biol. Chem.* **202,** 815 (1953).

Reproducibility and Validity of Sodium Sulfate Fractionation of Proteins in Plasma and Knee Joint Fluid

O. H. Gaebler, W. T. Beher, J. W. Sigler, and R. R. Galpin

Simple and rapid methods of determining plasma proteins, which yield results comparing favorably with those obtained by electrophoresis, have been sought by several investigators. The procedure of Milne seemed of particular interest to us, since it differs from the widely used one of Howe only with respect to the concentrations of sodium sulfate employed. The dual purpose of the present study was, first, to secure an additional series of normal values for serum proteins determined by the method of Milne, and second, to ascertain whether his reported agreement between salt fractionation and electrophoretic separation of serum applies to knee joint fluid. A component moving more rapidly than albumin was noted in all knee joint fluids examined, and was studied further by means of electrophoresis-convection (1).

MATERIALS AND METHODS

Blood samples were drawn from the cubital vein, during mid-morning, from 16 apparently normal staff members who were seated during venepuncture. About an hour after clotting, serum was separated by centrifugation. Analyses were made in duplicate or triplicate by the method of Milne.

Knee joint fluids were brought to the laboratory shortly after aspirations had been performed in the Arthritis Clinic of the Hospital. Veronal buffer, *p*H 8.6 and ionic strength 0.1, was used in electrophoretic studies.

From the Edsel B. Ford Institute for Medical Research, and the Arthritis Division, Henry Ford Hospital, Detroit, Michigan.

We are indebted to Dr. James C. Mathies for carrying out the electrophoresis-convection experiment; to Mr. R. B. Scott and Mr. Ernest J. Schoeb of the Research Laboratories, Parke, Davis and Company, for electrophoretic analyses; and to the Michigan Chapter, Arthritis and Rheumatism Foundation, for a grant in support of this study.

Received for publication July 24, 1954.

Each specimen was diluted 1:1 with this buffer and dialyzed against it for 16 to 24 hours before being run. The Aminco apparatus was used, and duration of electrophoresis was 120 minutes. Electrophoresis-convection had previously been applied, in this laboratory, to purification of alkaline phosphatase by Mathies, who carried out the experiment reported in this paper.

RESULTS

In Table 1 are presented the data on serum. The finding of Milne that there is no difference between results for males and females was confirmed. Our normal values also coincide with his, and, as already stated, represent values in persons who were seated for a few minutes in the course of their regular duties. Although Rowe in 1916 recognized that exercise and posture alter plasma protein values, and Wolfson and Cohn have quite recently stated that the change from a standing to a recumbent position

Table 1. Values for Fibrinogen, by the Method of Wu, and for Serum Proteins by the Sodium Sulfate Fractionation Procedure of Milne, in Normal Adult Male and Female Human Subjects

Subject	*Sex*	*Fibrinogen* (Gm. %)	*Serum proteins* (Gm. %)				*Serum proteins* (% total serum protein)			*Serum N.P.N.* (mg. %)
			Total	*Euglobulin*	*Pseudo-globulin*	*Albumin*	*Eu-globulin*	*Pseudo-globulin*	*Albumin*	
O. H. G.	M		7.22	1.76	0.86	4.60	24.4	11.9	63.7	32.6
M. J. S.	M	0.27	7.56	1.56	1.10	4.90	20.6	14.6	64.8	29.8
W. T. B.	M	0.31	7.60	1.81	1.07	4.72	23.8	14.1	62.1	29.6
R. S.	M		7.78	1.78	1.30	4.70	22.9	16.7	60.4	28.0
W. T. H.	M		7.88	2.06	1.26	4.56	26.2	16.0	57.8	27.8
P. D. B.	M	0.33	7.70	1.69	1.16	4.85	21.9	15.1	63.0	33.8
J. C. M.	M	0.36	7.40	1.86	0.92	4.62	25.1	12.4	62.5	26.8
H. H. S.	M	0.25	7.77	1.61	1.58	4.58	20.7	20.3	59.0	31.6
F. J. O.	M	0.23	6.91	1.81	0.92	4.18	26.2	13.3	60.5	28.9
E. H. W.	F	0.26	7.75	2.44	1.25	4.06	31.5	16.2	52.3	20.8
E. M. C.	F	0.28	7.46	1.51	1.42	4.53	20.2	19.0	60.8	24.2
B. M.	F	0.29	7.85	2.18	0.85	4.82	27.8	10.8	61.4	30.2
E. G.	F	0.31	7.16	2.04	0.97	4.15	28.5	13.5	58.0	25.4
B. C.	F	0.32	7.47	1.91	0.69	4.87	25.6	9.2	65.2	23.6
Mean, males		0.29	7.54	1.77[a]	1.13	4.63	..	..	..	..
Mean, females.....		0.29	7.54	2.02[a]	1.04	4.49	..	..	..	..
Mean, all subjects...		0.29	7.54	1.86	1.10	4.58	24.7	14.5	60.8	28.1
Standard deviation....		±0.04	±0.29	±0.25	±0.25	±0.27	±3.3	±3.0	±3.35	..

[a] Significance of difference in means, $t = 1.94$; $p > 0.05, < 0.1$.

Table 2. ANALYSES OF KNEE JOINT FLUIDS BY SODIUM SULFATE FRACTIONATION AND ELECTROPHORESIS

Sample number	*Albumin* (Gm.%)		*Pseudoglobulin by sodium sulfate* (Gm.%)	α_1 *plus* α_2 *globulins by electrophoresis* (Gm.%)	*Euglobulin by sodium sulfate* (Gm.%)	β *plus* γ *globulins by electrophoresis* (Gm.%)
	Sodium sulfate	*Electro-phoresis*				
1-L[a]	1.85	1.78	0.79	0.56	2.19	2.49
2-R[a]	1.98	2.00	0.70	0.70	2.12	2.12
3-L	1.40	1.91	1.52	0.55	1.95	2.41
4-R	1.76	2.14	1.04	0.62	2.07	2.10
5-L	1.35	1.99	1.14	0.52	2.06	2.04
6-R	1.64	1.89	0.87	0.70	2.15	2.08
7-L	1.18	1.92	1.44	0.57	2.08	2.20
8-R	1.65	2.00	1.17	0.63	2.02	2.18

[a] L left knee; R right knee.

has hydrostatic effects which may alter serum protein values 15 per cent, this information is still received with skepticism at times. In Table 1 fibrinogen values, determined by the method of Wu, are included for completeness. Specimens for this purpose were oxalated with 2 mg. of potassium oxalate per ml.

In Table 2 are presented the values for proteins in knee joint fluid. Actually, we analyzed 18 knee joint fluids by the method of Milne, but only 8, in which comparisons between the electrophoretic and salt fractionation results were made, are included in the table. These were all obtained at different visits from the same patient. In Samples 3 to 8, albumin values obtained by the sodium sulfate method were well below the electrophoretic ones, and pseudoglobulin considerably exceeded the sum of the α_1 and α_2 electrophoretic fractions. This suggests entrainment of albumin, when the high concentration of sodium sulfate required for precipitation of pseudoglobulin is used in the analysis of knee joint fluid. Whatman #50 filter paper was used throughout, since it has been reported (2) that this minimizes errors due to adsorption of albumin on filter paper. Results for euglobulin compared fairly closely with the sum of β and γ fractions, in six of the eight samples.

Results of electrophoresis-convection were simple. Pooled knee joint fluids from 4 patients were centrifugalized for 30 minutes at 5° and 3300 RPM to remove a flocculent precipitate. A 10 ml. sample (Sample 1) of the supernatant was diluted with an equal volume of phosphate buffer, *p*H 7.2 and 0.1 ionic strength, and dialyzed against four 4 liter portions of this buffer. The supernatant was still faintly turbid, and the solution was viscous. Electrophoresis-convection was carried out for 6 hours at

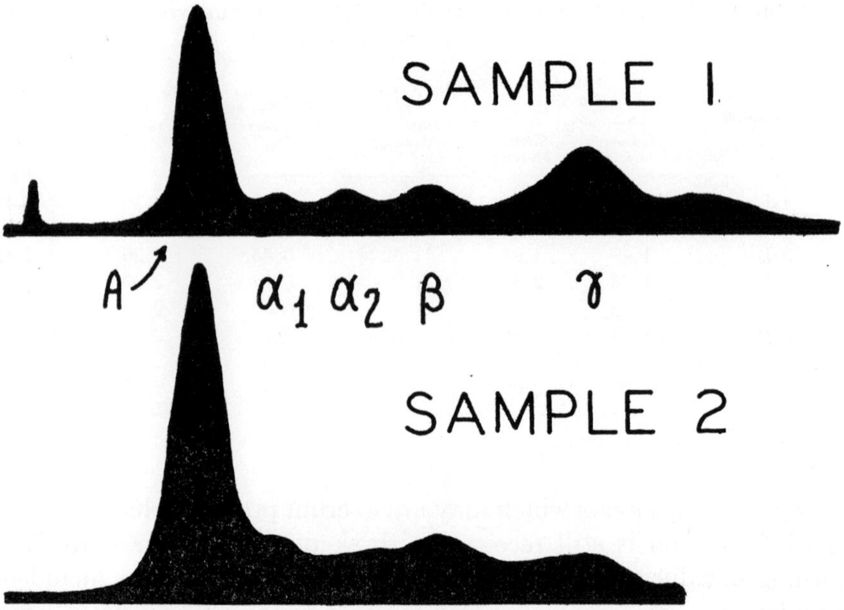

Fig. 1. Electrophoretic patterns (ascending boundaries) of pooled knee joint fluids (Sample 1) and fraction thereof (Sample 2) taken from lower chamber of electrophoresis-convection apparatus.

0.5 amp., the potential drop across the apparatus being 12 v. The bottom fraction was then sampled (Sample 2). The electrophoretic patterns before and after electrophoresis-convection are shown in Fig. 1. The fast moving component was not concentrated in the bottom fraction, as one had reason to expect, but disappeared. Adherence to the membranes of the apparatus is one of several possible explanations. In any case, use of this procedure to concentrate the component for study does not appear feasible. In the 8 samples, this component amounted to only 0.04–0.10 per cent of the total protein.

SUMMARY

Blood was drawn from 14 laboratory workers under conditions similar to those under which blood samples are taken from ambulatory clinic patients. The sera were analyzed for the various proteins by the method of Milne. Eighteen knee joint fluids were analyzed by the same method; and 8 fluids from one patient were also analyzed electrophoretically. Results for these 8 fluids, and for all of the sera, are presented in tabular form and discussed. A component moving faster than albumin was noted in all knee joint fluids. This could not be concentrated from a pooled lot from 4 patients by electrophoresis-convection, but disappeared instead.

REFERENCES

1. Cann, J. R., Kirkwood, J. G., Brown, R. A., and Plescia, O. J., *J. Am. Chem. Soc.*, **71**, 1603 (1949).
2. Harris, R. C., *J. Biol. Chem.*, **127**, 751 (1939).
3. Howe, P. E., *J. Biol. Chem.*, **49**, 93 (1921).
4. Mathies, J. C., *Science*, **115**, 144 (1952).
5. Milne, J., *J. Biol. Chem.*, **169**, 595 (1947).
6. Rowe, A. H., *Arch. Int. Med.*, **19**, 499 (1917).
7. Wolfson, W. Q., and Cohn C., *Rapid Chemical Micro Methods for the Analytical Fractionation of Serum Proteins*. Ann Arbor, Michigan, The Overbeck Co., 1951.
8. Wu, H., and Ling, S. M., *Chinese J. Physiol.*, **1**, 161 (1927).

Colorimetric Determination of Blood Arginase

Max M. Friedman and Edythe Becker

An extensive literature on arginase activity in tissues and tissue homogenates has accumulated in recent years. Roberts (1) has studied the arginase activity of liver, kidney, and epidermis of the Swiss mouse and of a transplantable squamous cell carcinoma. He found that liver had the greatest activity, followed by carcinoma, epidermis, and kidney. Sano (2) isolated an enzyme from rabbit intestinal mucosa which formed urea at *p*H 9.2 from D(−)arginine, but not from natural L(+)arginine. He called this enzyme "heteroarginase." Dounce *et al.* (3) found high concentrations of arginase in isolated nuclei from rat liver. Van Scott (4) found that normal skin (female breast) contained considerable arginase activity, predominantly in the epidermis. Liener and Schultze (5) found in acute uremia of newborn rats a significant increase of liver arginase activity. These workers also found a high degree of correlation between the arginase activity of the liver and the urea level of the blood.

Less attention has been directed towards the arginase activity of blood. Covolo and West (6), in a study of the arginase activity of red blood cells, found this activity quite constant in a given individual and slightly higher in women than in men. Of the various diseases studied, only in infectious mononucleosis was there found to be any increase in red blood cell arginase. Kochakian *et al.* (7) found the arginase activity of red blood cells higher in males than in females, and that the values for given individuals varied considerably from time to time. Their results were not in accord with the findings of the previous investigators (6). They also found much variation in pathologic conditions.

The presence of arginase has been reported in the red blood cells, but not in the plasma, of human blood (8). We attempted various procedures for hemolysis of the red blood cells in an effort to determine the blood

From the Department of Biochemistry, Pack Medical Foundation, New York, New York.
Aided by a grant from Mr. and Mrs. T. Ferdinand Wilcox.
We wish to thank the New York Regional Blood Program of the American Red Cross and William M. Markel, M.D., Administrator, for permission to collect specimens from donors.
Received for publication July 22, 1954.

arginase activity in patients with carcinoma. Only negligible enzyme activity was obtained with blood not previously hemolyzed, and this activity was increased by the addition of increasing amounts of distilled water to the blood. As will subsequently be shown, the maximum activity was obtained only with the use of saponin, upon which principle this method is based. The procedure adopted was similar to the colorimetric method of Van Slyke and Archibald (9, 10) with some modifications in its application to blood arginase. The enzyme is permitted to act on a buffered arginine substrate and the liberated urea is then measured colorimetrically. Since no enzyme other than arginase is present in the blood which is known to yield urea from arginine (9), we have adopted as *a unit of blood arginase that amount of activity which under the conditions of the described procedure will yield 1 micromole of urea (0.06 mg.) per milliliter of blood.*

REAGENTS

Manganese chloride ($MnCl_2 \cdot 4H_2O$), 20.0% solution.

Arginine substrate, to 9.0 gm. of L-arginine monohydrochloride (Merck), add 3.2 ml. of 9.0N NaOH (CO_2 free) and make to 50 ml. with water. Solution is 0.85M and *p*H 9.5.

Trichloroacetic acid, 15% solution.

Sulfuric-phosphoric acid mixture, 90 ml. conc. H_2SO_4 and 270 ml. 85% phosphoric acid are poured into water and made to 1000 ml.

Saponin, 0.05% solution.

α-isonitrosopropiophenone (*Eastman Kodak*), 3.0% solution in 95% ethanol.

Urea, stock, 67.3 mg. urea dissolved in 100 ml. water.

Urea, working standard, dilute urea stock solution by adding 1 part stock to 24 parts sulfuric-phosphoric acid mixture.

Arginine-trichloroacetic acid mixture, to 5.0 ml. of arginine substrate add 10.0 ml. of trichloroacetic acid and 5.0 ml. water.

PROCEDURE

Hemolysis

To 1.0 ml. of oxalated blood add 9.0 ml. saponin solution, mix well, and let stand 30 minutes at room temperature.

Activation

Add 0.5 ml. of 20% manganese chloride to the above solution and let stand 2 hours at room temperature. This is necessary for arginase activation by Mn^{++}. Two aliquots each of 2.0 ml. are transferred to test tubes marked T_1 (total urea) and T_2 (preformed urea). To T_1 add 1.0 ml. arginine substrate and incubate at 25° for exactly 10 minutes, followed immediately by 2.0 ml. of 15% trichloroacetic acid. To T_2 add 2.0 ml. trichloroacetic acid (to prevent enzyme activity), followed by 1.0 ml. arginine substrate. Shake both tubes, let stand 15 minutes, and filter. A reagent blank is prepared simultaneously by adding 0.1 ml. manganese chloride to 1.9 ml. saponin, 2.0 ml. trichloroacetic acid, and 1.0 ml. arginine substrate, shaking, and filtering. One blank may serve for any one series of determinations.

Urea Determination

To 2.0 ml. of the above filtrates (T_1, T_2, and blank) add 15.0 ml. sulfuric-phosphoric acid mixture to each, mix, and transfer 10.0 ml. portions into pyrex test tubes. To each add 0.5 ml. α-isonitrosopropiophenone, mix, and place in a boiling water bath for one hour in the dark. Test tubes should be fitted with a one-hole rubber stopper through which is passed a short heavy-walled capillary tube of 0.5–1.0 mm. bore. After removing from the boiling water bath place the tubes in a bath of 50–55°, transfer into warm curvettes, and read immediately in the colorimeter with a 540 mμ filter, the reagent blank set at 100 per cent transmission.

Preparation of Urea Curve

To 1, 2, 3, 4, 5, and 6 ml. of working urea standards as prepared under *reagents* are added respectively 8, 7, 6, 5, 4, and 3 ml. sulfuric-phosphoric acid mixture (total volume 9.0 ml.). To each tube is added 1.0 ml. arginine-trichloroacetic acid mixture and the urea is determined as described under *procedure*, with the addition of 0.5 ml. α-isonitrosopropiophenone, heat, etc. The blank consists of 9.0 ml. sulfuric-phosphoric acid mixture and 1.0 ml. arginine-trichloroacetic acid mixture, and is treated in the same manner as the standards.

Calculation

The urea working standards are so prepared that 1.0 ml. is equivalent to 10 blood arginase units as calculated from the aliquots of this procedure. A plot of the standard urea curve using the Leitz colorimeter and a 535 mμ filter is shown in Fig. 1. For subsequent determinations of blood arginase it is only necessary to subtract T_2 from T_1 and obtain the results directly in blood arginase units.

Discussion

The method described for blood arginase is based on the formation of urea by action of the enzyme on a buffered solution of arginine. After

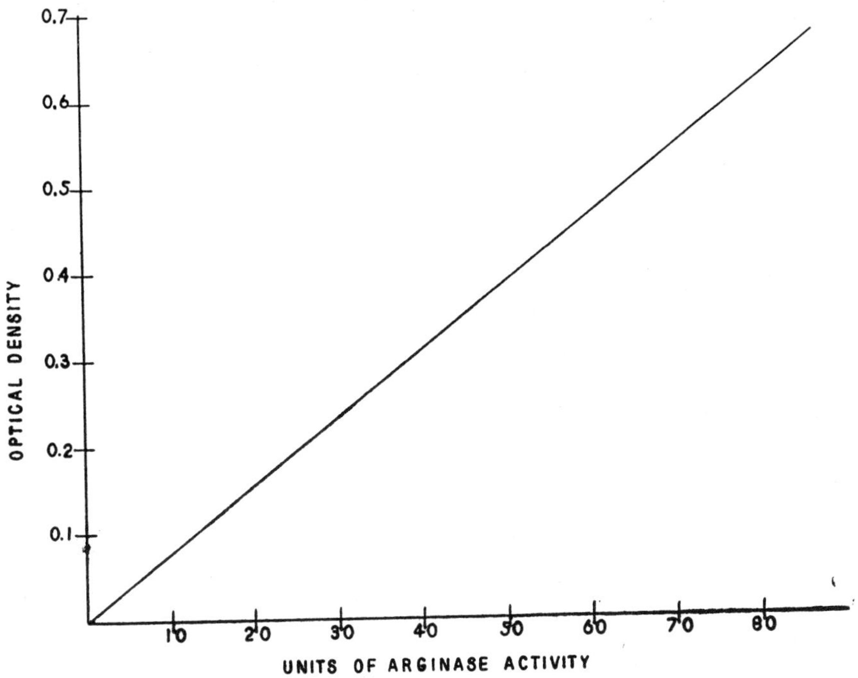

Fig. 1. Plot of standard urea curve in terms of arginase activity.

hemolysis of the red blood cells, the enzyme is activated for two hours at room temperature in the presence of 0.5 ml. of 20% manganese chloride. The conditions for incubation are those of Van Slyke and Archibald (9) using an arginine substrate of 0.85M at a *p*H of 9.5. For incubation 1 part of substrate is added to 2 parts of test solution giving a final arginine concentration of 0.28M. The incubation is allowed to proceed for 10 minutes at 25°. With this concentration of buffer it is not necessary to prepare a standard reference curve (9) since the urea formed is directly proportional to the amount of arginase activity. To further test this assumption a control experiment was performed using lyophilized beef liver arginase[1]. An aqueous solution of 1.0 mg. arginase per ml. was prepared, and diluted 1:20 with saponin. One milliliter of this solution now contained 0.05 mg. of lyophilized enzyme. To 1.0 ml. serum (arginase-free) was added 1, 2, 3, and 4 ml. of this diluted enzyme, made to 10 ml. with saponin, and the activity determined as described under *procedure.* The results are plotted in Fig. 2 and show a linear activity-concentration curve.

Since arginase is not present in human serum, but only in the red blood

[1] Worthington Biochemical Corporation, Freehold, New Jersey.

Table 1. Blood Arginase Activity as a Function of Time of Hemolysis with Water and Saponin

Sample No.	*Hemolysis* (min.)	*Water* (units)	*Saponin* (units)
1	15	17.0	33.2
	30	19.8	42.5
	180	18.0	39.0
2	30	25.3	53.5
	180	17.8	
3	30	14.3	36.0
4	30	24.0	56.8
5	30	24.0	63.2
6	15		48.0
	30		54.7
7	30		52.3
	60		52.0

cell, the procedure for hemolysis was investigated. Previous investigators (6, 7) hemolyzed the red blood cell with water and determined the arginase activity of the suspension. To expedite this step we attempted to use a lysing agent such as saponin and consequently found a marked increase in activity when compared to water alone. A series of determinations was run using 1 part of blood to 9 parts of water and 1 part of blood to 9 parts of saponin, and these were permitted to stand for varying periods of time for hemolysis. The results of these analyses are shown in Table 1. It is obvious from these data that with the use of saponin much larger amounts of arginase activity are obtained. The optimum enzyme activity was found with a 1:10 saponin dilution after 30 minutes standing, as adopted in this procedure. Rossiter (11) has also demonstrated that surface-active substances such as saponin liberate large amounts of active phosphatase from leukocytes in suspension, and Valentine and Beck (12) used saponin for the same purpose in the determination of acid and alkaline phosphatases of leukocyte suspensions.

Trichloroacetic acid was substituted for metaphosphoric acid (9) since it was found that the latter produced turbid supernatants on centrifugation or filtration.

As previously found (8), we could demonstrate no arginase activity in human sera. There was only negligible activity in freshly drawn blood determined without preliminary hemolysis.

For precise results it is also necessary to determine the preformed urea, since the activity is measured by the difference in urea before and after incubation. However, since the urea after incubation averages about ten times that of the preformed urea, it would be possible in the absence of

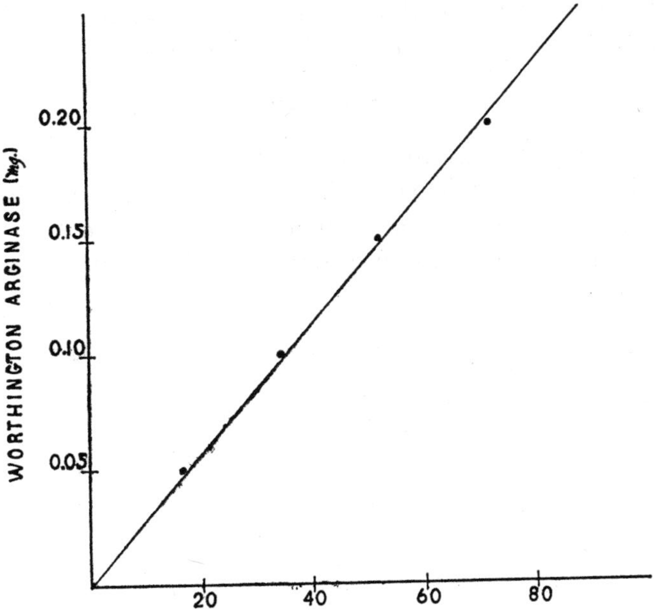

Fig. 2. Linear activity-concentration curve using lyophilized beef liver arginase.

Table 2. Distribution of Blood Arginase Values in Normal Adults

Arginase activity (Units)	*Number of subjects*
Below 30	0
30–40	18
41–50	33
51–60	29
61–70	11
71–80	8
Above 80	1

uremia to use an average value for urea as the control figure (T_2) with only a small error and thus simplify the procedure for clinical purposes. Also the preformed urea by any other method would be suitable.

RESULTS

A series of determinations was carried out on normal adults, which included 12 laboratory workers and 88 Red Cross blood donors. The distribution of results are shown in Table 2. The average value was found to be 51.7 units with a standard deviation of ± 12.4 units, and a range of

30.1 to 83.1 units. Most of the normal subjects were males and no attempt at this time was made to study sex differences.

SUMMARY

A colorimetric procedure for blood arginase has been described, based on hemolyzing the red blood cells with saponin and determining the urea formed by action of the enzyme on an arginine substrate.

The range of blood arginase in a series of normal human subjects has been presented.

REFERENCES

1. Roberts, E., *J. Biol. Chem.* **176,** 213 (1948).
2. Sano, M., *J. Biochem.* (Japan) **33,** 467 (1941).
3. Dounce, A. L., Tishkoff, G. H., Barnett, S. R., and Freer, R. M., *J. Gen. Physiol.* **33,** 629 (1950).
4. Van Scott, E. J., *J. Invest. Dermat.*, **17,** 21 (1951).
5. Liener, I. E., and Schultze, M. O., *J. Biol. Chem.* **187,** 743 (1950).
6. Covolo, G. C., and West, R., *J. Clin. Endocrin.* **7,** 325 (1947).
7. Kochakian, C. D., Keutmann, E. H., and Garber, E. E., *Conference on Metabolic Aspects of Convalescence, Trans. XVII Meeting,* **187,** (1948).
8. Weil, L., and Russell, M. A., *J. Biol. Chem.* **106,** 505 (1934).
9. Van Slyke, D. D., and Archibald, R. M., *J. Biol. Chem.*, **165,** 293 (1946).
10. Archibald, R. M., *J. Biol. Chem.*, **157,** 507 (1945).
11. Rossiter, R. J., *J. Physiol.*, **110,** 136 (1949).
12. Valentine, W. M., and Beck, W. S., *J. Lab. Clin. Med.*, **38,** 39 (1951).

Purification of Chromium (VI) for Use in the PBI Determination

W. Burkett Mason and Santo Coco

In connection with the determination of serum protein-bound iodine (PBI), it is occasionally advantageous to have available reagents with a very low iodine blank. Of the reagents required in a PBI procedure employing dialysis, wet combustion with H_2SO_4 and Cr (VI), volatilization of iodine after liberation with H_3PO_3, and estimation of iodine by means of the Ce (IV)–As (III) reaction, the Cr (VI) contributes most of the iodine blank.

Although CrO_3 and $Na_2Cr_2O_7$ can be obtained having as little as 5×10^{-9} Gm. I per Gm. Cr, the value is often much higher. Of various procedures undertaken for preparing Cr (VI) which is essentially free of iodine, conversion to chromyl chloride has proved most satisfactory. Using the method recommended by Fernelius (1), a batch of heavily contaminated CrO_3 containing 88×10^{-9} Gm. I per Gm. Cr, for example, was converted to crude CrO_2Cl_2 containing 1×10^{-9} gm. I per Gm. Cr, with a yield of 66 per cent. Studies utilizing I^{131} (as NaI) added to the initial CrO_3 solution confirmed the efficiency of the separation by indicating better than fiftyfold purification.

The crude chromyl chloride can be diluted with water and used with concentrated sulfuric acid for wet combustion of serum in the PBI determination. The digestion, however, had best be carried out in a well-ventilated hood because of the noxious fumes evolved.

SUMMARY

Chromium (VI) which is essentially free of iodine can be prepared by converting CrO_3 to CrO_2Cl_2. The crude chromyl chloride can be used with concentrated sulfuric acid for wet combustion of serum in the PBI determination.

REFERENCE

1. Fernelius, W. C., *Inorganic Synthesis*. New York, McGraw-Hill, 1946, Vol. II, p. 205.

From the Atomic Energy Project and Department of Biochemistry, School of Medicine and Dentistry, The University of Rochester, Rochester, New York.

This paper is based on work performed under contract with the United States Atomic Energy Commission at The University of Rochester Atomic Energy Project, Rochester, New York, and is covered in Report UR-242.

Received for publication October 18, 1954.

Iron Content of Tissues in Exogenous and Endogenous Hemochromatosis

Bernard Klein, Benjamin S. Gordon, and Irving Graef

Hemochromatosis is a disease marked by the pathologic appearance of large amounts of iron-containing pigment, hemosiderin, in various tissue cells, and is associated with periportal cirrhosis of the liver and pancreatic fibrosis. Three types of hemochromatosis have been recognized:

1. Idiopathic or endogenous hemochromatosis, wherein the intestinal "mucosal block" preventing excessive absorption of iron from the intestine is ineffective, and allows a gradual but persistent accumulation of surplus iron (1).
2. Exogenous hemochromatosis, in which multiple blood transfusions are said to be the underlying cause of excess iron accumulation (2).
3. Dietary hemochromatosis (3), in which extrinsic dietary factors are believed to be responsible for the breakdown of the mucosal block's regulation of iron absorption.

We have had the opportunity of studying several cases of the exogenous, or transfusion, type of hemochromatosis and analyzing the tissues at postmortem for iron. The results were compared with values obtained from the endogenous type for the purpose of differentiating chemically rather than histologically the two dominant forms of the disease. The pathologic and histologic aspects have been reported earlier (4). Cases of the third type were not available to us.

METHODS

A history of anemia of long duration was found in all exogenous cases studied. Multiple blood transfusions and hematinic therapy over a period of 1 to 8 years had been used unsuccessfully.

For comparison, the organs of several patients with long-standing

From the Laboratory and Medical Services, Veterans Administration Hospital, Bronx, N. Y.

Presented at the 126th National Meeting of the American Chemical Society, New York City, September 12–17, 1954.

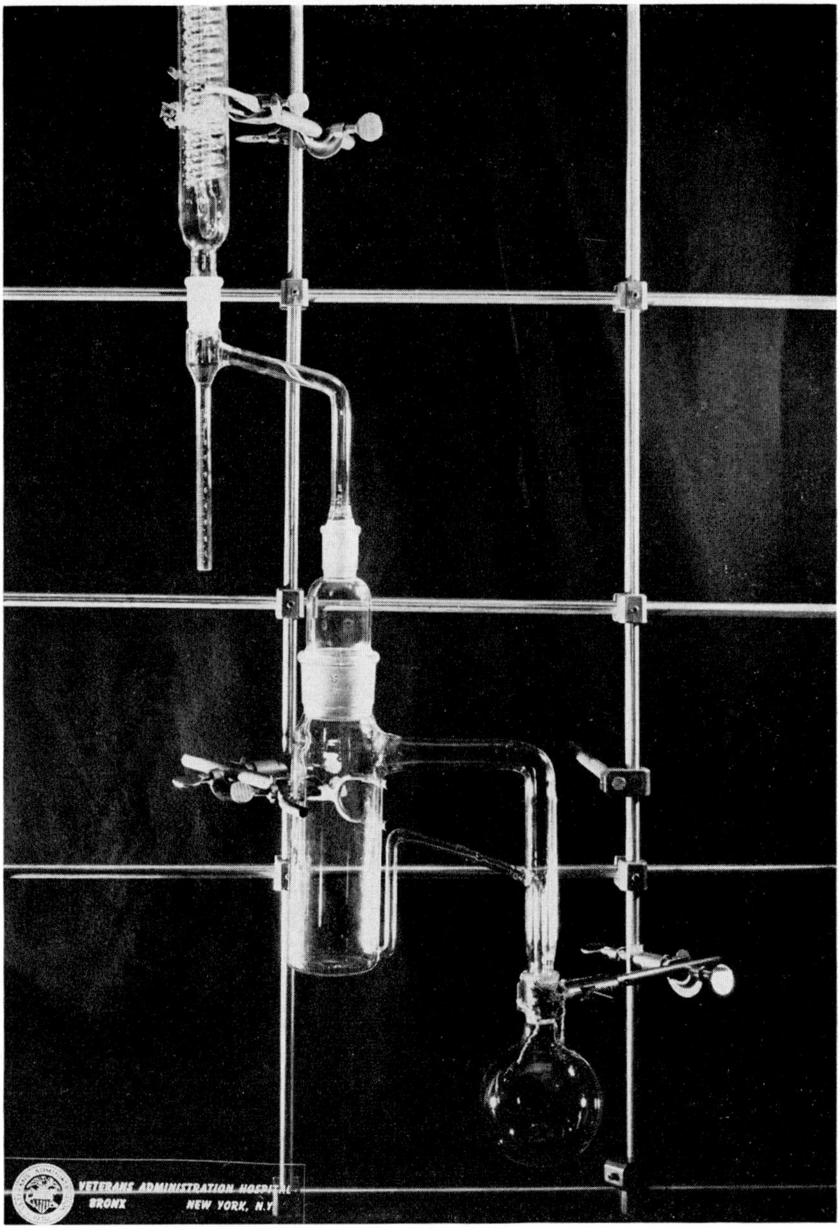

Fig. 1. Apparatus used for simultaneous drying and fat extraction of tissues by azeotropic distillation. The upper joint of the extraction chamber is 55/50; all other joints are 24/40.

anemia who had received multiple transfusions and who at autopsy did not reveal the anatomic features of hemochromatosis were analyzed for iron.

A representative 5–10 Gm. portion of tissue obtained at postmortem was washed free of blood with distilled water, blotted with cheesecloth, and placed in a 20 × 40 mm. thimble. Five to six such thimbles, comprising tissues from a single autopsy, were placed in the extraction chamber of the drying apparatus (Fig. 1) and subjected to simultaneous dehydration and extraction by azeotropic distillation with isopropyl ether. The distillation and extraction were continued for 1 hour after water was no longer given off after which the thimbles were removed to a vacuum desiccator and dried under reduced pressure for a half-hour after manometric pressure of the system had become constant. The contents of the thimbles were pulverized and stored in a desiccator.

The samples were analyzed for iron by digesting 0.10 to 0.20 Gm. of dried tissue with 2 ml. 1:1 sulfuric-perchloric acid mixture. In some cases a few drops of 20% hydrogen peroxide was added terminally to clear the digest. The cooled digest was diluted to 50 ml. and aliquots of 1–5 ml. were taken for analysis by the Wong thiocyanate procedure (5).

RESULTS

The iron content of tissues of 2 individuals without anemia or any metabolic iron disturbance, who had come to autopsy is given in Table 1. These serve as control values and are in keeping with the values obtained by Ramage and Sheldon (9) in their series of analyses of normal tissues.

Table 2 shows the iron content of tissues in 2 cases of endogenous hemochromatosis. Markedly increased amounts of iron are deposited and are the distinct chemical manifestation of the pathologic process.

Table 2 shows also the comparable values obtained in the analysis of tissues in 5 cases of exogenous (transfusion) hemochromatosis. Again the picture is that of excessive iron deposition with values in the same magnitude as the tissues analyzed by Ramage and Sheldon, but somewhat greater than the values obtained in our cases of the endogenous form. The tissue-iron values obtained in the series of anemia cases

Table 1. Iron Content of Normal Tissue

A #	*Liver*	*Heart*	*Spleen*	*Pancreas*
2303	1.61[a]	0.38	3.04	0.49
2248	0.14	0.49	2.38	0.53

[a] All results are expressed as mg. Fe/Gm. dry-fat-free tissue.

Table 2. Iron Content of Tissues in Hemochromatosis and Anemia

A #	*Kidney*	*Liver*	*Lung*	*Heart*	*Spleen*	*Pancreas*
Endogenous Hemochromatosis						
B39119	2.62[a]	4.88	4.77	0.74	..	10.4
B37926	1.49	12.6	5.8	0.84	..	12.5
Exogenous Hemochromatosis						
1115	4.68	23.7	2.63	2.78	7.11	18.4
1332	3.33	22.9	3.30	2.99	3.30	15.2
1032	4.92	41.2	4.08	6.77	..	21.0
1383	2.41	39.7	5.21	0.29	3.39	2.57
H	0.005	9.02	4.21	3.94	..	4.18
Refractory Anemias with Hemosiderosis						
1597	1.97	21.0	3.44	1.23	6.84	9.21
1598	3.43	32.3	..	0.29	..	..
480	..	..	4.18	..	..	8.35
1608	4.11	9.32	4.36	1.55	21.3	6.0

[a] All results are expressed as mg. Fe/Gm. dry fat-free tissue.

without fibrosis overlap, and are almost indistinguishable from the values obtained in the two true hemochromatotic types.

On the basis of results obtained, chemical analysis of tissues for iron does not decisively differentiate between the two varieties of the disease. There is considerable overlap.

DISCUSSION

Method

There are some points to be noted in the preparation of the samples for analysis. When dried by the customary process of oven-drying to constant weight, the tissues turned dark and hardened to a resin-like mass containing varying amounts of fat. This resulted in failure to get reproducible results on duplicate analyses of the same tissue, although in all other respects our technic when applied to blood and standard recovery studies was acceptable (average: 97.3 per cent). An improvement in the drying process was necessary. To this end, the drying-extraction apparatus of Kaye, Leibner, and Connor (6) was redesigned to permit the simultaneous dehydration and fat extraction by azeotropic distillation of representative portions of the organs from an entire autopsy in a single operation. After this treatment the organ fragments were colorless and easily powdered. Handling and weighing were simplified. The samples could be stored in a desiccator indefinitely. Duplicate analyses checked within 5 per cent.

Our data are therefore reported on a dry-fat-free basis and are in keeping both with the work of Pace and Rathbun (7), who showed that among laboratory animals the whole body fat varies from 1.5 to 35.8 per cent of body weight, and the plea of A. B. Hastings (8) that reports of tissue analysis be on a dry fat-free basis.

Results

From the results obtained in our series of tissue analyses, it can be concluded that in terms of tissue iron the exogenous and endogenous types of hemochromatosis are indistinguishable. Nodular pigment cirrhosis, hepatomegaly, and fibrosis with extensive pigment deposition were found in both at autopsy. Intracellular pigment was found in various tissue cells and in macrophages. The histologic criteria for diagnosis were satisfied.

Chemical findings however, did not in all instances coincide with the histologic picture. For example, in Case H, more hemosiderin was observed histologically in the pancreas, which contained 4.18 mg. iron/Gm. of tissue, than in the pancreas of A 1165, which contained 18.4 mg./Gm. Similarly, in the spleen of A 1115, with 7.1 mg. iron/Gm., less hemosiderin could be demonstrated histologically than in the spleen of A 1383, which had 3.39 mg. iron/Gm.

On the other hand, the 4 patients with various anemias which had been treated with iron therapy and multiple transfusions showed extensive hemosiderin deposits as well as increased tissue iron. Pathologically, none of the fibrotic stigmata seen in hemochromatosis were in evidence here. Here, too, clear-cut differentiation by chemical analysis of tissue cannot be made. These observations may possibly cast some light on the order and sequence of the pathologic manifestations of the exogenous form of hemochromatosis. After multiple transfusions, the iron released by the eventual breakdown of red blood cells by normal metabolic processes or otherwise, is stored in tissues because no excretory mechanism exists (10). Excess amounts are then taken up by the parenchymous liver cells, spleen, and other organs and fibrosis of the liver and pancreas ensues.

SUMMARY

1. Tissues from patients with the endogenous and exogenous (transfusion) forms of hemochromatosis were analyzed for iron content and their values compared.

2. Tissues from patients with long-standing anemia were analyzed for iron content.

3. The values obtained in all cases overlap and tissue-iron analysis cannot be used to differentiate the two forms of hemochromatosis.

REFERENCES

1. Granick, S., *Bull. N. Y. Acad. Med.* **25,** 403 (1949).
2. Schwartz, S. O., and Blumenthal, S. A., *Blood* **3,** 617 (1948).
3. Gillman, T., Mandelstam, J. and Gillman, J., *S. African J. Med. Sci.* **10,** 109 (1945).
4. Graef, I., Gordon, B. S., Newman, W., Olivetti, R. G., and Klein, B., *Am. J. Path.* **28,** 538 (1952).
5. Wong, S. Y., *J. Biol. Chem.* **77,** 409 (1928).
6. Kaye, I. A., Leibner, I. W., and Connor, E. B., *J. Biol. Chem.* **132,** 195 (1940).
7. Pace, N., and Rathbun, E. N., *J. Biol. Chem.* **158,** 685 (1945).
8. Hastings, A. B., *Harvey Lectures* **36,** 91 (1940–1941).
9. Ramage, H., and Sheldon, J. H., *Quart. J. Med.* **4,** 121 (1935).
10. Widdowson, E., and McCance, R., *Biochem. J.* **31,** 2029 (1937).

Clinical Significance of the Magnesium : Calcium Ratio

Technic for the Determination of Magnesium and Calcium in Biologic Fluids

Howard S. Friedman and Martin A. Rubin

The Schwartzenbach titration of calcium and magnesium has been applied principally in the field of determination of total hardness in water (1–4). Due to its particular application in this field where many contaminants are possible, Diehl, Goetz, and Hach have published a table of the principal interfering substances, their maximum tolerated concentrations, and the various inhibiting reagents which may be added to the titration to eliminate this interference. These considerations, however, have been found superfluous when the method or a modification is applied to biologic fluids, since these substances (for example, chromium, manganese, and so on) are either absent or are present in very small quantities.

Titration with Versene[1] has been done by, among others, Greenblatt and Hartmann. These investigators used a solid indicator, ammonium purpurate, which like eriochrome Black T, the Schwartzenbach indicator, forms a colored complex with calcium but not with magnesium. In our study it was desirable to obtain values for both calcium and magnesium in serum. Therefore a method was developed which permitted the determination of both ions in serum.

METHOD

Standards

Standards are prepared in concentrations comparable to those obtained in serum. All solutions are prepared from reagent-grade chemicals.

Received for publication August 26, 1954.

From the Chemo-Medical Institute, Georgetown University, Washington, D. C.

Presented as a requirement for the degree of Doctor of Philosophy, Georgetown University, Washington, D. C. (H.S.F.)

Present address: Tampa Municipal Hospital, Tampa, Fla. (H.S.F.)

[1] Trade name of ethylenediaminetetraäcetic acid; manufactured by Versenes, Inc., Framingham, Mass.

Magnesium

Transfer exactly 50.0 mg. magnesium powder to a 1000-ml. volumetric flask. Add 600 ml. of distilled water and 50 ml. of 0.1N hydrochloric acid. Shake gently until the powder is dissolved. Wash down the walls of the flask with distilled water and dilute to the mark. Mix well by inversion. This solution contains 4.12 mEq./L. magnesium.

Since the magnesium standard is made up from calcium-free magnesium metal, the versene solution is standardized with this standard alone, in terms of mEq./L. divalent ion. Most commercial calcium salts contain as much as 0.5 per cent magnesium.

Buffer Solution, pH 10 (4)

Mix 67.5 Gm. ammonium chloride and 570 ml. of concentrated ammonium hydroxide. Dilute to 1000 ml. with distilled water. Mix well and store in a tightly closed glass-stoppered bottle. Polyethylene ware may be used.

Indicator Solution

Dissolve 0.5 Gm. eriochrome Black T (Eastman Organic Chemicals or Versenes, Inc.) in 100 ml. of distilled water. This solution is stable for several months.

Stock Versene Solution

Dissolve 750 mg. of ethylenediaminetetraäcetic acid (or its equivalent of the di- or tetrasodium salt) in the minimum amount of 0.1N NaOH (about 80 ml. for the free acid, 40 ml. for the disodium salt, and distilled water for the tetrasodium salt) in a 1000-ml. volumetric flask, and dilute to the mark with distilled water. Mix well and store in a glass-stoppered borosilicate or polyethylene bottle. This solution is stable indefinitely.

Standard Versene Solution

Dilute 100 ml. of the stock Versene solution to 1000 ml. in a volumetric flask with distilled water. Titrate against the magnesium standard and adjust with distilled water or stock Versene solution so that 1 ml. magnesium standard will require 8.0 ± 0.3 ml. One ml. of the standardized solution will then be equivalent to approximately 0.5 mEq. of divalent ion.

Buffered Oxalate Solution (4)

To 35 Gm. ammonium chloride, add 1.5 Gm. ammonium oxalate and 3.5 ml. concentrated ammonium hydroxide. Dilute to 250 ml. with distilled water.

Procedures

Total Divalent Ions

Place 0.5 ml. of standard or unknown solution in a small Erlenmeyer flask. Add about 4 ml. of distilled water, 0.5 ml. buffer *p*H 10, and 2–4 drops of indicator solution. Titrate with standard Versene solution from a 5 ml. microburet (Koch type) until the solution turns from a pink to a pure blue color. This method is satisfactory with serum and spinal fluid.

Magnesium

Place 1 ml. serum or spinal fluid in a 15-ml. centrifuge tube. Add 2.5 ml. distilled water and 0.5 ml. buffered oxalate solution. Mix well and let stand for 30 minutes at room temperature. Centrifuge at 2500 rpm for 10 minutes. Transfer 2 ml. of the supernatant fluid to an Erlenmeyer flask, add reagents, and titrate as for total divalent ions.

Calculations

If, for example, Versene solution used was equivalent to 0.493 mEq./L. magnesium, this value becomes 0.986 mEq. per liter, as 0.5 ml. of sample is used. Thus 0.986 × ml. standard Versene solution = mEq./L. divalent or magnesium ions. The mEq./L. calcium ions is calculated by difference.

RESULTS

An initial series of 10 normal sera was tested in duplicate by Versene titration and by the Denis (8) and permanganate (9) methods for magnesium and calcium, respectively. The results are shown in Table 1. The Versene determination of magnesium checked with the Denis method within 0.1 mEq./L., approximately the standard error of the mean. The calcium values by Versene titration varied from the permanganate values by as much as 0.48 mEq./L., approximately 24 times the standard error of the mean.

A similar series was carried out with 10 spinal fluids. The results are

Table 1. Correlation of Serum Calcium and Magnesium Values by the Versene Titration and the Permanganate and Ammonium Phosphate Methods

Serum	Magnesium Versene (mEq./L.)	Magnesium NH_4HPO_4 (mEq./L.)	Calcium Versene (mEq./L.)	Calcium $KMnO_4$ (mEq./L.)	Versene/NH_4HPO_4	Versene/$KMnO_4$
1.	1.60	1.53	4.98	5.06	1.03	1.02
	1.61	1.59	4.97	5.08		
2.	1.35	1.31	5.60	5.62	1.01	1.00
	1.34	1.34	5.59	5.60		
3.	1.52	1.52	5.12	5.46	0.99	0.94
	1.52	1.55	5.13	5.40		
4.	1.00	1.09	4.46	4.40	0.93	1.01
	1.02	1.08	4.46	4.39		
5.	1.17	1.17	5.03	4.97	1.00	1.00
	1.18	1.17	5.01	5.02		
6.	1.89	1.87	4.36	4.84	1.00	0.91
	1.89	1.91	4.39	4.81		
7.	1.10	1.09	5.00	5.00	1.00	0.99
	1.08	1.09	5.00	5.04		
8.	1.35	1.27	5.51	5.58	0.97	0.98
	1.36	1.34	5.61	5.68		
9.	2.46	2.47	4.95	5.00	0.99	0.99
	2.46	2.47	4.94	4.99		
10.	1.42	1.43	4.87	4.98	1.00	0.98
	1.45	1.44	4.86	4.95		
Average	1.24	1.22	4.99	5.10	1.01	0.98

Table 2. Correlation of Spinal Fluid Magnesium and Calcium Values by the Versene Titration and the Permanganate and Ammonium Phosphate Methods

Spinal fluid	Magnesium Versene (mEq./L.)	Magnesium NH_4HPO_4 (mEq./L.)	Calcium Versene (mEq./L.)	Calcium $KMnO_4$ (mEq./L.)	Versene/NH_4HPO_4	Versene/$KMnO_4$
1.	2.0	2.2	2.3	2.4	1.10	1.05
2.	3.3	3.2	2.9	2.9	0.97	1.00
3.	1.8	1.8	2.4	2.5	1.00	0.98
4.	2.1	2.1	2.9	2.9	1.00	1.00
5.	1.7	1.6	2.1	2.1	1.06	1.00
6.	1.3	1.4	2.2	2.4	0.93	0.92
7.	3.1	3.1	2.3	2.3	1.00	1.00
8.	2.7	2.9	2.7	2.6	0.93	1.04
9.	2.6	2.6	2.4	2.5	1.00	0.96
10.	2.6	2.6	2.1	2.0	1.00	1.05
Average	2.32	2.35	2.43	2.46	0.99	0.99

shown in Table 2. The slightly better correlation is probably due to the fact that the end-point is more clearly discernible in spinal fluid titrations, because of the almost complete absence of proteins and chromogenic substances which tend to mask the indicator colors in the titration of serum.

Recovery experiments were performed on both serum and spinal fluid. The results showed good recovery, between 100 and 106 per cent. The correlation of the Versene titrations with the two standard methods was 0.94 for serum, 0.96 for urine, and 0.98 for spinal fluid. The method for urine is quite long and tedious and is not recommended for routine laboratory procedure.

CLINICAL APPLICATION

In an attempt to find some correlation between laboratory results and clinical entities, it was noted that in certain extreme conditions, such as terminal nephritis and diabetic coma, the normal ratio of magnesium to calcium in terms of mEq./L. appeared to be significantly altered. Accordingly, two sets of sera were analyzed for magnesium and calcium and the molar magnesium:calcium ratios were calculated. The first, or normal, set constituted the basis for the determination of the standard range of magnesium:calcium. An analysis of the literature dealing with normal values for serum calcium and magnesium revealed approximately the same range. The second set consisted of 100 pathologic sera, including repeated determinations on individuals comprising about 9 groups of systemic diseases. These were arbitrarily divided into 3 groups—those

Table 3. Statistical Analysis of Serum Magnesium and Calcium Values and the Mg/Ca Ratio in Normal and Pathologic Sera

	Normal (N = 10)	*Pathologic* (N = 100)			
		Low (21)	*Median* (43)	*High* (36)	*Total*
Magnesium mEq./L.					
Range	1.00–2.46	0.00–1.24	0.89–2.49	1.85–4.32	0.00–4.32
Average	1.24	0.52	1.57	2.57	1.71
S.E.	0.10	0.10	0.13	0.09	0.09
Calcium mEq./L.					
Range	4.36–5.61	1.72–6.50	3.07–5.85	2.71–6.35	1.72–6.50
Average	4.99	5.04	4.26	3.61	4.19
S.E.	0.20	0.25	1.00	1.10	1.00
Mg/Ca ratio					
Range	0.22–0.50	0.00–0.21	0.22–0.48	0.51–1.65	0.00–1.65
Average	0.30	0.10	0.37	0.75	0.44
S.E.	0.06	0.04	0.09	0.13	0.10

Table 4. Mg/Ca Molar Ratios According to Normal and Abnormal Magnesium and Calcium Values

Ratio	Ca normal				Ca abnormal				Total	
	Mg normal		Mg abnormal		Mg normal		Mg abnormal			
	No.	%	No.	%	No.	%	No.	%	No.	%
Normal	19	19	..	..	25	25	..	..	44	44
Abnormal	1	1	12	12	15	15	28	28	56	56
Total	20	20	12	12	40	40	28	28	100	100

with magnesium:calcium ratios below the standard range, those within the standard range, and those with values above the standard range. The results are shown in Table 3. The entire pathologic group was then arbitrarily divided again into 4 groups, as shown in Table 4.

The abnormal ratio obtained in the instance where both magnesium and calcium are normal (see Table 4) is due to the fact that the Mg/Ca ratios calculated from valves obtained from the literature, in which the ratios were calculated over the entire range of normal values, do not correspond to the observed ratios. The value in this case is 0.51, which may be considered on the borderline of the standard range, and thus may be excluded. We can then eliminate the first group from the discussion, since all of the ratios here are within the standard range. In the third group (Mg normal, Ca abnormal), we may say in general that the majority of this group have normal ratios, and that, while it may not detract from the clinical significance of the remainder of the group, patients with abnormally high or low calcium values generally fall under the clinical entities of nephritis, gastrointestinal disturbances, and parathyroid dysfunction. Over 50 per cent of the 25 patients in this group

Table 5. Normal and Abnormal Mg/Ca Ratios According to Systemic Groups

System or organ	Abnormal		Normal	
	No.	%	No.	%
Gastrointestinal	13	56.5	10	43.5
Renal	7	70.0	3	30.0
Endocrine	7	63.6	4	36.4
Hepatic	7	50.0	7	50.0
Biliary Tract	6	85.7	1	14.3
Cardiac	5	29.4	12	70.6
Gestational	4	100.0	..	..
Pulmonary	4	80.0	1	20.0
Hematologic	2	100.0	..	..
Averages		59.2		40.8

fall into these three categories and may generally be diagnosed by more specific means.

Of the two remaining groups, which comprise 40 per cent of the entire pathologic series, neither shows normal ratios nor normal magnesium values; about 30 per cent of the groups have normal calcium values. It is of interest to note that whenever the magnesium value is abnormal, the Mg/Ca ratio is also abnormal, and while it may be difficult at the present time to correlate changes in serum magnesium values with disease, it may be possible to show some correlation of the ratio. Table 5 shows all the abnormal values (ratios) grouped according to systems, along with the number of normal values obtained in each disease group in the entire series.

DISCUSSION

Clinicians, physiologists, and clinical chemists have long sought a relationship between serum magnesium concentration and various diseases with little or no success. A thorough search of the literature reveals only 1 instance in which the significance of the serum Mg/Ca ratio was examined. Jacoby and Friedel determined this value in experimental animals to which oxalic acid was administered both orally and parenterally. They found that, although there were extreme initial changes in the absolute concentrations of both magnesium and calcium, the normal ratio tended to be maintained over prolonged periods.

Of the 7 patients with nephritis who had abnormal ratios, 5, or half the total nephritic patients examined, had ratios higher than the standard range. In all the abnormal cases the deviations from the standard range were extreme, being 50 per cent or more.

Although the group with gastrointestinal diseases was heterogeneous, it may be said that they all had a common physiologic disturbance—decreased absorptive capacity in one region of the intestine or another. Of the 13 patients with abnormal ratios, 10, or 43 per cent of all patients in this series, had ratios above the standard range. The 3 instances of abnormally low ratios were in one individual, in whom extreme ascites had developed. Eight liters of abdominal fluid were removed at the first paracentesis.

Since the number of hematologic patients (multiple myeloma) is only 2, with neither showing an abnormal ratio, and since this disease is readily recognized by other laboratory and clinical examinations, the authors do not feel that these figures are significant.

Since, as has been pointed out by Rawson and Sunderman, the binding powers of the serum albumin and serum globulin for calcium are approximately equal, and since this may very well be true also for magnesium, we cannot explain the abnormal ratios observed in liver disease on the basis of disturbances in albumin:globulin ratios. Equal numbers of normal and abnormal values were found. Since hepatic diseases are rarely uncomplicated, it seems likely that those cases in which the ratio is abnormal were possibly complicated by other factors, most probably by some intra- or extrahepatic biliary obstruction.

Of the total of 7 patients with biliary tract obstruction, 6 had abnormal ratios, and all of these fell below the standard range. The 1 normal value was from a patient who had formerly had a low ratio, and had meanwhile undergone a cholecystectomy. It is significant that no deaths, serious complications occurred in any of these cases, as compared with the deaths in the nephritis and gastrointestinal groups.

The number of cardiac patients with abnormal ratios was 5, or about 29 per cent of the total cases in the series. The 12 standard values covered the entire standard range, with an average value of 0.38, which approximates the average of the entire median group. The average of the entire series of cardiacs is 0.46, which approximates the average of the entire series. It is therefore apparent that these results are not clinically significant.

Four abnormal values were observed in pulmonary involvement, all above the standard range. The single case giving a normal value was one of tuberculosis. This value was 0.43, approximating the average of the entire series. While it is difficult to ascertain the physiologic causes of variations of the Mg/Ca ratio in these instances, it may be pointed out that in emphysematous conditions great difficulty is experienced in breathing, i.e., in gaseous exchange. This usually leads to secondary phenomena, particularly tissue anoxia, which may bring about reversible or irreversible changes in cell membrane permeability and selectivity, which may account for the redistribution of magnesium and calcium throughout the body.

The ratios obtained in all patients in advanced pregnancy in which toxemia or edema had developed were abnormal; nevertheless, the majority of the ratios were not significantly removed from the standard range. A value of 1.32 was obtained in 1 patient who had severe hypoproteinemia, and the calcium value had fallen to an extremely low level. It is quite possible, however, that the ionized or physiologically active portion remained relatively unaffected.

Although 64 per cent of all endocrine disorders in this series were associated with abnormal ratios, nevertheless, it is felt that these diseases—diabetes, hypoparathyroidism, and hypothyroidism—can be diagnosed more readily by other laboratory and clinical methods.

SUMMARY

1. The Schwartzenbach method has been adapted for the simultaneous determination of calcium and magnesium in serum and spinal fluid. The method appears to be adaptable to all body fluids, including thoracic and abdominal transudates and exudates. Its use in the clinical laboratory is recommended because of the great saving of time, particularly in the determination of magnesium.

2. A series of 100 pathologic cases of various clinical entities has been analyzed by the new method and checked with the standard methods. A calculation and statistical analysis has revealed the Mg/Ca molar ratio to be of possible clinical significance.

REFERENCES

1. Schwartzenbach, G., *Helv. Chim. Acta.* **29,** 811 (1946).
2. Betz, J. D., and Noll, C. A., *J. Am. Water Works Assoc.* **42,** 49 (1950).
3. Connors, J. J., *J. Am. Water Works Assoc.* **42,** 33 (1950).
4. Diehl, H., Goetz, C. A., and Hach, A. C., *J. Am. Water Works Assoc.* **42,** 40 (1950).
5. Willson, A. E., *Anal. Chem.* **22,** 1571 (1950).
6. Greenblatt, J. J., and Hartmann, S., *Anal. Chem.* **23,** 1708 (1951).
7. Buckley, E. S., Gibson, J. G., and Bortolotti, T. R., *J. Lab. Clin. Med.* **38,** 75 (1951).
9. Clark, E. P., and Collip, J. B., *J. Biol. Chem.* **63,** 461 (1925).
8. Denis, W., *J. Biol. Chem.* **52,** 411 (1922).
10. Jacoby, M., and Friedel, H., *Biochem. Z.* **60,** 451 (1933).
11. Rawson, A. J., and Sunderman, F. W., *J. Clin. Invest.* **27,** 85 (1948).

the Clinical Chemist

EDITORIAL

The American Association of Clinical Chemists has promulgated a policy on legislation in a Resolution passed by the National Executive Committee in 1950 and reaffirmed three years later (1). These tenets still hold, and they were proposed in the best interest of those who require the services of clinical chemistry.

In this Resolution one of the clauses stipulates that the chemist should not be required to show proficiency in fields other than clinical chemistry to be permitted to practice his specialty. It is our conviction that disciplines such as hematology, microbiology, serology, and other such allied specialties, are separate sciences in spite of any overlap in the periphery. That they are frequently housed close to the chemistry laboratories, or even grouped in one laboratory, is fortuitous and the result of their historical development in the hospital.

The Attorney General in California has recently published an opinion (2) that "a technologist's license may not be issued to anyone not conforming to the requirement of five years general experience." This general experience refers to all the specialties above mentioned. We respectfully take issue with the Attorney General in California and should furthermore like to point out that real progress will be made by specialists in the respective disciplines and not by technologists whom his definition makes jacks-of-all-trades.

The American Association of Clinical Chemists is making every effort to attract competent chemists into our specialty. This will be most difficult if in the process it will first be necessary to train chemists as medical technicians. Should the California opinion become generally accepted the science of clinical chemistry and all who are dependent on its services will have received a serious setback.

MAX M. FRIEDMAN
National Secretary

REFERENCES

1. *Clinical Chem.* **5,** 65 (1953).
2. Opinions of the Attorney General. Hanna Legal Publications, Albany, Calif., **24,** 79 (1954).

FEDERATION MEETINGS: APRIL 10–16

The American Society of Biological Chemists, through Dr. Elmer Stotz, Program Chairman, has invited the American Association of Clinical Chemists to arrange a symposium on "Biochemistry of Disease" for the Federated Societies Meeting in San Francisco, April 10–16.

Dr. Marschelle H. Power has arranged the symposium for the A.A.C.C. The program is as follows:

"Porphyrins and Porphyrin Precursors in Human and Experimental Porphyria"—S. Schwartz, University of Minnesota, Medical School.

"Investigations of Diseases of the Thyroid Gland With Radioactive Iodine"—C. A. Owen, Jr., Mayo Clinic.

"Biochemical Studies in Relation to Comparative Susceptibility to Experimental Atherosclerosis"—L. Pilgeram, University of Illinois, College of Medicine.

"The Clinical Chemical Significance of Ionography"—H. J. McDonald, Stritch School of Medicine, Loyola University.

"Observations on Aldosterone In Human Urine"—J. A. Luetscher, Jr., School of Medicine, Stanford University.

MEMBERSHIP STATISTICS

The American Association of Clinical Chemists was founded by nine charter members on December 15, 1948. Since that date there has been a continuous increase in the membership. Table 1 is a summary compiled from the last five directories, including the 1955 Directory published in March, and contains a tabulation of the total members listed according to the years in which the individuals were admitted into the Association. In the past six years 16 members have died and 81 others have either resigned or been dropped for nonpayment of dues. The last year, 1954, saw an encouraging addition of new members, being only surpassed by 1949 and 1950. The steady increment over the years is evidence that the Association has yet to reach its full strength.

Table 1. Distribution of Members in the American Association of Clinical Chemists as Tabulated from the Directories of the Designated Dates. Listings Are According to the Year of Admission to Membership

	10/15/50	1/1/52	1/1/53	1/15/54	1/30/55
1948	9	8*	8	8	8
1949	166	154	152	129	121
1950	134	172	170	156	140
1951		81	75	69	65
1952			71	69	65
1953				83	81
1954				8	137
1955					12
Totals	309	415	476	522	629

* Jos Kahn, a charter member, died on December 30, 1951.

Table 2. Geographical Distribution as Percentages of Total Tabulated from the Directories of the Designated Dates

	10/15/50	1/1/52	1/1/53	1/15/54	1/30/55
N. Y.	28.2	25.1	22.9	21.2	19.0
Penn.	9.1	9.4	9.2	9.9	10.3
Calif.	8.4	10.1	10.5	10.3	9.2
Ill.	8.4	9.4	8.0	7.8	7.0
Mass.	11.3	9.6	9.5	7.7	6.6
Iowa	1.6	2.4	1.7	4.0	4.6
Md.	1.3	1.9	2.9	4.0	4.4
N. J.	3.2	3.6	4.6	4.2	3.5
Ohio	3.2	3.1	2.9	2.7	3.0
D. C.	1.0	1.2	1.9	2.9	2.8
Tex.	1.3	1.9	1.9	1.7	2.8
Mich.	2.9	2.7	2.9	2.1	2.5
Mo.	2.9	2.4	2.3	2.3	2.5
Other	17.2	17.1	17.0	18.9	21.6
Total	309	415	476	522	629

Table 2 shows the geographic distribution in percentage of total membership as tabulated from Association files. This table may be confined to the "department of useless information" except that it bears out the fact that where a local section exists the membership is significantly higher than where there is none.

IN MEMORIAM

Adolph Bernhard, 64, director of the Biochemical Laboratories at the Lenox Hill Hospital in New York City, died at the hospital on December 1, 1954 after an extended illness.

He received a B.S. from the Polytechnic Institute of Brooklyn and an M.A. from Columbia University in 1922. He was appointed chief biochemist to Lenox Hill Hospital in 1915 and served there continuously until his death.

He was a member of the American Chemical Society, Sigma Xi, The Society for Experimental Biology and Medicine, the New York Academy of Sciences, and was a Fellow of the American Association for the Advancement of Science. He had published over 60 papers in clinical biochemistry.

Adolph Bernhard was one of the first to be admitted to membership in the American Association of Clinical Chemists and was active in the organizational stages. At that time he made available to his colleagues the benefit of his long experience in clinical chemistry. He was invited to lecture in Glasgow in October, 1954, to the Scotland and Northern Ireland Region of the British Association of Clinical Biochemists, but could not accept due to ill health.

He is survived by his wife and a daughter.

AMERICAN BOARD OF CLINICAL CHEMISTRY

The American Board of Clinical Chemistry has authorized preparation and distribution of a *Directory of Certified Clinical Chemists*. This directory is now being distributed to chemists listed therein and to numerous university departments of chemistry and biochemistry. Heads of hospital departments or other laboratories engaged in clinical chemistry can secure a copy of the Directory by writing to the Secretary-Treasurer, Dr. O. H. Gaebler, Henry Ford Hospital, Detroit 2, Michigan.

A copy of the *Instructions to Applicants for Certification*, as approved by the Board at its annual meeting in 1954, is also available without cost. Chemists wishing to apply for certification should secure this information at once, since considerable time is required to process a formal application.

ASSOCIATION NOTES

Membership Certificates

Members and associate members may obtain a membership certificate that is suitable for framing. Anyone interested in ordering same should send a check for four dollars to the National Treasurer, Dr. Louis B. Dotti, St. Luke's Hospital, New York 25, N. Y. Please state how you wish your name inscribed and the degrees to be included.

Membership Requirements

Information concerning requirements for membership in the Association may be obtained by writing to the National Secretary, Dr. Max M. Friedman, Lebanon Hospital, New York 57, N. Y. Present subscribers to *Clinical Chemistry* will have subscription included in 1956 dues.

Members in Arrears

Members who have not paid their annual dues by March 15 will be removed from the membership roster. In the past a longer period of grace was permitted, but with our commitments for the journal this cutoff date is necessary. However, for this year only, those still in arrears will be reinstated if payments are received before May 1, 1955.

Ballots

Members of the Association have received a directory and a ballot for the election of officers to the Executive Committee of 1955–56. These ballots must be returned to the National Secretary by May 1, 1955, to be counted in the final tabulation.

Local Sections

There are at present seven chartered local sections in the Association. These include, in the order of their formation, Metropolitan New York, Boston, Philadelphia, Southern California, Chicago, Washington-Baltimore-Richmond, and Midwest. Other areas are now in the process of organizing such local sections, and Greater Kansas City has already applied for section status. All local sections are invited to submit copy of news of their activities for publication in CLINICAL CHEMISTRY.

REPORTS FROM THE SECTIONS

Metropolitan New York

A. Saifer

The Section held a successful symposium and exhibit on "Recent Advances in Instrumentation" during January 21 and 22, 1955, at the New York Medical College. A symposium on "Physical Methods in Clinical Chemistry" was attended by an overflow audience of more than 400 people. The speakers included Robert J. Slater of Cornell University Medical College on "Paper and Zone Electrophoresis"; Charles L. Fox, Jr. of the New York Medical College on "Flame Photometry"; and Solomon A. Berson of the Bronx V. A. Hospital on "Radioisotopes as Tracers." Kurt G. Stern of Polytechnic Institute of Brooklyn was chairman.

A "Round Table on Instrumentation" was held the following morning. The participants included Joseph Greenspan, Process and Instruments, Brooklyn, N. Y.; Sergei Feitelberg, Mt. Sinai Hospital, N. Y.; and Alfred Henley, American Instrument Company, Silver Spring, Md. The subjects covered were flame photometers, radioisotope equipment, and electrophoresis instrumentation. Julius J. Carr of the Mount Sinai Hospital was chairman.

More than 30 companies participated in the exhibits. Space does not permit the mention of all whose efforts made this possible. Special thanks should be extended to the New York Medical College for making its facilities available, and to William Gruen of Instrumentation Associates for carrying the major efforts in organizing the exhibits.

Washington-Baltimore-Richmond

Marian E. Webster

The first meeting of the 1954–55 year was held on November 18, 1954, at the Walter Reed Army Medical Center. A symposium on measurements of thyroid function and their interpretation was the topic for the evening.

Recent advances in the analysis of protein bound iodine was discussed by Max Sherer, Cancer Institute of the National Institutes of Health. James C. Syner, Walter Reed Army Hospital, could not be present to talk on the measurement and evaluation of basal metabolic rate data, but the abstract of his paper was read by Lt. Col. Irving Gray and commented on by J. I. Sherman. Herschel J. Wells concluded the symposium with a discussion of the use of I^{131} uptake in the measurement of thyroid function.

The second meeting of the year was scheduled for January 6, 1955, and was devoted to a discussion of recent advances in the laboratory control of diabetes mellitus. The third meeting was held on March 3, at which hematologic technics and their interpretation was discussed. The final meeting will be held on April 21. The program will be announced.

The American Instrument Company, A. S. Aloe Company, and Fisher Scientific Company have generously contributed funds to the Washington-Baltimore-Richmond Section in order to assist in the scientific program for 1955. These funds assure the success of the scientific meetings.

Southern California

Clyde A. Dubbs

"The (California) Clinical Laboratory Technology Act does not provide for the licensing of technologists in special fields." This opinion, rendered August 27, 1954, by the Attorney General of California, means that the clinical chemist is still legally restrained from directing a clinical chemistry laboratory unless he also has additional general experience in all the clinical laboratory fields.

The law now makes no specific provision for *special technologists* who can direct laboratory work in their special fields, although Section 1264 of the Act does provide that "licenses under this chapter may cover work in any one basic science, or may cover proficiency in the entire field of clinical laboratory work." Nevertheless the Attorney General stated that this "general provision of Sec. 1264 is in conflict with Sec. 1260, which requires that technologists have five years of experience embracing the various fields."

It is believed that this conclusion does not conform to the intentions and expectations of clinical chemists and others who supported the 1951 law.

The first symposium of the current year was held November 2, 1954, at the Hollywood Presbyterian Hospital. The subject, "Calcium and Phosphorus Metabolism in Relation to Bone Disorders," was discussed by William R. Bergren, George N. Donnell, and Mary Mulloy, staff members of the Childrens Hospital and the University of Southern California Medical School.

The second symposium, on the "Determination, Origin and Significance of Corticosteroids" was held on December 7 at the Cedars of Lebanon Hospital, Los Angeles. The speakers were Robert Commons, University of Southern California Medical School; Orville J. Golub, Bio-science Laboratories; and Harry Sobel, Cedars of Lebanon Hospital.

A special dinner on January 4, 1955, at the Carolina Pines Restaurant was devoted to a discussion of the California Attorney General's opinion on specialized technologist licensure and its consequences; and to discussion of the inter-laboratory accuracy survey program of the Southern California Section.

LETTER to the editor

To the Editor:

In *The Clinical Chemist 6:* 61 (1954) Henry J. Goeckel of Cranford, N. J., asks our organization to give serious consideration to the development of comprehensive, reliable standard specimens for the specific use of the average institutional and community laboratory for checking the accuracy of their biochemical procedures. He also suggests that such standards be assayed by a sufficient number of our large research-type institutional laboratories to establish the limits of accuracy of the *Standard Methods* and that such standard samples be readily available to any interested laboratory.

The inconsistency of publishing a book of standard methods (with more to follow) without making available standard analyzed samples, is a problem that we in the New York Section have wrestled with over the past two years. We feel that we have arrived at a partial solution to this important problem by the use of sterile bovine ultrafiltrate as a general laboratory standard. This is a water-clear solution which contains all the constituents of bovine blood (except proteins and sterols) at approximately their original concentrations and, unless contaminated, it remains stable over many months under ordinary refrigeration and use. It is treated exactly as if it were a blood specimen and reports from some 12 laboratories scattered over the country have given excellent reproducibility of values with a variety of methods and instruments. As soon as a few additional results are achieved, we are planning to make a complete statistical analysis of the results and to publish them in CLINICAL CHEMISTRY.

While it is our hope then to make these samples available through various laboratory supply dealers, it should be stressed that we are not endorsing the products of any manufacturer or dealer. In fact, it is our purpose and function to check and evaluate all such proposed standards. We are at the present time looking into the matter of testing some protein- and sterol-containing standards which have been recently brought to our attention, since these constituents are not covered by the ultrafiltrate standard.

While this report is somewhat premature, we feel that our readers should be informed that our organization is taking constructive steps in attempting to improve the accuracy of clinical laboratory procedures.

Sincerely yours,

ABRAHAM SAIFER

Secretary Metropolitan-New York Section

ABSTRACTS

Editor: Ellenmae Viergiver. *Contributors:* Joseph A. Annino, Gladys J. Downey, Clyde A. Dubbs, Alex Kaplan, Margaret M. Kaser, Miriam Reiner, Herbert Thompson

A method of insulin bio-assay and its application to human plasma fractions. F. C. Goetz, P. M. Beigelman, and G. W. Thorn (*Harvard Medical School and Peter Bent Brigham Hospital, Boston, Mass.*).

Concentrated human plasma protein preparations were assayed for insulin activity by a modification of the method of Yenerman, Cornfield, Bates, and Anderson [*Federation Proc.* **12,** 162 (1953)]. Hypophysectomized, alloxanized male mice were given the test material by intraperitoneal injection with simultaneous administration by gavage of 300 mg. dextrin. Blood glucose was determined by the Nelson-Somogyi procedure [*J. Biol. Chem.* **153,** 375 (1944); **195,** 19 (1952)] in 0.02 ml. samples collected after 4, 30, and 65 minutes. Near-complete suppression of the hyperglycemia was produced by 4–5 milli-units of insulin with equivocal results with 1–2 milli-units. No insulin activity could be demonstrated in 0.25–1.0 ml. of human plasma, but it was present in 0.25 ml. or more of a 5-fold concentration of globulin.—*Proc. Soc. Exp. Biol. Med.* **86,** 484 (1954).

M.K.

Electrophoretic fractionation of serum protein in multiple sclerosis. J. Bernsohn and L. S. G. Cochrane (*Veterans Administration Hospital, Hines, Ill.*).

Electrophoretic separations of the serum proteins of 27 patients with multiple sclerosis were carried out for 70–80 minutes in a Tiselius apparatus in Veronal buffer, *p*H 8.6 and 0.1 ionic strength, after dialysis for 24 hours against the buffer at 3° and with a protein concentration of approximately 1 per cent. Area and mobility measurements were made on the ascending boundary. Protein determinations were made by the micro-Kjeldahl method. There was no difference between the mean total serum protein concentrations of the patients and of 16 normal subjects, but the albumin fraction averaged 55 per cent in the multiple sclerosis cases and 60.2 per cent in the controls, while the mean figures for α_2-globulin were 12.4 per cent and 8.9 per cent, respectively. These differences were statistically significant ($p < 0.001$). There were no significant quantitative variations in the other globulin components. In 15 patients the α_2-globulin exhibited a double peak.—*Proc. Soc. Exp. Biol. Med.* **86,** 540 (1954).

M.K.

Aluminum hydroxide as an adsorbing agent for urinary gonadotropins R. F. Malburg and J. R. Goodman (*Paraplegia Laboratory, Veterans Administration Hospital, Long Beach, Calif.*)

A procedure is described for adsorbing urinary gonadotropins with aluminum hydroxide. The reagents are inexpensive and commonly available and the method is simple and rapid. Results obtained with this procedure were in agreement with those obtained with the usual alcohol-precipitation method.—*J. Clin. Endocrinol. & Metab.* **14,** 666 (1954).

E.V.

Jaundice and xanthochromia of the spinal fluid. L. B. Berman, L. W. Lapham, and E. Pastore (*Medical Services and Neurological Service, Boston City Hospital; Dept. of Medicine and Dept. of Biochemistry, Boston University Medical School; and Dept. of Neurology, Harvard Medical School; Boston, Mass.*)

Bilirubin concentration was determined in serum and in spinal fluid from 20 jaundiced patients. Detectable amounts were present in the spinal fluid, including those specimens from patients with jaundice of recent onset. The concentration in the spinal fluid ranged from 1:10 to 1:100 of the serum values. Although the data did not show a linear relationship between serum and spinal fluid bilirubin, there was a trend in that direction, the higher spinal fluid values occurring when the serum values were high.—*J. Lab. & Clin. Med.* **44,** 273 (1954).

E.V.

The use of glycogen as a substrate for the determination of serum amylase. H. S. Friedman (*Tampa Municipal Hospital, Tampa, Fla.*)

Glucose liberated from a buffered glycogen substrate is measured in a barium zinc filtrate by the Somogyi-Nelson copper reduction method. The procedure is said to be simple, rapid, and accurate. The glycogen substrate is more stable than starch substrate and is easier to prepare.—*J. Lab. & Clin. Med.* **44,** 308 (1954).

E.V.

Blood levels of absorbed labeled fat and chylomicronemia. W. W. Burr, Jr., C. Dunkelberg, J. C. McPherson, and H. C. Tidwell (*Southwestern Med. School, Univ. of Texas, Dallas, Tex.*)

Chylomicron counts were compared with the blood levels of absorbed fat containing palmitic acid-1-C^{14}. The similarity of the results obtained by these two methods suggests that the same function is being measured. Thus, chylomicron counts and the areas under the curves from them may be used as a satisfactory relative measure of the changing blood levels of absorbed fat and as a means of following the active process of fat absorption.—*J. Biol. Chem.* **210,** 531 (1954).

E.V.

A method for the estimation of inulin in plasma and urine containing dextran. J. R. K. Preedy (*Coll. of Physicians & Surgeons, Columbia Univ., and Presbyterian Hosp., New York, N. Y.*)

A modification of the method of Roe et al. (*J. Biol. Chem.*, **178,** 839 [1949]) is presented. Proteins in plasma or urine diluted to contain 15–55 mg. of inulin are precipitated with zinc chloride and sodium hydroxide. Dextran is precipitated from the protein-free filtrate by ethanol. The dextran-free supernatant is evaporated to dryness. The residue is treated with resorcinol-thiourea reagent and hydrochloric acid solution, and the color intensity compared with standard inulin solutions.—*J. Biol. Chem.* **210,** 651, (1954).

E.V.

The determination of 17,21-dihydroxy-20-ketosteroids in urine and plasma. R. H. Silber and C. C. Porter (*Merck Inst. for Therapeutic Research, Rahway, N. J.*)

A procedure is described which is applicable to routine clinical use, and which can be completed within a working day. It involves (a) a 15-second extraction with chloroform, (b) a 10-second washing with dilute alkali, (c) a 15-second extraction of an aliquot of the chloroform extract with alcoholic phenylhydrazine-sulfuric acid reagent, and (d) measurement of the optical density in microcuvettes in the Beckman spectrophotometer after heating the samples to 60° for 30 min. Concentrations as low as 6 μg. per 100 ml. can be determined.—*J. Biol. Chem.* **210,** 923 (1954).

E V.

A rapid colorimetric method for the determination of isonicotinic acid hydrazide in blood plasma: II. Application to blood plasma from human tuberculosis patients. B. Prescott, S. Katz, and G. Kauffman (*U.S. Dept. of Health, Education, and Welfare, Public Health Serivce, Natl. Inst. of Health, Natl. Microbiological Inst., Bethesda, Md., and D.C. General Hosp., Washington, D.C.*)

A simple and rapid procedure for the determination of isoniazid in blood plasma is presented which employs 4-pyridylpyridinium dichloride as indicator.—*J. Lab. & Clin. Med.*, **44,** 600 (1954).

E.V.

A rapid method for the estimation of morphine. J. M. Fujimoto, E. Leong Way, and C. H. Hine (*Sch. of Med. and Pharmacy, Univ. of California, San Francisco, Calif.*)

A method is described which is highly specific, requires no specialized apparatus, and can be carried out in less than 90 min. The morphine is extracted from a highly alkalinized solution with *n*-butanol and interfering substances are removed in subsequent extraction steps. A colorimetric phenol reagent is used for the final estimation in a buffer extract. Optical density is measured at 675 mμ.—*J. Lab. & Clin. Med.*, **44,** 627 (1954).

E.V.

Paper electrophoresis with automatic scanning and recording. G. R. Cooper and E. E. Mandel, with technical assistance of R. H. Owings and J. Fetner (*U.S. Dept. of Health, Education & Welfare, Emory Univ. Sch. of Med., and Grady Memorial Hosp., Atlanta, Ga.*)

An automatic scanning and recording apparatus is described which furnishes electrophoretic patterns closely comparable to those obtained by means of the standard Tiselius apparatus.—*J. Lab. & Clin. Med.* **44,** 636 (1954).

E.V.

Blood ACTH in man: "active" and "activable" fraction. G. Morruzzi, C. A. Rossi, L. Montanari, and M. Martinelli (*Univ. di Bologna, Italy*)

Blood ACTH has been assayed in 6 normal subjects and in 6 patients with hypocorticism, a condition reported to have an increased level of blood ACTH. Two different technics were used: (1) the direct method of injecting plasma directly into hypophysectomized rats and assaying ACTH by the adrenal ascorbic acid depletion method; (2) mixing the plasma with 4 volumes of glacial acetic acid and processing with oxycellulose, the eluate being assayed as above. Two fractions of ACTH have been found in human blood. One, called "active" ACTH, is a labile and ultrafiltrable fraction which is found mainly in normal subjects. The other, called "activable" ACTH, is detectable only after treatment with oxycellulose. This form occurs mainly in the blood of human subjects with hypocorticism, but is present normally in the blood of other species of animals. —*J. Clin. Endocrinol. & Metab.* **14,** 1144 (1954).

M. R.

Indirect method for determination of serum inorganic sulfate by flame spectrophotometry. R. D. Strickland and C. M. Maloney (*Veterans Administration Hospital, Albuquerque, N. M.*)

Serum inorganic sulfate determination is of value as an early indication of renal insufficiency because significant increase above the normal range of 0.3–1.0 mEq./l. may occur before any retention of inorganic phosphate, blood urea nitrogen, or creatinine can be detected. To 9 ml. of uranyl acetate solution (4 Gm. $UO_2Ac_2 \cdot 2H_2O$/l.) in a 15-ml. conical bottom centrifuge tube, add 3 ml. of serum. Cover the tube with Parafilm and mix thoroughly by shaking. Centrifuge and filter the supernatant liquid. Pipette 4 ml. of the filtrate into a test tube and add 1 ml. of solution containing 5 mEq. $BaCl_2$/l. (20 mEq./l. if a very high sulfate determination is anticipated). Prepare a blank using 2 ml. of filtrate and 0.5 ml. of water to correct for interfering substances determined as "barium."

Let stand 1 hour and filter to remove $BaSO_4$. The barium remaining in the sample and in the blank is determined with the Beckman B Spectrophotometer with oxygen (15 lb./sq. in.) and acetylene (1.5 lb./sq. in.) at 873 mμ and slit width of 1.0 mm. From a standard curve determine barium and compute mEq. of sulfate as the difference between mEq. of barium added and the amount remaining in the filtrate after sulfate precipitation. The standard curve is prepared following this procedure and using a standard sodium sulfate solution (20 mEq./l. so diluted that a series of solutions varying in concentration from 0.0 to 20 mEq./l. are obtained. Time required is approximately 90 minutes and the error is small. In advanced renal insufficiency, inorganic sulfate may reach 20 mEq./l.—*Am. J. Clin. Pathol.* **24,** 1100 (1954).

H. E. T.

A spectrophotometer adapter for reading paper strips. D. M. Schultz, R. L. Dryer, and M. A. Holdcraft (*Indiana University School of Medicine, Indianapolis, Ind.*

Details and illustrations are presented for the construction of an adapter for reading paper strips obtained in electrophoresis or chromatography with the Coleman Junior spectrophotometer. The device could be used with slight modification on other instruments of a similar type. With this adapter inserted in the cuvette well, the spectrophotometer becomes a satisfactory and convenient substitute for a densitometer. The curves obtained have been quite comparable to those derived by other methods of direct photometry and, in general, lend themselves easily to planimetry.—*Am. J. Clin. Pathol.* **24,** 1110 (1954).

H. E. T.

Barbiturate studies: II. Correlation between clinical condition and blood barbiturate levels. I. Sunshine and E. R. Hackett (*School of Medicine, Western Reserve University, Cleveland, Ohio*).

Blood barbiturate levels in patients who had received excessive dosages were determined by the procedure of Goldbaum [*Anal. Chem.* **24,** 1604 (1952)] and correlated with the patients' clinical condition. For phenobarbital the blood levels associated with varying stages of drug effect were: Stage I, awake, competent, and mildly sedated, 2.4–3.6 mg./100 ml.; Stage II, sedated, reflexes present, prefers sleep, 4.2–4.6 mg./100 ml.; Stage III, comatose, reflexes present, 5.0–6.2 mg./100 ml.; Stage IV, comatose, areflexive, 7.7–9.2 mg./100 ml.; Stage V, comatose, circulatory and/or respiratory difficulty, 20.6 mg./100 ml., with death of the patient (1 case). For phenobarbital, decrease in the blood level to one half the original level requires 3 days. Data are also given for secobarbital, amobarbital, butabarbital, and pentobarbital, in which the blood levels of barbiturate in each stage of the drug effect are all lower than for phenobarbital. *Am. J. Clin. Pathol.* **24,** 1133 (1954).

H.E.T.

Application of densitometry to paper chromatography of barbiturates. A. J. McBay and E. J. Algeri (*Harvard Medical School, Boston, Mass.*).

Using the Beckman DU spectrophotometer, densitometry was successfully applied to paper chromatograms of the location and identification of barbiturates. The method has been applied to chromatograms of extracts of stomach contents, liver, blood, and urine, as well as to those of pure materials.—*Am. J. Clin. Pathol.* **24,** 1139 (1954).

H.E.T.

Transphosphyralation as a source of error in assay of serum acid phosphatase. R. B. Barrueto, M. M. D. Reynolds, B. S. Walker, and H. M. Lemon (*Boston University School of Medicine, Boston, Mass.*).

In a study of the method of Andersch and Szcypinski [*Am. J. Clin. Pathol.* **17,** 571 (1947)], in which the substrate used is nitrophenylphosphate, a small transfer of phosphate was found to take place. However, this does not affect the usefulness of the method as a clinical laboratory test.—*Am. J. Clin. Pathol.* **24,** 1144 (1954).

H.E.T.

Two methods for the determination of glycogen in liver. J. van der Vies (*N. V. Organon, Oss, Holland*).

A 200 mg. sample of liver is homogenized in 20 ml. of 5% trichloroacetic acid· The glycogen content may be determined rapidly by adding 3 ml. of Lugol solution to 2 ml. of liver extract and reading the optical density at 650 mμ. The amount of glycogen is read from a calibration curve, which must be prepared using glycogen of the same origin as the sample to be estimated.

The glycogen may be determined more accurately by hydrolyzing 2 ml. of the above liver extract with 2 ml. of 10N KOH at 100° for 1 hour. After cooling, 1 ml. of glacial acetic acid is added to neutralize the alkali and the solution is diluted to 20 ml. Two milliters of this solution is added slowly to 4 ml. of anthrone reagent (0.5 Gm. anthrone dissolved in 250 ml. of 95% (W/V) H_2SO_4 in a test tube placed in cold water. Color is developed by heating at 100° for 10 minutes. After cooling, the density is read in a photometer within 2 hours.—*Biochem. J.* **57,** 410 (1954).

A.K.

Influence of smoking on urinary pepsinogen excretion. S. Bornstein and S. Eichen (*Veterans Administration Hospital, Montrose, N. Y.*).

Urinary pepsinogen was determined by the method of West, Ellis, and Scott [*J. Lab. Clin. Med.* **39,** 159 (1952)] with a casein substrate [Goodman, Sandoval, and Halstead, *J. Lab. Clin. Med.* **40,** 872 (1952)]. Twenty white male office and professional hospital workers between 18 and 45 years of age, who smoked 20 or more cigarettes per day, were each examined 5 times. The control group consisted of 20 nonsmokers. Considerable diurnal and day-to-day variation was found in the controls. The average urinary excretion of pepsinogen for the smokers was 43 units per hour compared with a value of 30 for the controls, a difference which had a p value of 0.03 by the "t" test. A group of 5 smokers had an average excretion of 47 units per hour when they smoked during tests as compared with 43 units when they abstained. No information is given concerning the length of the experimental periods, but the statements are made that the immediate effect of smoking, although of statistical significance, is not of appreciable magnitude and that there is a prolonged effect on pepsin secretion.—*Proc. Soc. Exp. Biol. Med.* **86,** 619 (1954).

M.K.

Conjugated steroids: V. Hydrolysis of total ketosteroids in urine. I. B. Oneson and S. L. Cohen (*University of Minnesota Medical School, Minneapolis, Minn.*)

An improved method of hydrolysis is presented which results in an increase of about 15 per cent in the total steroids of urine as compared with hydrochloric acid hydrolysis. The hydrolysate contains larger amounts of ketosteroid sulfates and about 20 per cent of the total steroids as the beta type. The procedure is similar to that previously described for ketosteroid sulfates [Cohen and Oneson, *J. Biol. Chem.* **204,** 245 (1953)]. Acidified urine (pH 2–3) is extracted with butyl alcohol. The extract is washed with water and evaporated to dryness at a temperature not exceeding 60°. Portions equivalent to 100–200 ml. of urine are hydrolyzed by heating for 10 minutes on a steam bath with 10 ml. of 1,4-dioxane. containing 10% of concentrated hydrochloric acid.—*Proc. Soc. Exp. Biol. Med.* **86,** 728 (1954).

M.K.

BOOK REVIEWS

Organic Analysis (Vol. 2)

J. Mitchell, Jr., I. M. Kolthoff, E. S. Proskauer, and A. Weissberger (Eds.) Interscience Publishers, Inc., New York, 372 pp., $8.50

This is the second of the excellent series, *Organic Analysis,* designed to present reliable and critical information on general methods of direct analysis of organic systems. It stresses chemical and instrumental technics for analysis through functional groups.

The topics of Volume 2, and their authors, are:

"Microdetermination of Carboxyl Groups (Neutralization Equivalent)," by Al Steyermark.

"Determination of Esters," by R. T. Hall and W. E. Shaefer.

"Determination of Nitro, Nitroso and Nitrate Groups," by W. W. Becker and W. E. Shaefer.

"Application of Lithium Aluminum Hydride to Organic Analysis," by T. Higuchi.

"Coulometric Methods," by W. Donald Cooke.

"Application of Polarography to Organic Analysis," by Philip J. Elving.

"Methods Based on Reaction Rate," by T. S. Lee.

"Phase Solubility Analysis," by W. J. Mader.

"Countercurrent Distribution," by J. R. Weisiger.

This volume also contains the indices to Volume I and II.

Legal Medicine, Pathology and Toxicology (ed. 2)

T. A. Gonzales, M. Vance, M. Helpern, and C. J. Umberger. Appleton-Century-Crofts, Inc., New York, N. Y., 1349 pp., $22.00

This noted text and reference book has been revised and brought up to date in this enlarged second edition, which contains almost twice the number of pages than the original, first published in 1937. As before, the text is well illustrated with photographs of actual cases taken from the files of the Office of the Chief Medical Examiner of New York City. The statistical data incorporates cases through 1951.

The first 40 chapters are devoted to pathology as applied to this type of work. New subject matter has been added to include autopsy findings in enbalmed bodies, cardiac contusions, sports injuries, serologic applications (Rh-Hr factors), radioactive compounds, new drugs, poisonings, and operative and postoperative deaths.

The entire section, 365 pages, on analytic toxicology has been rewritten. This section contains much data and formerly unpublished methodology of the Microchemical-Physical Laboratory of the Medical Examiner's Office. The hospital chemist would have to critically evaluate the methodology for application to the needs of an active hospital laboratory. In the main, the methodology and instrumentation are applicable to large state and city laboratories dealing chiefly with such analytical problems, who have enough funds for the purchase of the specialized instrumentation. In isolated portions of this section, the chemist can find the rapid and simple chemical procedures that one could apply to the occasional requests from the emergency wards of the general hospitals, but the major portion of the procedures enumerated are too time consuming and require apparatus not usually found in hospital laboratories. On reading this section, one is left with the feeling that there is great need for a critical compilation of the fundamental, rapid, and specific methodology for use as part of the toxicologic procedures encountered in an active hospital chemistry laboratory. Here, speed and accuracy are essential for the immediate treatment of the patient.

As a reference book for pathologists and chemists concerned with forensic toxicology this text is essential to the laboratory library. The clinical chemist, with careful adaptation of the published procedures can establish an efficient routine which can be of practical help to his toxicologic problems. The descriptive toxicology (diagnosis and treatment), is unexcelled.

Electrometric pH Determinations: Theory and Practice

Roger G. Bates. John Wiley and Sons, Inc., New York, 331 pps. $7.50

Dr. Roger G. Bates, chemist at the National Bureau of Standards, has written this book to make some order out of the widespread confusion about the principles of *p*H determinations. The rapid advances in *p*H meters have overshadowed the basic principles and the meaning of the *p*H numbers which are so easily obtained and used.

The first six chapters of this book are devoted to the presentation of the theoretical and experimental basis for a practical electrometric scale of acidity and compares the various possible scales as to usefulness and validity. The author shows that, although the *p*H value is a thermodynamic quantity, the actual value and measurements depend upon certain basic assumptions. There is a full discussion of the standard *p*H scale and the National Bureau of Standards *p*H standards, which are rapidly being adopted throughout the world. Dr. Bates stresses the importance of accurate and reliable standard solutions and gives detailed instructions for the preparation of these solutions.

A separate chapter is devoted to a discussion of scales of acidity and basicity in nonaqueous solutions. The last four chapters discuss the many experimental and practical aspects of *p*H measurement. The instrumentation is presented fully and clearly. The selection and preparation of electrodes and salt bridges are described and errors pointed out, and the care and handling of the instruments are outlined. Complete chapters are devoted to the discussion of the glass electrode and to automatic *p*H control as used in industry.

This book is recommended as a natural adjunct to the laboratory *p*H meter.

CLINICAL CHEMISTRY

Articles to Appear in Forthcoming Issues

CANNAN, R. KEITH: Proposal for the Distribution of a Certified Standard for Use in Hemoglobinometry.

GOTTFRIED, SIDNEY P., POPE, RUSSELL H., FRIEDMAN, NATHAN H., AKERSON, IRVING B., and DI MAURO, SALVATORE: Serum Beta-Lipoproteins of Normal, Atherosclerotic, and Lipemic Individuals: Changes in Concentration, Stability and Mobility upon Incubation at 6.5° and 37.5°, as Determined by Paper Electrophoresis.

MANDEL, EMANUEL E., GORSUCH, THOMAS L., and COOPER, GERALD E.: A Study of Seromucoid in Hepatobiliary Disease.

NADEAU, GUY and JOLY, L. P.: A Convenient Apparatus for the Continuous Dehydration of Histologic Material.

NATELSON, SAMUEL and MENNING, CAROL M.: Improved Methods of Analysis for Oxygen, Carbon Monoxide, and Iron on Fingertip Blood.

PERALTA, OSCAR and REINHOLD, JOHN G.: A Method for Rapid Estimation of Amylase Activity of Serum by Means of Turbidimetry.

SAIFER, ABRAHAM and ZYMARIS, MICHAEL C.: Effect of Shaking on the Accuracy of Salt Fractionation Methods for Serum Albumin.

Proposal for the Distribution of a Certified Standard for Use in Hemoglobinometry

Prepared by the Division of Medical Sciences, National Academy of Sciences-National Research Council

R. Keith Cannan

THERE IS PROBABLY NO PROCEDURE more commonly used in clinical laboratories than hemoglobinometry and few that are less satisfactory in their results. The deficiencies may reside, in part, in inadequacies of the chosen method. In larger part, however, they result from manipulative errors in the measurement and processing of the samples of blood. The latter involve questions of technical proficiency which are entirely within the control of the analyst himself. When, however, he converts his observations—gasometric or photometric readings, measurements of specific gravity, etc.—to grams of hemoglobin in 100 ml. of blood, he must depend upon his own calibration or a calibration supplied by an instrument maker, both procedures involving a conversion factor taken from the literature. To be satisfied that the calibration remains valid for the instrument, reagents, and technical routines in use in his laboratory, he should periodically undertake a precise and time-consuming series of standardizations. If a uniform hemoglobin standard were available nationally and a single method of analysis widely practiced, the individual laboratory would then have assurance not only that its results would be comparable from month to month, but that they would also be comparable with those from other laboratories employing the same standard. Inconsistencies in results that persisted under these conditions could then be clearly attributed to technical and manipulative errors.

Chairman, Division of Medical Sciences, National Academy of Sciences-National Research Council.

Presented in part at the meeting of the American Association of Blood Banks, Washington, D. C., September, 1954.

The purpose of this report is to describe a plan for the distribution of a certified hemoglobin standard and to advocate the wide adoption of a recommended analytic procedure. The use of both the new procedure and the standard is recommended. At the same time it is pointed out that the standard may be employed for the calibration of other methods of hemoglobin analysis in laboratories that do not choose to adopt routinely the advocated photometric procedure.

In 1941 the British Medical Research Council instituted an extensive study of the problem of standardizing hemoglobinometry and emerged with (a) a recommended analytic procedure, (b) a simple hemoglobinometer for general use, and (c) a certified national hemoglobin standard for distribution to cooperating laboratories (1, 2, 3, 4).

In the United States the initiative was taken by the Army Medical Service Graduate School with a limited field trial (5) of a cyanmethemoglobin solution proposed by Dr. David L. Drabkin. The success of the Army plan so impressed the Hematology Study Section of the National Institutes of Health that it requested the National Research Council to explore the possibility of establishing a National Hemoglobin Standard for general use throughout the country.

To this end the Academy-Research Council established an *ad hoc* panel under the Subcommittee on Blood and Related Problems of the Division of Medical Sciences. This panel has sought the cooperation of the College of American Pathologists, the American Society of Clinical Pathologists, the American Association of Blood Banks, the Department of Defense, the Veterans Administration, the National Institutes of Health, and the National Bureau of Standards. It has also maintained close liaison with the Committee on Hemoglobinometry of the Medical Research Council of the United Kingdom and with the National Research Council of Canada.

The panel gave serious consideration to the British plan, but decided that, in respect to simplicity and adaptability, the cyanmethemoglobin method (6, 7, 8, 9, 10, 11) adopted by the U. S. Army would be more suitable for use in the United States and Canada. It was agreed that the choice of a solution of some form of hemoglobin as a standard for hemoglobinometry was both logical and direct. In contrast to a glass standard, it would have the advantage of adaptability to a variety of photometric instruments and cuvettes. Among the forms of hemoglobin well adapted to photometry, cyanmethemoglobin has outstanding advantages. It has been shown that solutions of this pigment are stable for years when preserved at refrigerator temperatures (12). The absorption band of cyanmethemoglobin in the region of 540 mμ is broad rather than sharp, so that its solutions are suitable for use in filter type photometers as well as in narrow band spectrophotometers (13, 7). Finally, all forms of hemoglobin likely to be found in blood, with the exception of sulfhemoglobin, are quantitatively converted to cyanmethemoglobin upon the addition of a single reagent (7).

RECOMMENDATIONS

On the basis of these considerations, the panel reached agreement on the following recommendations:

1. Standard of Reference

There shall be a Standard of Reference in the form of a preparation of crystalline human hemoglobin prepared by the method of Drabkin (14, 15, 16). The acceptable criteria for this preparation shall be that a solution containing 1 milliatom of hemoglobin iron per liter shall have a millimolar extinction coefficient of 11.5 at a wave length of 540 mμ, when measured as cyanmethemoglobin (13, 7). Certification of this Standard of Reference shall rest upon the results of spectrophotometric measurements and of analyses for iron made independently by the National Institutes of Health, the Army Medical Service Graduate School, the National Bureau of Standards, and Dr. Drabkin's laboratory at the University of Pennsylvania.

Professor King of the Postgraduate Medical School in London will also characterize the Standard of Reference both chemically and spectrophotometrically and compare the results of its use with determinations of hemoglobin employing the British standard.

2. Iron Content of Hemoglobin

The iron content of hemoglobin shall be accepted to be 0.335 per cent (17). This value for iron is the traditional figure used in this country and is in substantial agreement with that adopted by the British. It corresponds with an equivalent weight for hemoglobin of 16,700 per atom of iron and with an oxygen capacity of 1.34 ml. per gram of hemoglobin (17).

The adoption of an agreed figure for the iron content is necessary in order that the spectrophotometric measurements in terms of iron may be translated into grams of hemoglobin. Should any change be made in the future in the accepted values for the extinction coefficient of cyanmethemoglobin and the iron content of hemoglobin, results based on the use of the above standard may be readily recalculated.

3. Standard for Distribution

There shall be a Standard for Distribution in the form of a certified solution of cyanmethemoglobin which shall be prepared directly from the Standard of Reference. The Standard for Distribution shall be packaged as three separate solutions containing certified concentrations of approximately 20, 40, and 60 milligrams of hemoglobin in the form of cyanmethemoglobin per 100 ml.

These three solutions will correspond to 1:250 dilutions of blood containing approximately 5, 10, and 15 Gm., respectively, of hemoglobin per 100 ml. After bottling, samples of these standard solutions will be spot-checked for correctness of optical density by the four analytic laboratories that have been designated above. The batch will then be certified and distributed to cooperating laboratories by designated national agencies.

4. Adoption of Cyanmethemoglobin Method

In conjunction with the use of the proposed standards, it is recommended that clinical laboratories consider the adoption of the cyanmethemoglobin method of hemoglobin determination described by Drabkin.

The use of the cyanmethemoglobin method follows from the concept that it would be logical to adopt a method of analysis which converts hemoglobin into the same pigment as that used in the standard. It does not, however, preclude the use of the cyanmethemoglobin standard for the calibration of other methods of hemoglobin analysis which may be in routine use in some laboratories. However, it should be realized that such a procedure may lead to some loss of accuracy.

The cyanmethemoglobin method employs a single solution containing potassium ferricyanide and potassium cyanide, which converts the hemoglobin in blood quantitatively to cyanmethemoglobin. The ferricyanide converts the hemoglobin iron from the ferrous to the ferric state to form methemoglobin, which then combines with potassium cyanide to produce the stable pigment cyanmethemoglobin. These two reactions are rapid and stoichiometric.

There should be no reluctance to employ this standard and reagent because they contain cyanide. The concentration of cyanide in the reagent that is proposed for use is only 52 mg. of potassium cyanide per liter. Its lethal dose for man approaches four liters (18). Most clinical laboratories use for the determination of uric acid, a reagent containing 50 Gm. of this salt per liter. In view of this and of the fact that laboratories of clinical pathology are disciplined in the use of such dangerous materials as isotopes and virulent pathogens, it would seem that the handling of the proposed reagent constitutes a quite negligible hazard.

The panel also agreed to undertake a field trial of one year's duration using the Standard for Distribution described above. It is now felt that the plans for this field trial have progressed to the point where the participation of laboratories desiring to cooperate may be invited. The standards will be prepared by Dr. David L. Drabkin and distributed without charge to clinical laboratories on application, provided they will agree to meet certain minimum requirements for participation, as follows:

1. To conduct and report at three-month intervals, for one year, measurements of the actual photometric readings of the three standard solutions in the photometer routinely in use for hemoglobin measurements in that laboratory.
2. To cooperate in answering a simple questionnaire designed to furnish information on the influence of various factors on the results of the hemoglobin determinations which will assist the panel in its long range plans for making this standard available on a national scale.
3. To cooperate in the analysis and reporting of (a) an unknown solution of cyanmethemoglobin, and (b) an unknown sample of blood.

The Standard for Distribution, consisting of the three solutions described above, will be packaged as a single unit. Details of the procedure for the determination of hemoglobin as cyanmethemoglobin, as well as details of the procedure for calibrating another method in terms of the cyanmethemoglobin standard, will be furnished with the standard.

Distribution will be made to civilian laboratories by the College of American Pathologists, 203 North Wabash Avenue, Chicago, Illinois; to military and government laboratories by the Army Medical Service Graduate School, the Navy Bureau of Medicine and Surgery, the Air Force Surgeon General's Office, and the Veterans Administration* and to laboratories in Canada through the Division on Medical Research, National Research Council, Ottawa, Ontario, Canada. Cooperating laboratories are requested to apply to the distributing agency with which they are most closely associated. Because of limitation in the number of sets of the standard available, distribution will be determined by priority of application and willingness to comply with the conditions listed above. Application for standards will assume acceptance of these conditions. It is estimated that the Standard will be ready for distribution by April 15, 1955.

---

* Veterans Administration, Central Office, Room 871.

This plan has been drafted by the *ad hoc* Panel on the Establishment of a Hemoglobin Standard of the Division of Medical Sciences, National Academy of Sciences-National Research Council.

REFERENCES

1. King, E. J., and Gilchrist, M., *Lancet* **2,** 201 (1947).
2. King, E. J., Gilchrist, M., and Matheson, A., *Brit. Med. J.* **1,** 250 (1944).
3. King, E. J., Gilchrist, M., Wootton, I. D. P., Donaldson, R., Sisson, R. B., Macfarlane, R. G., Jope, H. M., O'Brien, J. R. P., Peterson, J. M., and Strangeways, D. H., *Lancet* **2,** 789 (1947).
4. King, E. J., Wootton, I. D. P., Donaldson, R., and Sisson, R. B., *Lancet* **2,** 971 (1948).
5. Crosby, W. H., Munn, J. I., and Furth, F. W., *U. S. Armed Forces Med. J.* **5,** 693 (1954).
6. Stadie, W. C., *J. Biol. Chem.* **41,** 237 (1920).
7. Drabkin, D. L., and Austin, J. H., *J. Biol. Chem.* **112,** 51 (1935–6).
8. Evelyn, K. A., and Malloy, H. T., *J. Biol. Chem.* **126,** 655 (1938).
9. Sunderman, F. W., *Am. J. Clin. Path., Tech. Suppl.* **7,** 1 (1943).
10. Collier, H. B., *Can. Med. Assoc. J.* **50,** 550 (1944).
11. King, E. J., Gilchrist, M., and Delory, G. E., *Lancet* **1,** 239 (1944).
12. Drabkin, D. L., personal communication.
13. Drabkin, D. L., and Austin, J. H., *J. Biol. Chem.* **98,** 719 (1932).
14. Drabkin, D. L., *J. Biol. Chem.* **164,** 703 (1946).
15. Drabkin, D. L., *Arch. Biochem.* **21,** 224 (1949).
16. Drabkin, D. L., *J. Biol. Chem.* **185,** 231 (1950).
17. Hüfner, G., *Arch. Anat. u. Physiol., Physiol. Abt.,* page 130 (1894).
18. Sollmann, T. H., *Manual of Pharmacology* (ed. 7), Philadelphia, Saunders, 1948, p. 713.

Rapid Estimation of Amylase Activity of Serum by Turbidimetry

Oscar Peralta and John G. Reinhold*

THE CHOICE OF RAPID METHODS for estimation of serum amylase activity is limited (1). Such methods depend upon the change in color of starch with iodine brought about by splitting of the starch by the enzyme. It is often difficult to establish an end point visually by this reaction in partially digested starch solutions, especially by those whose experience with the method is limited. Furthermore, the use of solutions of elemental iodine in laboratories in which microanalytical methods for iodine are applied introduces a considerable hazard of contamination to the latter.

Favorable experience with the turbidimetric method of Waldron for measuring the amylase activity of pancreatic juice suggested that this procedure might be adapted to the rapid estimation of amylase activity of serum. The present paper describes such a method and offers evidence that it is capable of detecting elevation of amylase activity in serum.

This approach to the estimation of amylase activity of serum has received little attention. A turbidimetric method for measurement of serum amylase activity was described by Jacobsson and Hansen, who used dextrin as a substrate. Their method called for a 30-minute period of incubation and removal of protein before turbidimetric measurement of dextrin concentration. The method to be described requires less time

From the William Pepper Laboratory of Clinical Medicine and the Gastrointestinal Section (Kinsey-Thomas Foundation) of the Medical Clinic, Hospital of the University of Pennsylvania, Philadelphia, Pa.

* Latin American Fellow in Gastroenterology from Chile, sponsored by the Kellogg Foundation and the American College of Physicians. Present address: Calle Hernan Cortes 3432, Santiago, Chile.

The authors wish to acknowledge the assistance in various ways of the following in the development and trial of the method described: Misses Lola Allen, Sonya Graboyes, Edythe Gershman, Shirley Matis, Joan McNichol, Doris Thompson, Ruth Winger, and Dr. Frank Dituri.

Received for publication December 27, 1954.

and fewer manipulations than that of the Scandinavian workers. Another method of applying turbidimetry to estimation of amylase activity of pancreatic secretion is that of Guth, Komarov, and Shay.

The basis of the turbidimetric method for measurement of amylase activity is the decrease in the absorbency of a buffered starch suspension caused by the splitting of the starch by the enzyme during a timed interval and at a controlled temperature.

REAGENTS

Stock Starch Suspensions

Fifty grams of acid-digested cornstarch (Argo Laundry Starch has proved satisfactory) are crushed to a powder (in a mortar, if necessary). A preservative (5) of 1.5 Gm. of methylparahydroxybenzoate and 0.3 Gm. of propylparahydroxymethylbenzoate may be mixed with the starch powder, although it is not essential. Water, 150 ml., is added and the resulting thin paste poured slowly into 850 ml. of boiling water in a beaker while stirring rapidly with a mechanical stirrer. The mixture is heated just to boiling on an asbestos-covered electric hotplate, the stirring being continued. 10 Gm. of sodium chloride are added. When cool, the starch suspension is transferred to a wide-mouth bottle and stored, well stoppered, at room temperature.

If the starch suspension thickens, aliquots for preparation of diluted starch suspension are removed by means of a spoon or spatula.

A more convenient source of substrate is the liquid starch suspension widely distributed under the trade name "Zippy." Standardized preparations of this product contain 10% starch and are without the blue dye present in starch sold for household use.[1] The pine oil included as a preservative does not interfere. Although the blue dye present in household starch does not demonstrably affect the action of amylase, and acceptable results may be obtained with liquid laundry starch as purchased in the market, the dye complicates the standardization of the substrate and dye-free preparations are preferred.

Diluted Starch Suspension

Sufficient stock starch suspension is added to the buffered NaCl diluent in a stoppered cylinder to give a reading of approximately 325

[1] Available from the Hartman-Leddon Company, Philadelphia, Pa.

scale divisions on a Klett-Summerson photocolorimeter or a transmittance of 25 per cent if other photoelectric photometers are used. Usually a dilution of 1 part of stock starch suspension to 10 parts of buffered NaCl diluent approximates the desired concentration. The diluted starch suspensions remain usable for as long as 5 days. The starch always must be completely dispersed by thorough mixing before use.

Buffered Sodium Chloride Diluent

13.0 Gm. of NaCl, 5.9 Gm. of KH_2PO_4, and 15.9 Gm. of Na_2HPO_4 (anhyd.) are dissolved in water and diluted to 1000 ml. The *p*H is 7.2.

METHOD

All tests are done in duplicate.

1. Measure 5 ml. of diluted starch suspension into a cuvette and place it in a water bath at 38° for approximately 5 minutes.
2. Measure 1 ml. of serum into a tube of about 15 ml. capacity. Mix the warm starch suspension and serum by pouring the starch into the serum and then pouring back and forth 2 times before returning the mixture to the cuvette. Start a timer, which has been set at 5.5 minutes, immediately after the starch and serum have been mixed. Adjust the zero setting of the photometer by means of a cuvette containing distilled water.
3. Exactly 0.5 minutes after mixing, measure the absorbency (A_1). Replace the cuvette in the water bath.
4. Exactly 5 minutes later, mix and again measure the absorbency (A_2). Readjust the zero setting if necessary before making the reading.

CALCULATION

Convert A_1 and A_2 into percentages by means of the standard curve. The amylase activity is expressed as a velocity constant, k.

$$k = \frac{1}{5} \times 2.3 \log \frac{C_1}{C_2} \times 10{,}000 = 0.46 \log \frac{C_1}{C_2} \times 10{,}000$$

C_1 and C_2 are the initial and final concentrations expressed as percentages. To obtain whole numbers, k is multiplied by 10,000. Table 1 shows k values corresponding to the various ratios of C_1/C_2.

STANDARDIZATION

Measure the volumes of buffered NaCl solution and diluted starch suspension shown in Table 2 into cuvettes of uniform diameter. Place

Table 1. Values of "k" Corresponding to Various Final Concentrations of Starch Substrate

Initial concentration = 100 per cent

Final concentration (%)	k ($\times 10^4$)
99	20
98	40
97	61
96	82
95	103
94	124
93	145
92	166
91	188
90	210
89	232
88	255
87	277
86	300
85	324
84	349
83	373
82	397
81	422
80	448
79	472
78	496
77	522
76	548
75	574
74	601
73	628
72	655
71	682
70	712
69	741
68	770
67	800
66	830
65	860

If the initial reading does not correspond to 100 per cent on the standard curve, plot the initial absorbency of the diluted starch suspension (plus serum) on the abscissa corresponding to 100 per cent. Then draw a line parallel to that given by the 3 standards. Convert the absorbency of A_2 to percentage by means of the new line.

Percentages between those shown in the table may be converted to k values by interpolation.

Table 2. Volumes for Standardization

Standard No.	*Buffered NaCl* (ml.)	*Diluted starch suspension* (ml.)	*Per cent of initial concentration*
1	1	5	100
2	2	4	80
3	3	3	60

the cuvettes in the water bath at 38° for 5 minutes. Mix the contents thoroughly and measure the absorbency. Plot absorbencies against percentages. The line obtained is nearly straight.

HIGH AMYLASE ACTIVITIES

The quantity of starch provided in the substrate is not sufficient to enable accurate measurement of high amylase activities. If the change in absorbency exceeds 0.12 (60 scale divisions on the Klett-Summerson photocolorimeter), the test should be repeated, using 0.5 ml. of serum or less.

Micro Method

Serum samples of 0.2 ml. are combined with 1.0 ml. of diluted starch suspension and the absorbencies are measured in micro cuvettes. Smaller samples may be used if appropriate cuvettes are available.

COMMENTS

Studies of amylopsin and of serum amylase showed that starch suspensions cleared more rapidly when the enzyme acted at 38° than at the lower temperature used by Waldron. Since the main purpose of introducing the new method was to shorten the time required for estimation of amylase activity, the higher temperature was adopted.

The activity of amylase is favored also by high concentrations of substrate and it diminishes rapidly as the concentration of substrate decreases. It is advantageous, therefore, to use a short time interval, and the 5-minute reaction time serves not only to expedite the analysis but makes possible a more sensitive measurement of enzyme activities than would be obtained by longer incubation times.

The buffer solution is that described by Guth, Komarov, and Shay. The *p*H is not critical. Measurements are made at 660 mμ so as to enable maximal concentrations of starch to be used while still making possible measurements within a favorable absorbency range of the photometer. This wave length also avoids interference by pigments of serum and diminishes the contribution of turbidity in the serum.

RESULTS

The results obtained by the rapid turbidimetric method have been compared with those of the Somogyi saccharogenic method (6). Reducing substances were measured by the Nelson-Somogyi method (7, 8), as described by one of the authors (9). Figure 1 shows that speci-

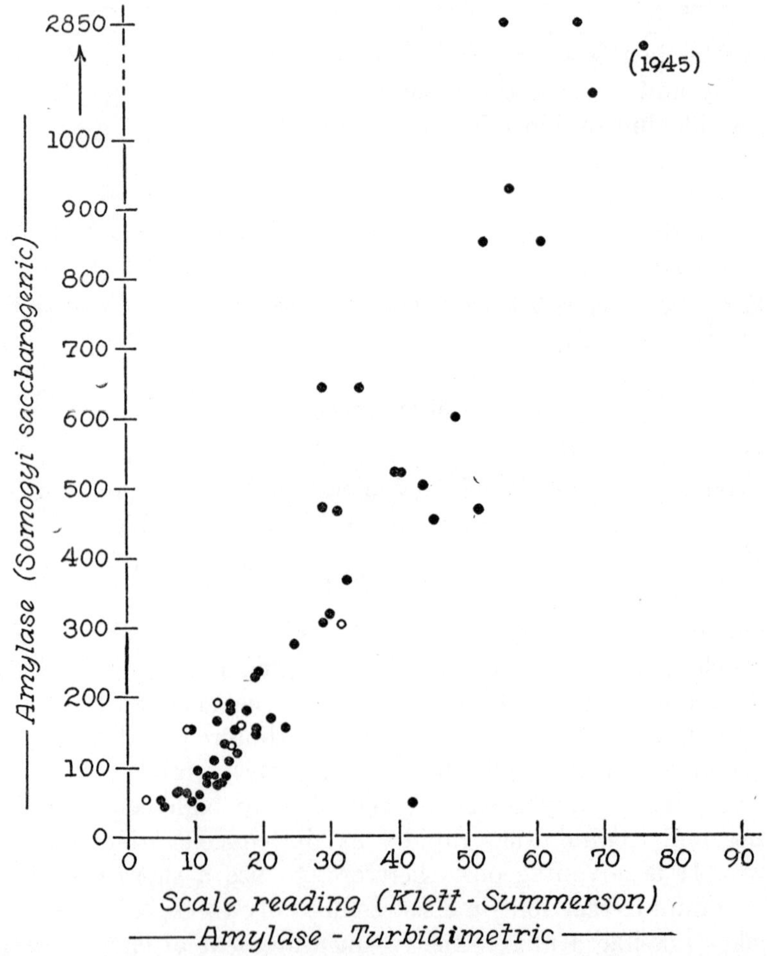

Fig. 1. The correlation between amylase estimated by the turbidimetric method and the Somogyi saccharogenic method. Where symbols are paired, each represents a single determination. Open circles show the results of determinations made by the micro technic, using 0.2 ml. of serum and 1 ml. of diluted starch suspension. All the abnormal values, with one exception (see text), were associated with pancreatic disease and are clearly differentiated from those of the control group.

Figures on the abscissa are scale readings of the Klett-Summerson photocolorimeter; those on the ordinate as glucose, in mg./100 ml.

mens having high activities by the standard method also had significantly increased values by the turbidimetric method. However, those having excessively high activities did not show a proportionate increase by the turbidimetric method unless smaller amounts of serum—0.5 ml. or 0.05 ml. for macro and micro techniques, respectively—were used.

Activities of serum amylase have been measured in 41 healthy individuals by use of the turbidimetric method. These included laboratory workers, staff physicians, and blood donors. The distribution of values is shown in Fig. 2.

The turbidimetric method has been applied to serum during the past 6 months in the laboratories of the authors, especially when emergencies required prompt reports. In only 1 instance out of approximately 50 trials did the results differ from those of the standard Somogyi method. The exception was attributed not to a failure of the method but to a technical error by an intern working alone at night, who lacked actual experience with the method. A recurrence of this error was traced to contamination of the serum by blood cells.

SUMMARY

The method of Waldron for turbidimetric measurement of amylase activity of duodenal contents has been adapted to measurement of

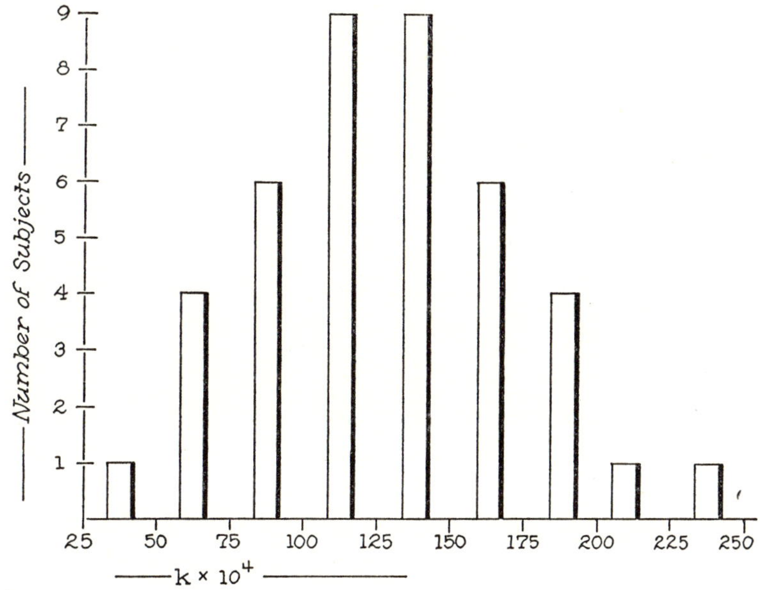

Fig. 2. Distribution of k ($\times 10^4$) values of a group of 41 healthy control subjects whose serum amylase activities were measured by the turbidimetric method.

amylase activity of serum. The speed and simplicity of the method make it suitable particularly when results are needed quickly.

Comparison of the results obtained by the turbidimetric method with those of a saccharogenic method showed that high amylase activities could be established dependably by the turbidimetric method.

REFERENCES

1. Gomori, G., *Am. J. Clin. Pathol.* **24,** 99 (1954).
2. Waldron, J. M., *J. Lab. Clin. Med.* **38,** 148 (1951).
3. Jacobsson, L., and Hansen, H., *Scan. J. Clin. and Lab. Invest.* **4,** 134 (1952).
4. Guth, P., Komarov, S. A., and Shay, H., *Am. J. Physiol.* **173,** 461 (1953).
5. Wenger, R. G., *Clin. Chemist* **6,** 10 (1954).
6. Somogyi, M., *J. Biol. Chem.* **125,** 399 (1938).
7. Nelson, M., *J. Biol. Chem.* **153,** 375 (1944).
8. Somogyi, M., *J. Biol. Chem.* **160,** 61 (1945).
9. Reinhold, J. G., in Reiner, M. (Ed.), *Standard Methods of Clinical Chemistry*, New York, Acad. Press, 1953, p. 65.

Improved Methods of Analysis for Oxygen, Carbon Monoxide, and Iron on Fingertip Blood

Samuel Natelson and Carol M. Menning

THE TENDENCY OF CERTAIN premature and new born infants to become cyanotic necessitates a rapid and convenient method for the determination of oxygen, iron, and carbon monoxide on minute quantities of blood. These procedures are necessary to distinguish between cardiac anomalies, methemoglobinemia, lung abnormalities, and other conditions that result in anoxia to tissues (1–6).

The procedures described herein for oxygen and carbon monoxide use an improved form of a microgasometer, described previously (7, 8), in which both gases are estimated manometrically. A photograph of the instrument with an inset showing the method of sampling is shown in Fig. 1.

For the estimation of oxygen in blood the usual technic for liberating the O_2 by ferricyanide, removing the CO_2 with alkali, and absorbing the oxygen in sodium hydrosulfite is used (9–11). For carbon monoxide the same steps are followed using a special reaction chamber (Fig. 2). The CO is absorbed in cuprous chloride–ammonia complex (12, 13).

Iron is estimated as the thiocyanate by a modification of a method previously described (8) after wet ashing the blood (14). The use of small quantities of blood permits the use of relatively large amounts of perchloric and sulfuric acids so that digestion is rapid.

From the Department of Biochemistry of the Laboratories of Rockford Memorial Hospital, Rockford, Illinois.

Supported in part by a grant from the Bureau of Maternal and Child Health, Illinois Department of Public Health, Division of Preventive Medicine through the Rockford Health Department.

Presented in part at the meeting of the Federation of American Societies for Experimental Biology, Chicago, 1953.

Received for publication October 26, 1954.

REAGENTS AND METHODS

Estimation of Oxygen Capacity and Content

Reagents

Simultaneous deaeration of reagents is carried out for approximately 10 minutes just before use, by transferring the reagents to small containers (Fig. 3). Reduced pressure is obtained by means of a water aspirator and a glass manifold. As the reagents are layered with oil, they remain air-free. During the 10-minute deaeration process, the bottles or vials are tapped occasionally to facilitate the displacement of air.

Potassium Ferricyanide: 1.2% in distilled water. Transfer a portion of this solution to a 20 ml. short form vial and cover with a layer of caprylic alcohol. After deaeration the reagent is removed for the procedure by taking up, in order, caprylic alcohol, the reagent, and then caprylic alcohol. Contamination of this reagent with mercury should be avoided.

Saponin Solution: 0.5% in distilled water. Transfer a portion to a 20 ml. vial, cover with mineral oil, and add mercury to about 2 cm. high in vial. Deaerate just before use.

Potassium Hydroxide: 1N. Keep in a polyethylene bottle. Transfer a portion to a 20 ml. vial and cover with mineral oil. Mercury is added to a height of 2 cm. in vial.

Sodium Hydrosulfite Solution: Place 1 Gm. sodium hydrosulfite placed in a vial or test tube and cover with mineral oil. Add 5 ml. of 1N KOH and 2 ml. of mercury. The powder will dissolve as the solution is being deaerated. If not completely dissolved, deaerate while tube is in a 60° water bath. It is best that this solution be prepared daily.

Preparation of Microgasometer

Draw approximately 1 ml. of water into the 3 ml. bulb and expel. Repeat. Draw 0.1 ml. of 1N lactic acid into the instrument, retreat to the 3 ml. mark, and then expel the acid. The gasometer is thus left acid which eliminates the need for an acid ferricyanide reagent.

Collection of Sample

Prick the fingertip or heel and allow the blood to flow into a heparin-lined tube, 1.5 mm. bore, as described previously (7, 8). Discard the first drop by wiping with a cotton pledget, insert the tip of the fire-polished tube into the cut, and allow the blood to flow directly into the tube until approximately 10 cm. (0.1 ml. approx.) has been collected.

Oxygen Capacity: Transfer the blood to the bottom of a silicone-lined,

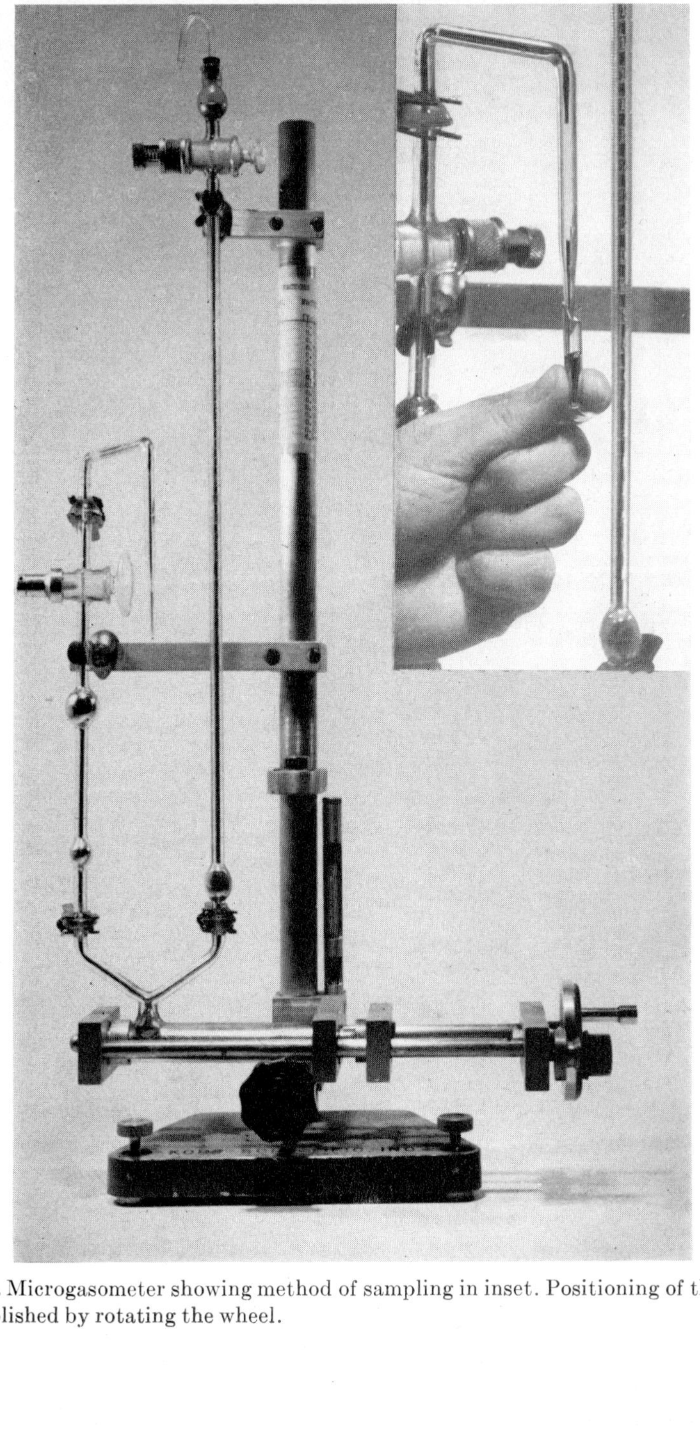

Fig. 1. Microgasometer showing method of sampling in inset. Positioning of the mercury is accomplished by rotating the wheel.

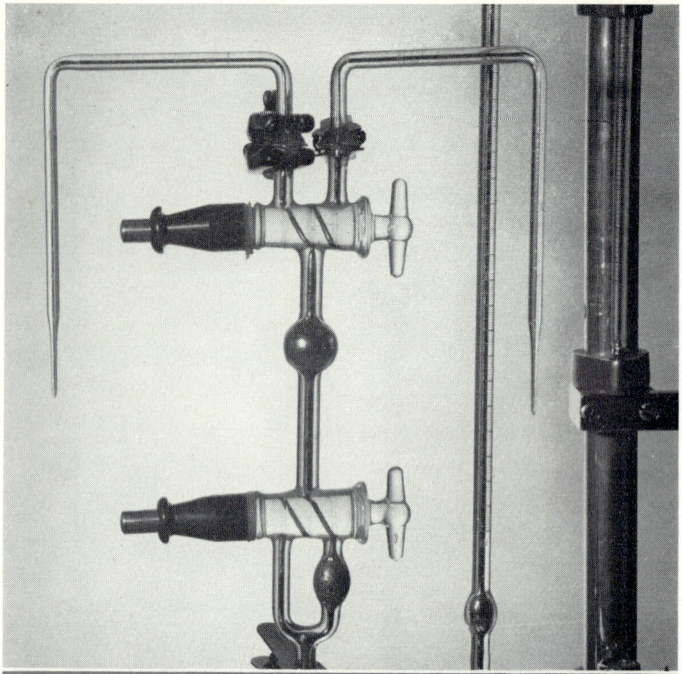

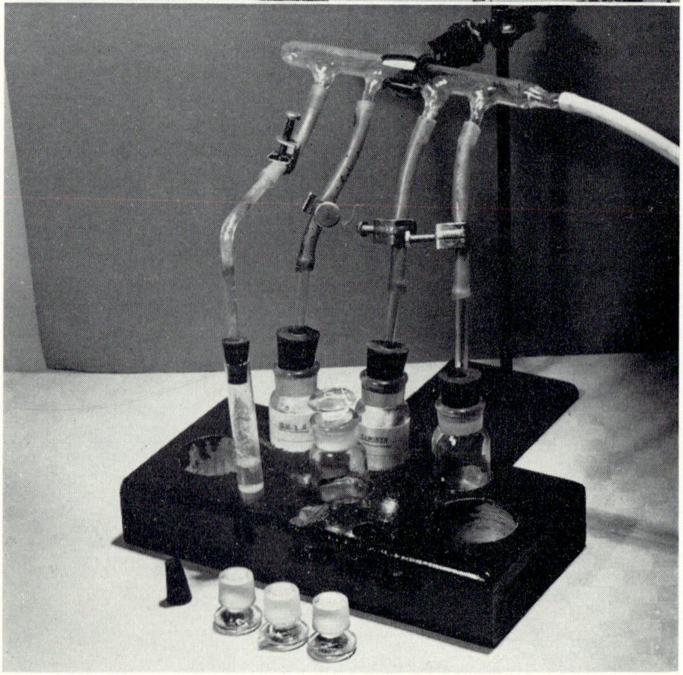

Fig. 2. Reaction chamber for CO estimation. Two-way stopcock at top permits rinsing of the instrument while the gas bubble is trapped at right above stopcock. Lower stopcock is not used in this determination.

Fig. 3. Simultaneous deaeration of reagents for oxygen and carbon monoxide estimation with the water aspirator.

3 ml. test tube (10 × 75 mm.) that has been cut to half its height. The blood is saturated with oxygen by beating the tube with the fingers, as for shaking, for about three minutes. As an alternative, a slow stream of O_2 or air is passed through the blood from a fine-tipped glass tube. Just before performing the analysis the blood is again shaken to resuspend the cells. Approximately 0.05 ml. is transferred to a 0.5 ml. tube half filled with mercury. This tube is made by cutting in half the 1 ml. test tube (6 × 50 mm.). An additional tube and sample should be used for duplicate determinations.

Oxygen Content: This is best done if the gasometer, which is portable, is placed within a few minutes walking distance of the patient. Collect the blood in the same manner as for O_2 capacity and transfer about 0.05 ml. directly into the 0.5 heparinized tube containing mercury covered with a layer of mineral oil. Insert the collecting tube so that its tip extends below the mineral oil and allow the blood to layer under it, leaving some in the collecting tube. The blood sample has not been exposed to air except for the minute surface at the narrow collecting tip. For the duplicate, wipe the tip of the collecting tube and layer another sample. The collecting tube should rest in a horizontal position so that subsequent sampling is representative, the cells settling laterally in the tube. If settling is marked, the tube may be rolled on the table to resuspend the cells. When both determinations are to be done on the same sample it is best to do the O_2 content first using the remaining blood for the O_2 capacity.

Procedure

Sampling of the reagents into the gasometer is done by advancing the mercury so that a bubble protrudes from the end of the capillary tip, dipping the capillary tip into the sample to be taken up, retreating with the plunger until the required amount has been sampled, and then following the sample with mercury or caprylic alcohol without withdrawing from the solution. The procedure is necessary to exclude air.

First, 0.03 ml. of whole blood is drawn up followed by a mercury plug. Next 0.02 ml. caprylic alcohol, 0.03 ml. of ferricyanide reagent, and 0.02 ml. caprylic alcohol are drawn up in that order. Finally, 0.1 ml. saponin solution is taken into the instrument followed by mercury until the sample and all the reagents are drawn to the 0.12 mark beyond the stopcock, which is then closed. All reagents are drawn into the lower bulb by retreating with the plunger and mixed well. If any mercury has remained in the tube, it is removed by vigorous shaking with the shaking rod or by advancing and allowing the bubble of released gas to get above the mercury and retreating to permit the mercury to drop down. The plunger is retracted until the mixture is below the 3 ml. mark and allowed to remain there for three minutes, with occasional shaking. To be certain that all O_2 has been released, a reading is taken on the manometer when the caprylic alcohol meniscus is at the 0.12 ml. mark. The mercury is lowered again and then brought back to check the reading. When two consecutive readings check, the O_2 liberation is complete.

The screw is advanced to release the pressure. The stopcock is opened and 0.03 ml. of 1N KOH is introduced followed by mercury to bring all the KOH beyond the stopcock, which is then closed. The plunger is retracted to the 3 ml. mark, the mixture shaken, and the caprylic alcohol meniscus brought back to the 0.12 ml. mark. The pressure on the manometer (P_1) is read.

The pressure is released and 0.03 ml. of hydrosulfite reagent is introduced, followed to the 0.12 ml. mark with mercury, and the stopcock closed. The reaction chamber is evacuated to the 3 ml. mark and the caprylic alcohol meniscus brought back to the 0.12 ml. mark. The pressure (P_2) is read. At this point the precipitated methemoglobin (brown) should turn to the red of hemoglobin. If this is not the case the hydrosulfite reagent is at fault. The analysis is not lost since 0.03 ml. of freshly prepared hydrosulfite may be added and the reading (P_2) taken.

Calculations

$$(P_1 - P_2) \times \text{factor (Table 4)} = O_2 \text{ in vols./100 ml.}$$

$$O_2 \text{ in vols./100 ml.} \times 0.446 = O_2 \text{ in mM/l.}$$

Estimation of Carbon Monoxide Saturation of Blood

Preparation of the Sample

The sample is collected as for oxygen capacity and placed in the silicone-lined test tube. A stream of CO (HOOD) is passed through the blood by means of a tube drawn to a fine tip. The CO is generated by dropping conc. H_2SO_4 on formic acid contained in a suction flask, by means of a dropping funnel and a one-holed rubber stopper. The gas is passed through a tube containing soda lime and then calcium chloride (anhyd.) to remove acids and water.

Reagents

The reagents are the same as for O_2 estimation with the following additional ones.

Cuprous Chloride-Ammonia Reagent: 15 grams of cuprous chloride is added to 25 Gm. of ammonium chloride and made to 100 ml. with water. 30 cm. of fine copper wire, which has been cleaned with sandpaper and thoroughly rinsed in distilled water, is added. The copper wire is used in short lengths. Excess copper wire must always be present. The mixture is covered with a layer of mineral oil. The solution is allowed to stand overnight, or warmed to 60° until the solution becomes colorless. Some excess cuprous chloride will remain at the bottom. Transfer some of the supernatant to a vial containing mercury and mineral oil and deaerate by suction. The original solution is stable indefinitely.

Ammonium Hydroxide Buffer: To 25 Gm. of ammonium chloride add 100 ml. of water and 50 ml. of concentrated ammonium hydroxide. Transfer some to a vial containing mercury.

Air-free Water: Add water to a bottle containing mercury and mineral oil and deaerate as above. This is used for washing and approximately 100 ml. of such water should be kept on hand.

Procedure

For CO estimation the cuprous chloride solution may not be mixed with the other reagents used for removal of O_2 and CO_2. For this reason, a two-way stopcock is needed. Figure 2 shows the reaction chamber used. The bottom two-way stopcock is not required for this determination. This was left open so that it led into the chamber below the stopcock.

The procedure for O_2 determination is followed exactly as described. However, the time required for complete release of CO is much longer than that for O_2. Thus, after addition of the ferricyanide, five minutes must be allowed for liberation of all the gases. After the oxygen has been removed, 0.1 ml. of caprylic alcohol is introduced into the instrument followed by mercury. The residual gases (CO, N, and the rare gases) are pushed up to the capillary tube on the right by turning the stopcock 180° and advancing the plunger until the gas bubble is pushed above the stopcock with a little caprylic alcohol acting as the seal. The pipet at the right contains mercury so that the gas is trapped between caprylic alcohol and mercury. The stopcock is turned to its original position and all the reagents are expelled. The machine is rinsed twice with air-free water and the mercury pushed to the tip of the pipet.

The bubble of gas is now returned to the instrument by rotating the stopcock and drawing the bubble followed by a little mercury into the instrument and again returning the stopcock to its original position. Then 0.1 ml. of ammonia buffer followed by 0.1 ml. of water is drawn into the gasometer, followed by mercury until the reagents are beyond the stopcock. The stopcock is closed and evacuation made to the 3 ml. mark. Shake for one minute, bring to the 0.12 ml. mark, and read (P_3). The pressure is released by advancing the mercury. The stopcock is opened and 0.03 ml. of the cuprous chloride reagent followed by mercury is entered. The stopcock is closed, evacuation made to the 3 ml. mark, and then returned to the 0.12 mark after 1 minute shaking. The pressure (P_4) is read. The blank is determined by rinsing the instrument with water and then adding 0.1 ml. of ammonia buffer followed by 0.1 ml. of water and the mercury until the reagents are beyond the stopcock and the pressure read. Finally, 0.03 ml. of the cuprous chloride reagent is added as in the determination, and the second pressure read. The difference between the two readings is the blank to be used in the calculations.

Calculations

$$(P_3 - P_4 - \text{blank}) \times \text{factor (Table 4)} = \text{CO in vols./100 ml.}$$

$$\text{CO in vols./100 ml.} \times 0.446 = \text{CO in mM/l.}$$

Estimation of Iron in Whole Blood and Serum

Reagents

Iron Standard: 0.5 mg./ml. Add 100 ml. of distilled water to 3.51 Gm. reagent grade ferrous ammonium sulfate ($(NH_4)_2SO_4 \cdot FeSO_4 \cdot 6H_2O$). Add 10 ml. saturated potassium persulfate and dilute to 1 L. Stable at room temperature.

Saturated Potassium Persulfate: 8 Gm./100 ml. Stable at room temperature.

Sodium Thiocyanate (25%): Dissolve 25 Gm. NaSCN in a minimum of distil ed water. Add 2 ml. acetone and dilute to 100 ml. Store in refrigerator.

Perchloric Acid (70%): This analytical reagent contains 0.5–2.0 μg. Fe/ml.

Procedure

Iron in Whole Blood: 0.02 ml. of oxalated blood, or blood freshly drawn, is washed into 0.2 ml. of dist. H_2O. Use a constriction pipet (7) or an Accupipet[1] and a 13 × 100 mm. Pyrex culture tube which has been marked at 4 ml. Add 0.2 ml. conc. H_2SO_4 and 0.2 ml. 70% $HClO_4$.

[1] American Hospital Supply Corp., Evanston, Ill.

Digestion is carried out on a medium heated hot plate with tubes set at approximately a 15° angle to avoid bumping. The tubes are heated until clear. After cooling, approximately 1 ml. of H_2O and 0.2 ml. of saturated $K_2S_2O_8$ are added. After 1 minute, 0.4 ml. NaSCN solution is added and the mixture diluted to the 4 ml. mark with dist. H_2O. The reagent blank is similarly prepared.

For the standard, 0.02 ml. of the iron standard (10 μg.) is pipetted *from the same pipet* used for the blood. This cancels any pipet calibration error. If reaction is cloudy after cooling, it is due to incomplete digestion and is caused by precipitation of $KClO_4$.

The Klett-Summerson colorimeter with the #52 filter or the Coleman spectrophotometer (470 mμ) have been used for the readings.

Calculations:

$$\frac{\text{Reading of the unknown}}{\text{Reading of the standard}} \times 50 = \text{Fe mg./100 ml.}$$

Iron in Serum or Plasma: 0.5 ml. clear unhemolyzed serum or plasma is mixed with 0.5 ml. conc. H_2SO_4 and 0.5 ml. $HClO_4$ (70%) in a Pyrex tube (16 × 125). Digest on a medium heated hot plate until clear. 5 ml. H_2O and then 1 ml. NaSCN reagent are added and the solution mixed. 3 ml. colorless amyl alcohol is then added, mixing vigorously by hand for 30 seconds. After centrifugation the supernatant amyl alcohol layer is read in a colorimeter (#52 filter for Klett-Summerson, 495 mμ Coleman spectrophotometer).

The working standard is prepared by diluting the stock standard (500 μg./ml.) 1:250. 0.5 ml. (1 μg.) of the working standard is used. Distilled water in place of serum or plasma is used for the reagent blank.

The same procedure can be used for smaller samples. For 0.05 ml. serum aliquots using the Coleman spectrophotometer, Model 14, 3 ml. cuvettes with 5 cm. light path is used. 0.2 ml. aliquots can be assayed with the Klett-Summerson colorimeter using 2 ml., 4 cm. light path cuvettes. For these reduced amounts of sample, all reagents are reduced proportionally, except the amyl alcohol. 3.5 ml. is used with the Coleman cuvette and 2.5 ml. with the Klett-Summerson. The standard and reagent blank are also reduced accordingly.

In this determination the reagents used contain a significant amount of iron, making the reagent blank an important determination. To determine the amount of iron in the reagents read the color developed in the blank against colorless amyl alcohol. All reagents should be accurately measured.

Calculation:

$$\frac{\text{Optical Density of unknown}}{\text{Optical Density of standard}} \times 200 = \text{Fe } \mu\text{g./100 ml.}$$

This formula is the same for all quantities of serum or plasma.

RESULTS

The validity of the oxygen procedure was checked by comparing the results obtained for the O_2 capacity of the blood of 32 normal individuals with that of the iron content of the same blood. It has been established that the Fe to O_2 holding capacity of hemoglobin is 1 Fe to 1 O_2 (15) or 1:1 when both are expressed in mM/l. of blood.

In our experiments on normal adults we observed a range of 100–160 μg. of Fe/100 ml. of serum, which is in agreement with the reported values for plasma Fe (16). Since the whole blood Fe content is of the order of 55,000 μg./100 ml. it is apparent that the plasma Fe interference in the normal individual is outside the range of experimental error.

The values in the column for hemoglobin (Table 1) were obtained by the conventional colorimetric measurement (17). In this procedure the cells are hemolyzed in alkaline solution and the density of the color read. Cell debris, chromophoric substances other than hemoglobin present in blood such as bilirubin (particularly in the newborn), carotene, and lipids all serve to influence the reading. Further, an absolute standard is difficult to prepare in view of the instability of oxyhemoglobin (18). One usually prepares a standard curve based on iron or oxygen determinations. The standard curve used was the one supplied with the hemoglobinometer, as an outside reference. On the basis of the data in the O_2

Table 1. Mean Values for Blood Constituents for Apparently Healthy Adults and Newborns

Subject	*Cases*	*Fe*[a] (mM/l.)	*Av. dev.* (±)	*O_2*[b] (mM/l.)	*Av. dev.* (±)	*Hemoglobin* (Gm./100 ml.)	*Av. dev.* (±)	*Hemoglobin*[c] *(Fe equiv.)* (mM/l.)	*Hematocrit value* (%)	*Av. dev.* (±)
Adult males	8	9.51	0.45	9.56	0.52	15.36	0.62	9.35	48.7	3.3
Adult females	8	8.28	0.18	8.17	0.53	13.10	1.04	7.98	41.8	3.3
Newborn males	8	10.01	0.78	9.97	1.07	16.01	2.49	9.75	54.4	6.6
Newborn females	8	9.49	0.74	9.67	0.63	15.89	1.10	9.68	50.4	4.8

[a] Fe, mM/l. × 5.585 = Fe, mg./100 ml.
[b] O_2, mM/l. × 2.24 = O_2, vol/100 ml.
[c] Hemoglobin value × 0.0609.

or Fe column this curve yields significantly lower values. The column showing the average deviation indicates a much broader range of values from individual to individual, than observed in the O_2 or Fe column. We believe this to be due to variations of these artifacts from individual to individual.

The hematocrit values (percentage red cells by volume) were estimated by a method previously described. They are only qualitatively related to the hemoglobin content in that the size and number of cells is not directly proportional to the hemoglobin content. The hemoglobin and hematocrit values both indicate roughly that the values obtained for O_2 are in the correct range. For convenience of comparison the hemoglobin values have been converted to "iron equivalent" by using the value 0.340 as the percentage of iron in hemoglobin (19).

Table 1 shows the results obtained in this study. These are divided into groups for adult males and females and newborn males and females. Wherever duplicate values for a particular determination differed by more than 3 per cent, the results were discarded except for O_2 capacity when a difference of 5 per cent in duplicates was accepted.

The columns for average deviation for each column are a measure of the variation from individual to individual. These columns are of interest in indicating the range of values to be expected in the particular group of individuals studied. To determine whether the O_2 method is valid it is necessary to demonstrate that, within the range of experimental error, the values obtained by the O_2 method are the same as those obtained by the iron method. The t test was therefore applied using the simplified procedure described by Varnum (20). The mean value for the Fe column, 32 cases, is 9.323. For O_2 it is 9.343. The variance (σ^2) for the Fe column is 0.3468 and the variance for the O_2 column is 3.3267, the sum of the variances being 3.674. Applying this to the chart of Varnum one obtains a necessary mean difference (D) of 0.023 to be exceeded for a significant difference of the means at the 5 per cent level. The actual difference of the means is 0.020.

While one would be justified in saying that the difference between the two columns is not convincing one cannot say that they are essentially identical. There is a suggestion that the oxygen values tend to be high. This may be due in part to oxygen dissolved in the plasma. Calculating the percentage difference between the Fe and O_2 values obtained for each of the 32 cases and averaging the percentage difference, one obtains a mean difference of 1.2 per cent with a standard deviation of ± 0.33. This seems to indicate more clearly that within the range of the experimental error of the methods the values for O_2 and Fe are in agreement.

Table 2. Values for Blood Constituents in Three Anoxic Premature Infants and One Case of Sickle Cell Anemia

Case	*Diagnosis*	*Fe* (mM/l.)	O_2 (mM/l.)	*Hemoglobin* (Gm./100 ml.)	*Hematocrit value* (%)
1	Prematurity (anoxic)	8.33	8.66	12.9	45
2	Prematurity (anoxic)[a]	8.42	8.62	12.3	42
3	Prematurity (anoxic)	8.52	8.63	12.9	48
4	Sickle cell anemia	5.70	6.12	8.6	23

[a] Expired at 48 hours of age, lungs poorly expanded.

Table 2 lists the values obtained on the blood of 3 premature infants selected because they exhibited periods of cyanosis. The hematocrit values are lower than those usually observed, probably because these infants were receiving fluids parenterally. A case of untreated (not transfused) sickle cell anemia is included in the table. These cases are of interest in that the premature is claimed to have large amounts of fetal hemoglobin (5) and that certain types of anemias are characterized

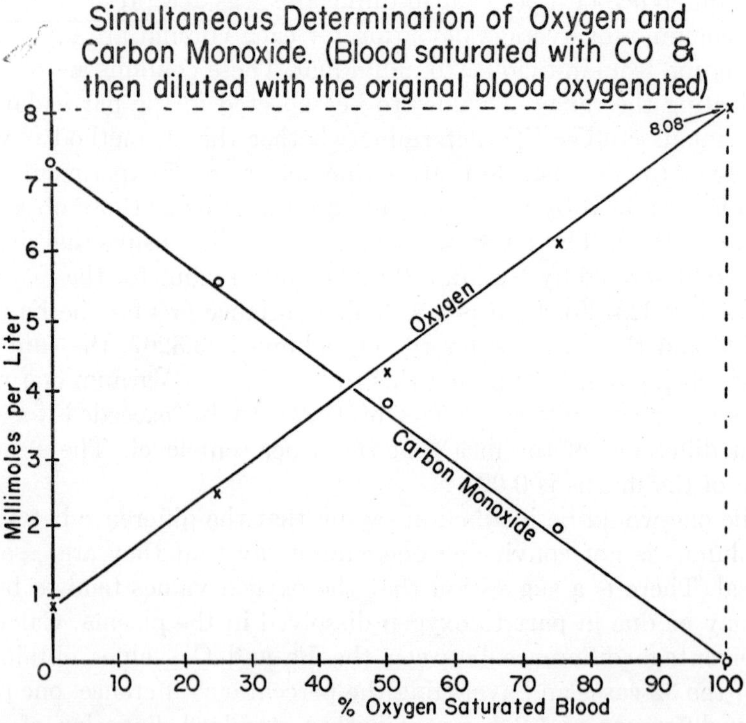

Fig. 4. Determination of oxygen and carbon monoxide content on the same sample with the microgasometer.

Table 3. COMPARISON OF PERCENTAGE OXYGEN SATURATION OF FINGERTIP AND ARTERIAL BLOOD

	Fingertip blood[a]	*Arterial blood*
O_2 Content (vol.%)	16.7	17.8
O_2 Capacity (vol.%)	20.1	20.3
O_2 saturation (%)	83	88

[a] Patient six years after operation for tetralogy of Fallot.

by the presence of a "fetal type" hemoglobin (21, 22). The O_2 capacity obtained is somewhat high for the amount of Fe found in the blood. Fetal hemoglobin has been crystallized and characterized as differing from hemoglobin of the normal adult (5). While this may be related to the differences observed, one must also consider the possibility that the lower hematocrit values, especially in the case of sickle cell anemia, with the higher proportion of plasma, may have exaggerated the effect of the dissolved O_2. The number of cases, is not adequate for statistical interpretation. It can be said, however, that in these 4 cases the hemoglobin did not exhibit a lowered ability to hold O_2.

Figure 4 shows the results obtained on blood saturated with CO and then analyzed for O_2 and CO content simultaneously, as it was diluted with blood from the same individual saturated with O_2. The points shown are compared with theoretical lines drawn from the original and final composition. Each point represents an average of four determinations. The distance of the points from the theoretical lines drawn indicates the expectable error.

The question is often raised as to whether the percentage O_2 saturation of blood taken from the fingertip is a true measure of the percentage O_2 saturation of arterial blood. Actually the results were always lower

Table 4. FACTORS FOR CALCULATING OXYGEN OR CARBON MONOXIDE CONCENTRATION IN VOLUMES/100 ML.

Temp. (°C.)	*Factor*	*Temp.* (°C.)	*Factor*
18	0.494	27	0.478
19	0.492	28	0.476
20	0.490	29	0.475
21	0.488	30	0.473
22	0.486	31	0.472
23	0.485	32	0.470
24	0.483	33	0.468
25	0.481	34	0.467
26	0.480	35	0.465

in our series on fingertip blood but not by a consistent percentage when the arterial blood of the same individual was studied. A typical case is listed in Table 3. The lower values obtained from finger puncture are probably indicative of the fact that while fingertip blood is largely arterial blood, there is sufficient contamination from venous blood to render the results invalid for the accurate estimation of the percentage saturation of arterial blood. Air contamination is not the problem it would seem to be since the results obtained from fingertip blood were consistently lower than that obtained from arterial blood.

Fingertip blood percentage O_2 saturation values are useful, however, in following the course of certain individual conditions. For example, in premature infants, marked changes take place as the infant goes into or comes out of a condition of cyanosis. Because of the ease of obtaining fingertip blood practical use may be made of this procedure, if allowance is made for its limitations.

SUMMARY

Improved gasometric methods of analyses for oxygen and carbon monoxide in fingertip blood are described. The accuracy of the method for oxygen is evaluated by comparison with the iron concentration of the blood. The accuracy of the method for carbon monoxide is evaluated by analyzing samples of blood saturated with carbon monoxide serially diluted with the same blood saturated with oxygen.

Technics are described for obtaining the blood for analysis from fingertip puncture.

REFERENCES

1. Barcroft, H., Gibson, Q. H., and Harrison, D. C., *Methhaemoglobinemia in Haemoglobin*, New York, Interscience, p. 223 (1949).
2. Dunham, E. C., *Premature Infants*, Washington, D. C., Fed. Sec. Agency, Childrens Bureau Publication No. 325, pp. 33–52 (1948).
3. McCarthy, E. F., *J. Physiol.* **102,** 55 (1943).
4. Paul, W. D., Burnham, E., Schottelius, D., and Routh, J. I., *Fed. Proc.* **12,** 253 (1953).
5. Roughton, F. J. W., and Kendrew, J. D., *Haemoglobin*, New York, Interscience, pp. 261–287 (1949).
6. Taussig, H. B., *Pediatrics* **1,** 307 (1943).
7. Natelson, S., *Am. J. Clin. Path.* **21,** 1153 (1951).
8. Natelson, S., Crawford, W. L., and Munsey, F. A., *Immature Infant*, Publication of Bureau of Maternal and Child Health, Ill. Dept. Pub. Health and Rockford Bd. of Health (1952). Available free from: Medical Director, Endo Products, Richmond Hill 18, N. Y.
9. Roughton, F. J. W., and Scholander, P. F., *J. Biol. Chem.* **148,** 541 (1943).
10. Van Slyke, D. D., and Neill, J., *J. Biol. Chem.* **61,** 523 (1924).
11. Van Slyke, D. D., and Sendroy, J. Jr., *J. Biol. Chem.* **73,** 127 (1927).

12. Scholander, P. F., and Roughton, F. J. W., *J. Biol. Chem.* **148**, 551, (1943).
13. Van Slyke, D. D., and Stadie, W. C., *J. Biol. Chem.* **49**, 1 (1921).
14. Snell, F. D., and Snell, C. T., *Colorimetric Methods of Analysis*, New York, Van Nostrand, p. 307 (1949).
15. Michaelis, L., in *Annual Reviews of Biochem.*, Stanford Univ. Calif., Vol. XVI, p. 28 (1947).
16. Tompsett, S. L., and McAllister, R. A., *Analyst* **74**, 315 (1949).
17. Sheard, C. and Sanford, A. H., *J. Lab. Clin. Med.* **14**, 558 (1929).
18. Sunderman, F. W., MacTate, R. P., MacFadyen, D. A., Stevenson, G. F., and Copeland, B. F., *Am. J. Clin. Path.* **23**, 520 (1953).
19. Bernhardt, F. W., and Skeggs, L. J., *J. Biol. Chem.* **147**, 19 (1943).
20. Varnum, E. C., *Prod. Eng.* **24**, No. 2, 215 (1953).
21. Sansone, G., and Cusmano, F., *Boll. Soc. Ital. Biol. Sper.* **26**, 1343 (1950).
22. Sansone, G., and Cusmano, F., *Boll. Soc. Ital. Biol. Sper.* **26**, 1680 (1950).

Effect of Shaking on the Accuracy of Salt Fractionation Methods For Serum Albumin

Abraham Saifer and Michael C. Zymaris

A COMMONLY USED PROCEDURE proposed by Kingsley, (1), for separating the serum globulins from the soluble albumin fractions after salt fractionation, is shaking with ether and centrifugation. Among the salts most frequently used for the separation and determination of serum albumin are sodium sulfate (2), sodium sulfite (3), and mixtures of the two (4).

It has long been recognized that many protein solutions can be "denatured" by prolonged shaking at an air interface (5, 6) and this phenomenon is accelerated when such solutions are shaken in the presence of certain salts, such as sodium chloride or magnesium sulfate (6, 7, 8). Denaturation is defined for purposes of this discussion as the loss of solubility of albumin.

Several investigators (4, 9, 10) have stated that the shaking of albumin solutions in the presence of ether and of the salt used for the precipitation of the serum globulins (e.g., sodium sulfite) may lower the albumin values obtained. Wolfson *et al.* (9, 10) proposed the use of ether containing suitable surface-active agents (e.g., Span 20) for the centrifugal separation of globulins without alteration of the albumin values obtained. However, none of the above investigators have presented quantitative data on the conditions influencing serum albumin denaturation. It is the purpose of this paper to supply the experimental data required to eliminate this potential source of error for the accurate determination of serum albumin, α-globulins, and A/G ratios.

The results obtained by the salt fractionation technic described here,

---

Received for publication November 26, 1954.

From the Biochemistry Department, Division of Laboratories, Jewish Chronic Disease Hospital, Brooklyn, N. Y.

under conditions *least* favorable to albumin denaturation, compared closely with those determined electrophoretically for 42 different sera from both healthy subjects and patients.

EXPERIMENTAL

Reagents and Apparatus

1. Ether, reagent grade.
2. Ether-Span reagent. A mixture of 1 ml. of Span 20[1] with 99 ml. of ether is filtered through Whatman #1 filter paper and made up to the original volume with ether. It should be kept cold.
3. Sodium sulfite, 28%.
4. Biuret reagent (11).
5. Sodium sulfate, 23%. Store at 37°.
6. Sodium-sulfate–sodium-sulfite solution (4).
7. Albumin standard. A 25 per cent solution of human serum albumin[2] is diluted with 0.85% NaCl to give a concentration of about 5 per cent. The solution is then dialyzed overnight in a cellophane bag against running tap water. After dialysis, the solution is brought back to its original volume and enough NaCl is added to bring the salt concentration to 0.85 per cent. Total nitrogen and nonprotein nitrogen were determined by the Kjeldahl nitrogen method. The value obtained was used as the standard for all subsequent albumin determinations. The standard is preserved with a few crystals of thymol and remains stable for a 6-month period or longer if kept refrigerated.

Determination of Albumin with the Ether-Span Procedure

The chemical procedure described in this paper is essentially that used by Wolfson and Cohn (10) for the separation of human albumin using 26.9% sodium sulfite. The electrophoretic fractionation of human serum was performed with the portable Aminco electrophoresis apparatus using the technic previously described (12). The salt fractionation method is as follows:

Pipette 12.0 ml. of 28% sodium sulfite into a 15 mm. × 125 mm. o.d. test tube. Add 0.5 ml. of the standardized albumin solution (or serum) and mix the contents thoroughly by inversion. Then add 2 ml. of ether-Span reagent. Stopper the test tube and mix twenty times by gentle

[1] Atlas Powder Co., Wilmington, Del.
[2] Red Cross, Squibb & Son, N. Y.

inversion. (The tube is turned upside down and then back to its original position with stopper upright for *one* inversion.) Remove the stopper and centrifuge for 10 minutes at 2000 rpm. If the centrifugate is not perfectly clear, repeat the separation step with more ether-Span.

The precipitated globulins are packed at the ether–water interface in the form of a button. By carefully tilting the tube, the protein button disengages itself from the side of the tube permitting the withdrawal of a 5 ml. aliquot of the centrifugate. Biuret reagent (5 ml.) is then added to 5 ml. of the sample and the contents of the tube are mixed thoroughly by inversion.

After a 30 minute incubation period, the colors are read in a photoelectric colorimeter using a 540 mμ filter, adjusting the zero reading with a reagent blank which is carried through the procedure using 0.5 ml. of 0.85% NaCl in place of the albumin standard or serum.

A comparative study of the albumin values obtained with the electrophoretic and chemical methods for both normal and pathologic sera was performed and the results obtained are shown in Table 1.

Effect of Time of Shaking Using Tubes of Various Sizes

1. Wolfson-Cohn Procedure (10) with Pure Albumin

The procedure described above was carried out with 0.5 ml. aliquots of the standard albumin solution. The tests were run, in duplicate, in tubes of the following three sizes: 15 mm $\times$ 125 mm. o.d.; 16 mm. $\times$ 150 mm. o.d.; and 20 mm. $\times$ 150 mm. o.d. After all the components were introduced, the free air space in each tube is that shown in Fig. 1A. The tubes were shaken in one of two ways, either by gentle inversion, or by vigorous manual shaking for the indicated lengths of time. The effects on the albumin values are shown in Fig. 1A.

The exact procedure as described above was repeated using ether in place of ether-Span. The results obtained in these runs are given in Fig. 1B.

Table 1. Comparison of Albumin Results Obtained with Chemical and Electrophoretic Methods for Normal and Pathologic Sera

	Albumin (Gm./100 cc.)					
	Electrophoretic data			*Wolfson-Cohn procedure with ether-Span*		
	Mean	*S.D.*	*Range*	*Mean*	*S.D.*	*Range*
18 Normal sera	4.22	±0.36	3.68–4.92	4.10	±0.23	3.75–4.58
24 Pathologic sera	3.45	±0.66	1.50–4.39	3.47	±0.71	1.50–4.70

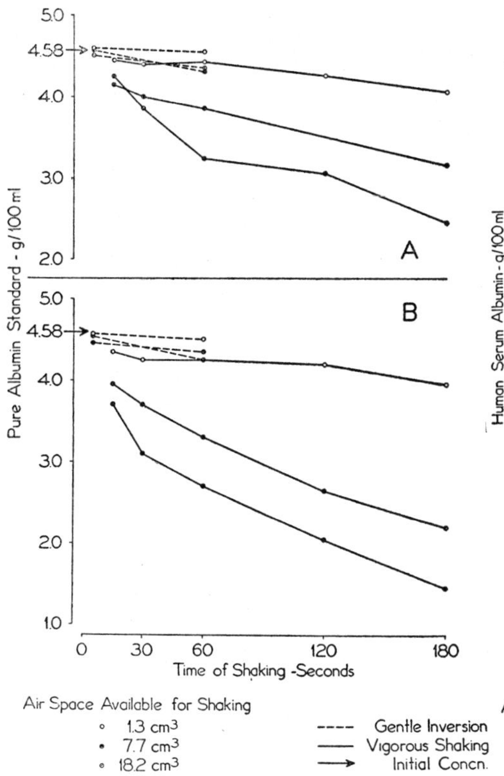

Fig. 1.

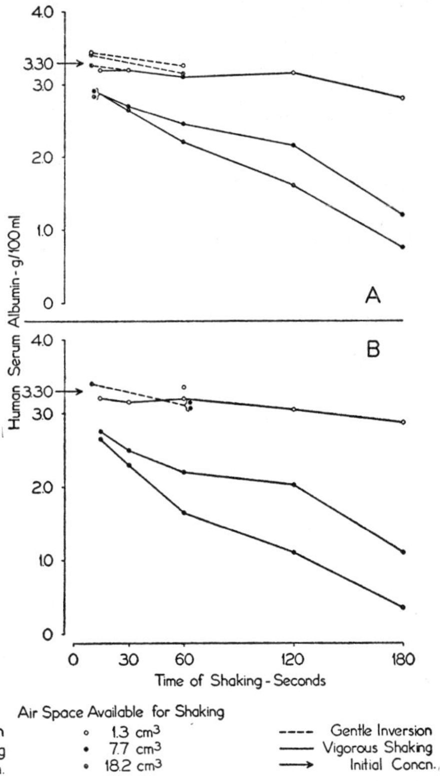

Fig. 2.

Fig. 1. *A*, Effect of shaking time on a 4.58% pure albumin standard in 26.8% Na_2SO_3 solution separated with the aid of ether-Span in tubes of various sizes. *B*, Effect of shaking time on a 4.58% pure albumin standard in 26.8% Na_2SO_3 solution separated with the aid of ether in tubes of various sizes.

Fig. 2. *A*, Effect of shaking time on a 3.30% human serum albumin (measured by electrophoresis) in 26.8% Na_2SO_3 solution separated with the aid of ether-Span in tubes of various sizes. *B*, Effect of shaking time on a 3.30% human serum albumin in 26.8% Na_2SO_3 solution separated with the aid of ether in tubes of various sizes.

2. Wolfson-Cohn Procedure with Serum Albumin

The procedures employing both ether and ether-Span were run as described in above, except that a pooled serum sample of known albumin content (as determined electrophoretically) was used in place of the albumin standard. The results are shown in Fig. 2.

3. Reinhold Procedure (4) with Serum Albumin

The albumin content of the same pooled serum samples was determined with the Reinhold procedure, except that tubes of different sizes were

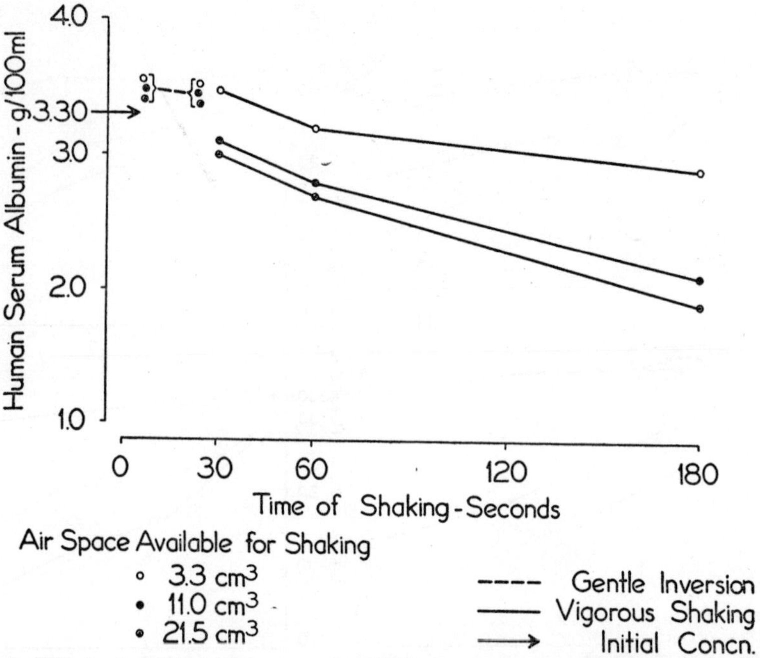

Fig. 3. Effect of shaking time on a 3.30% human serum albumin in 19.5% Na_2SO_4–6.6% Na_2SO_3 solution (4) separated with the aid of ether in tubes of various sizes.

used and the contents were shaken with ether for the length of time indicated in Fig. 3 instead of the 20 seconds recommended in the original procedure.

4. Pure Albumin, Serum Albumin, and Human Serum with 21.2% Na_2SO_4

The procedure used was the same as that described by Wolfson and Cohn (10) for the estimation of albumin plus α-globulins and human serum, except for the variation in shaking times and tube sizes noted in Figs. 4A and 4B.

RESULTS

Wu and Ling (6) showed experimentally in 1927 that the degree of denaturation obtained by shaking an egg albumin solution is markedly increased with time or with an increase in the size of the container. The magnitude of this effect for solutions of standardized pure human albumin in 26.8% sulfite is shown for the 3 minute shaking time in Fig. 1 where there is a decrease of about 44 per cent for ether-Span and about 67 per cent for pure ether below the initial albumin concentration. As is shown in Fig. 2, the magnitude of the denaturation effect for the albumin con-

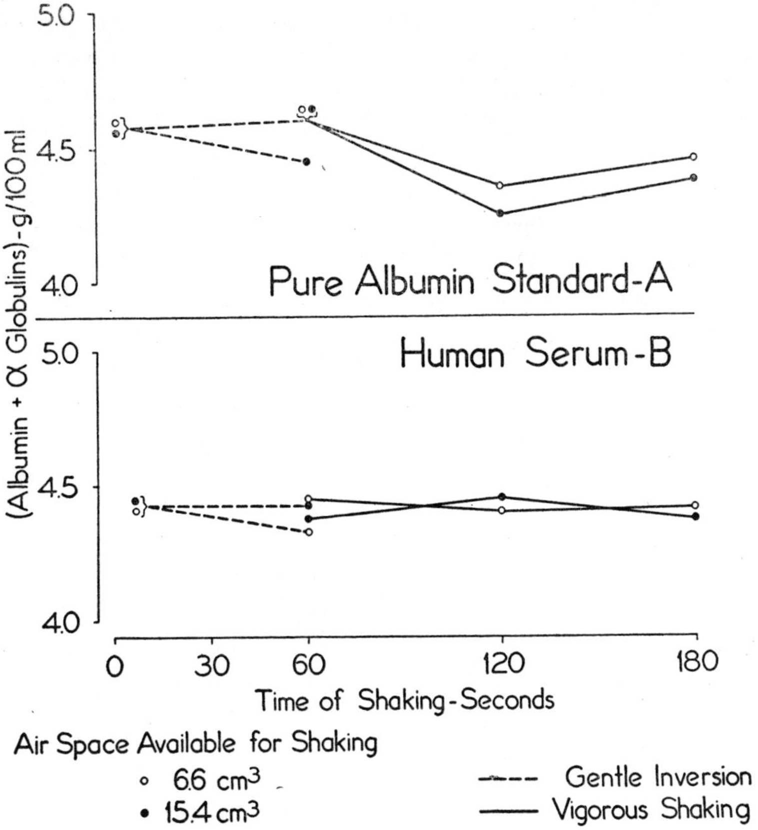

Fig. 4. *A*, Effect of shaking time on a 4.58% pure albumin standard in a 21.2% Na_2SO_4 solution separated with the aid of ether in tubes of various sizes. *B*, Effect of shaking time on human serum albumin plus alpha globulins in a 21.2% Na_2SO_4 solution separated with the aid of ether in tubes of various sizes.

tent of pooled human serum is even greater than that for the pure albumin solution—a 77 per cent decrease for ether-Span and a 88 per cent decrease for pure ether. The exact albumin concentration of the pooled serum sample was determined by electrophoretic analysis.

The data in both Figs. 1 and 2 indicate that the denaturation effect can be reduced both by decreasing the time of shaking and by using gentle inversion in place of vigorous shaking for any given size tube. The amount of denaturation can be further reduced to a relatively insignificant value by decreasing the space available for shaking to a minimum. In this latter case even a 3 minute period of vigorous shaking decreases the albumin concentration by less than 15 per cent. For the small tube, with a 1.3 cm.^{3} free air space, gentle inversion of less than 30 seconds will reduce the denaturation error to 2 per cent or less—within the experimental error of the biuret method itself. The main advantage of ether-Span over ether as a reagent for the rapid centrifugal separation of albumin from the precipitated globulins, is the enhanced ability of this reagent to effect this process with a minimum of shaking and not its small protective action against denaturation.

The data in Fig. 3 show that the albumin content of the pooled human serum sample, as determined with the sodium-sulfate–sodium-sulfite reagent of Reinhold (4), decreases about 44 per cent after shaking 3 minutes in the largest size tubes. Again, as in the case of the Wolfson-Cohn procedure (10), this decrease can be reduced to within the experimental error of the photometric method by employing small tubes with a free air space of 3.3 $cm.^3$ or less and by gentle shaking for less than 30 seconds.

The data in Fig. 4 indicate that albumin denaturation does not occur to any appreciable extent with ether shaking in the presence of 21.2 per cent sodium sulfate with either an increase in the time of shaking or with increase in the tube size. This holds true whether a pure albumin solution (as in Fig. 4A) or human serum albumin is used (as in Fig. 4B). This fact is of importance in the accurate determination of the total α-globulin content of serum with the Wolfson-Cohn procedure (10) as this is determined as a difference of two large numbers so that any slight error in the albumin procedure will introduce a significant error in the α-globulin values.

With proper precautions with respect to tube size, the use of ether-Span and with a minimum of gentle shaking, the values obtained with the Wolfson-Cohn procedure (10) give mean values for both normal and pathologic sera which check with the electrophoretic method. As can be seen from the data in Table 1, the two methods check with an average error of about 3 per cent for both normal and pathologic sera. The mean value obtained for 18 normal sera with the chemical method is 4.10 gm./100 cc. with a standard deviation of $\pm.23$. The mean value for the same 18 sera as determined electrophoretically is 4.22 gm./100 cc. ±0.36 S.D. Since the chemical albumin values were determined in duplicate on two separate aliquots of serum, the dispersion from the mean as measured by the standard deviation is somewhat less for this method than for the single-run electrophoretic procedure.

DISCUSSION

Excellent comprehensive review articles on the subject of protein denaturation have been published by Neurath *et al.* (13), by Anson (14, 15), and by Putnam (16). Protein denaturation has been defined (13, 16) as any nonhydrolytic change of the unique structure of native proteins, giving rise to definite changes in chemical, physical, or biologic properties, such as decreased solubility. Wu (17) proposed that the phenomenon be looked upon as a change from the unique and specific rigid structure of the native protein to the much more randomly arranged denaturated form. Anson (15), while stating that no rigid definition of denaturation is possible at present, suggests that the process involves the breaking of a considerable number of looser bonds within the molecule, i.e., hydrogen bonds, salt bonds, and van der Waals bonds, making the protein more like a simple peptide chain. While the term "denaturation" may be divided experimentally into three distinct steps—denaturation, flocculation, and coagulation—it has been employed loosely in this presentation to include all three stages resulting in the loss of albumin solubility.

Numerous studies have appeared in the literature with regard to protein denaturation by means of heat, concentrated acids and bases, alcohol, urea, guanidine salts, alkyl sulfates, x-rays, ultraviolet radiation, surface actions, etc. (13–17), but only those of Ramsden (5) and Wu and Ling (6) have dealt directly with protein denaturation during the shaking process. The latter investigators have made especially careful studies on the effects of surface active substances, salts and nonelectrolytes, *p*H, and temperature on the rate of coagulation during the shaking process. Their experimental findings show that shaking egg albumin solutions in the presence of ether *decreases* the amount of coagulation and that the presence of high concentration of sodium chloride or foaming of the protein solutions has little influence on the denaturation of albumin.

Denaturation by shaking results from "rolling up" the surface film and unlike heat denaturation cannot be separated into distinct stages. The effect of temperature on the rate of coagulation by shaking of human serum albumin has not been studied in the present investigation. However, Wu and Ling (6) have shown that for egg albumin the temperature coefficient for a 10° rise (25° to 35°) is only 1.09. Changes of this magnitude are seldom encountered in the laboratory and would be largely offset by their simultaneous effect on both standards and unknowns as well as the cooling effect due to increased ether evaporation at higher temperatures.

Our own experimental findings with respect to human serum albumin have confirmed, in general, those of Wu and Ling (6) for egg albumin. It was found that albumin denaturation was caused mainly by prolonged shaking in the presence of high concentrations of sodium sulfite, whereas ether alone had no effect, while solutions of sodium sulfate exerted a protective action as previously reported by Boyer, Ballou, and Luck (18).

While previous investigators (4, 9, 10) have given due attention to the time of shaking as a potential factor for albumin denaturation, little stress has been placed on the importance of the available air space as a cause of protein denaturation. When proper precautions are taken with respect to *tube size* as well as the technic of shaking, results are obtained for serum albumin with either the Wolfson-Cohn (10) or Reinhold (4) method which check closely with the more expensive and time-consuming electrophoretic method.

Accurate albumin values are not only important clinically in a wide variety of disease states (19) for both diagnostic and prognostic purposes, but are especially important where it is desired to determine accurately other protein fractions—such as α-globulins—by means of salt fractionation technics.

SUMMARY

1. The important factors causing albumin denaturation in the presence of sodium sulfite when shaking with ether or ether-Span, are the method and time of shaking, and the free air space available for shaking.

2. Gentle inversion with ether-Span for 30 seconds or less, and a free air space of about 1.3 cm.^{3} gave results with the Wolfson-Cohn procedure (10) which were in close agreement with the electrophoretic method in 42 normal and pathologic sera.

3. There is little or no albumin denaturation from shaking with ether in the presence of 21.2% sodium sulfate as used in the procedure of Wolfson-Cohn (10) for albumin plus α-globulins.

ACKNOWLEDGMENTS

The authors wish to acknowledge the aid of Dr. Bruno W. Volk, Director of Laboratories, who permitted part of the experimental work in this paper to be performed under Grant No. B-285 of the U. S. Public Health Service dealing with the general subject of "Protein Studies in Chronic Diseases." We also wish to thank Miss Renee Eisner for editing and typing the manuscript.

REFERENCES

1. Kingsley, R., *J. Biol. Chem.* **133,** 731 (1940).
2. Kingsley, R., *J. Lab. Clin. Med.* **27,** 840 (1942).
3. Campbell, W. R., and Hanna, M. L., *J. Biol. Chem.* **119,** 15 (1937).

4. Reinhold, J. G., *Standard Methods of Clinical Chemistry*, New York, Academic, 1953, vol. 1, p. 88.
5. Ramsden, W., *Proc. Roy. Soc. (London)*, *B*, **72**, 156 (1903).
6. Wu, H., and Ling, S. M., *Chinese J. Physiol.* **1**, 407 (1927).
7. Popják, G., and McCarthy, E. F., *Biochem. J.* **40**, 789 (1946).
8. Jager, B. V., Schwartz, T. B., Smith, E. L., Nickerson, M., and Brown, D. M., *J. Lab. Clin. Med.* **35**, 76 (1950).
9. Wolfson, W. Q., Cohn, C., Calvary, E., and Ichiba, F., *Am. J. Clin. Path.* **18**, 723 (1948).
10. Wolfson, W. Q., and Cohn, C., *Rapid Chemical Micromethods for the Analytic Fractionation of Serum Proteins*, Ann Arbor, Mich., Overbeck Co., 1951, p. 7.
11. Weichselbaum, T. E., *Am. J. Clin. Path.* **16**, 40 (1946).
12. Saifer, A., Rabiner, A. M., Oreskes, I., and Volk, B. W., *Am. J. Med. Sci.*, **225**, 287 (1953).
13. Neurath, H., Greenstein, J. P., Putnam, F. W., and Erikson, J. O., *Chem. Revs.* **34**, 157 (1944).
14. Anson, M. L., *Advances in Protein Chem.* **2**, 361 (1945).
15. Anson, M. L., "The Denaturation of Proteins." In *Les Proteines*, Institut International de Chimie Solvay., Bruxelles, R. Stoops, 1953, p. 201.
16. Putnam, F. W., *The Proteins: Chemistry, Biological Activity and Methods*. New York, Academic 1953, vol. 1, part B, p. 807.
17. Wu, H., *Chinese J. Physiol.* **5**, 321 (1931).
18. Boyer, P. D., Ballou, G. A., and Luck, J. M., *J. Biol. Chem.* **162**, 199 (1946).
19. Ardry, R., *Ann. biol. clin. (Paris)* **10**, 575 (1952).

Convenient Apparatus for the Continuous Dehydration of Histologic Material

Guy Nadeau and L. P. Joly

USUAL METHODS OF DEHYDRATING histologic material, such as repeated passages through weak to strong solutions of alcohol, are rather time consuming, and the time lost in the recovery of the solvent has compelled most laboratories instead to discard it after use. Such a practice can amount to enormous expense of material. Automatic devices reduce to a minimum the personnel and the time required for their operation, but they can hardly be afforded by small organizations.

The apparatus (Fig. 1) described in this paper was devised at the request of the Department of Pathology and is an example of how the special technics of a chemistry department may be used advantageously to solve problems of other laboratory sections.

The method and apparatus involve the continuous extraction of water from specimens by ethanol which, in turn, is dehydrated by distillation over quicklime. Soxhlet extractors cannot be used with advantage since in such apparatus the specimens are immersed in hot solvent and may be readily coagulated. This can be avoided, however, by having the solvent cooled before it reaches the samples.

COMPONENTS

The apparatus, which may be held to a single stand with the aid of extension clamps, consists mainly of the following parts:

1. One 2-liter, 3-necked, round-bottom flask. This flask is placed far enough from the base of the stand to allow easy dismantling and cleaning without having to move the rest of the assembly.
2. An ascending column of about 22 mm. O.D., insulated with asbestos

From the Faculty of Science, Laval University; and from the Hosps. du Saint-Sacrement and Saint-Michel-Archange, Quebec, Canada (G.N.).
Received for publication January 7, 1955.

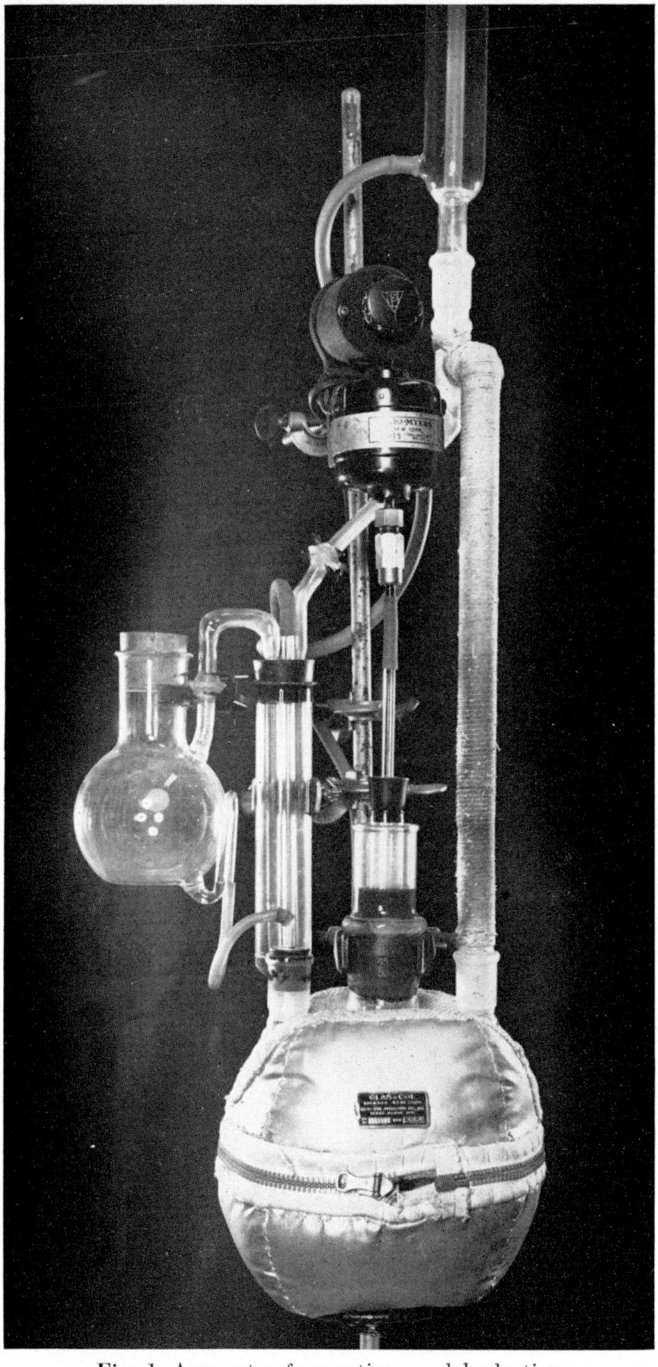

Fig. 1. Apparatus for continuous dehydration.

thread to reduce the loss of heat by radiation and increase the rate of distillation.

3. An efficient condenser for the ethanol vapors. The top inlet is protected against air moisture with a calcium chloride tube (not shown in illustrations).

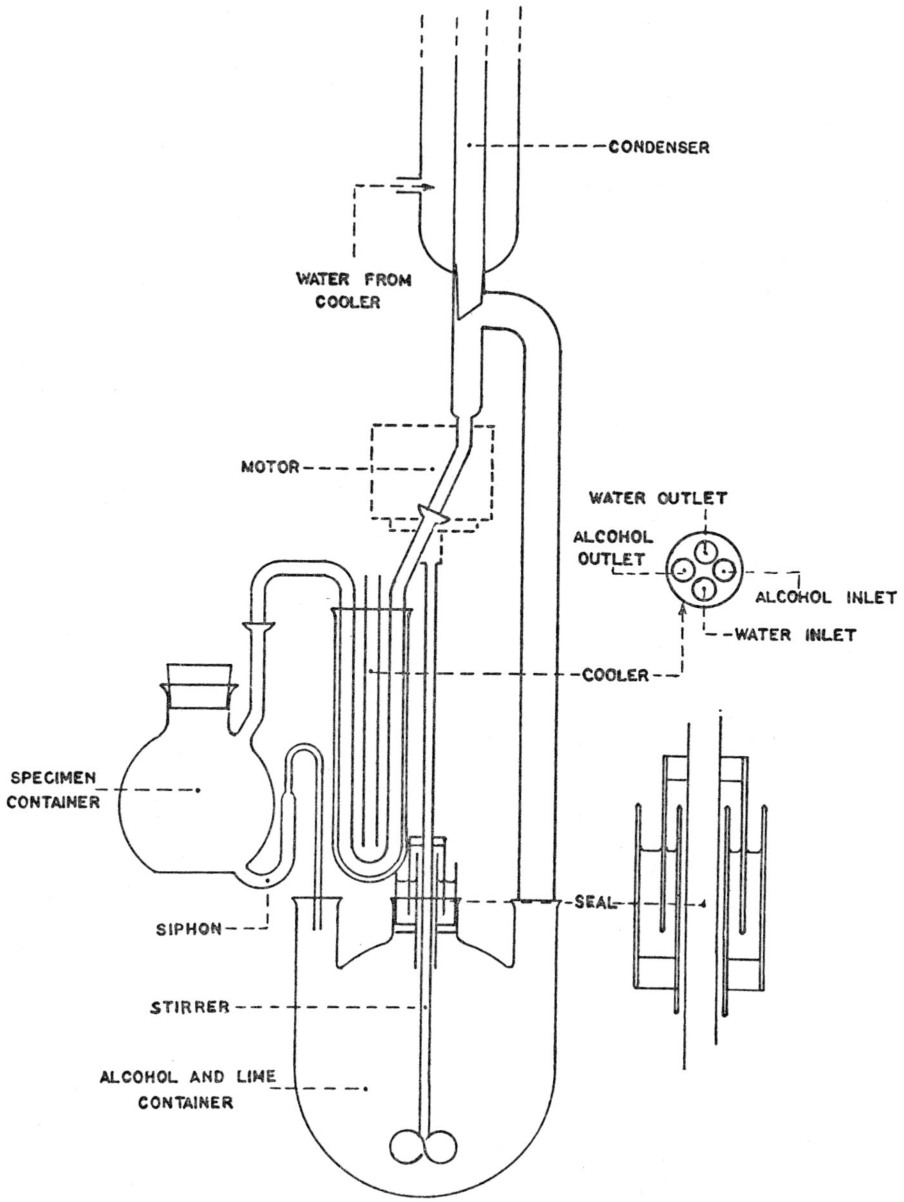

Fig. 2. Diagram of assembly and manner of operation.

4. A cooler built from a large test tube (about 35 mm. O.D.), a U-shaped tube for the solvent, an inlet and an outlet for the water, the former reaching the bottom of the device.
5. One 500-ml., wide-mouth specimen container, to which has been added a 12-mm. O.D. glass inlet and a 5-mm. O.D. glass outlet siphon. (The ratio of both diameters should be as described to avoid undue suction of the solvent from the cooler). It should be kept in mind that the height of the siphon will regulate the rate of renewal of solvent in the container.

Additional Features

An efficient stirrer is added to eliminate the bumping due to solid quicklime. It should be actioned by a variable speed motor. Glass seals may be obtained from various manufacturers or conveniently assembled (Fig. 2). Mercury was first used, but on account of unavoidable spattering and vapor formation, was advantageously replaced by a viscous, alcohol-insoluble polymer (equal parts of Indopol H-25 and H-100).

Distillation of the solvent is effected with an electric heating mantle (Glas-Col). A supporting ring is placed under the whole apparatus.

The use of ball-and-socket type joints (See Figs. 1 and 2) in the assembly reduces the hazards of breakage through torsion or vibration.

OPERATION

The 3-necked flask is lowered and 1.2–1.3 liters of ethanol are added, with about 50 gm. of quicklime (calcium oxide, lumps, technical) to insure smooth stirring.

To avoid bumping, the stirrer is started as soon as the heating mantle is plugged in. More power will be required at the beginning to stir the sludgy mass.

Small specimens may be individually wrapped in gauze for further identification. The interval of time allotted for each bath will depend upon the rate of distillation of alcohol and the height of the siphon (20 minutes in the apparatus described). It can be easily adjusted after a few trials. The time necessary for proper dehydration will be set by experience, but it has been found that a 2-hour period is quite sufficient for biopsy specimens of average size.

CLEANING

The lime has to be replaced from time to time, according to the rate of turnover of material. Most of the pure solvent may be recovered from the disconnected siphon in another container. The 3-necked flask is lowered and washed thoroughly with water (hydrochloric acid will dissolve any residue), followed by absolute ethanol.

COMMENT

This compact (12″ × 12″ × 25″ without condenser), inexpensive, and easily built device has now been in constant use for nearly a year without mechanical failure. It has reduced the time necessary for the dehydration of specimens to one fourth, and the expense of ethanol to one fifteenth, of the previous figures.

the Clinical Chemist

MEMORANDUM

SUBJECT: Recognition of Specialists in Other Fields

FROM: Dr. Edward L. Turner, Secretary
Council on Medical Education and Hospitals
American Medical Association
535 North Dearborn Street
Chicago 10, Illinois

DATE: June 18, 1954

At the December, 1953, meeting of the Board of Trustees of the American Medical Association, the Committee on Specialists in Other Fields indicated that it believed the subject of the relationship of American medicine to professional nonmedical groups in the health field was of such importance that a small *ad hoc* committee could not do justice to the problem. The Committee recommended that the Board of Trustees and the Council on Medical Education and Hospitals and its staff, in association with the appropriate councils and bureaus of the American Medical Association and relevant professional groups undertake a detailed investigation of all facets of the problem and that following the receipt by the Committee of a report from the Council on its findings and recommendations, the Committee on Specialists in Other Fields will submit its recommendations to the Board of Trustees. The Board concurred in this recommendation of the Committee and reported to the House of Delegates in December, 1953. Following adoption of the report by the House of Delegates, the Board of Trustees voted to request the Council on Medical Education and Hospitals to study this matter and to report back to the Board at the earliest opportunity as to a possible plan of procedure, the recommendation of the Committee including personnel needs, cost, and so on.

The Council on Medical Education and Hospitals has been making a careful analysis of the various facets of this problem and recognized the need for aid from allied professional organizations. An expression of

This memorandum is being published with the consent of Dr. Edward L. Turner.

opinion on the part of various medical organizations will be of great assistance to the Council in formulating the recommendation it should prepare for the Committee on Specialists in Other Fields. The following material has been prepared in order to present the general trends and to seek your counsel and advice.

The rapid increase in knowledge over the past three decades has led to the necessity for the development of many subgroups or specialty areas in what were formerly covered by larger general fields of interest in medicine. For example, in the field that was once just medicine we now recognize, besides the general internist, allergists, neurologists, psychiatrists, dermatologists, gastroenterologists, cardiologists, chest specialists and other experts. Similarly, in the surgical area there are now such specialties as thoracic surgery, urology, neurosurgery, plastic surgery, proctology, ophthalmology, otolaryngology, and orthopedics in addition to the general surgeon. Even in some of the narrower specialty areas such as radiology, we now see further subdivision such as has been brought about by the recognition of diagnostic roentgenology and therapeutic radiology.

In some of the specialty areas in other fields essential to adequate modern diagnosis, prevention, and therapy, similar increments of knowledge have been taking place which have necessitated varying degrees of specialization and widespread recognition of the need for such developments.

The area of microbiology may be utilized as a specific example of one of the fields that has seen great advances during recent years in its various disciplines such as (a) virology, (b) mycology, (c) bacteriology, (d) parasitology, and (e) immunochemistry. The rate of progress in this over-all field has been tremendous, and the field of microbiology in general is a very broad one, encompassing many other disciplines than medicine. Medical microbiology, on the other hand, has a unique place in the diagnosis, prevention, and therapy of disease, with all its areas of concern constantly assuming roles of ever-greater importance.

In order to qualify as a competent medical microbiologist it is necessary that an individual have the broad background and training of general microbiology essential to adequate understanding of this field. Since in order to obtain such training it is necessary that a potential medical microbiologist spend a long period of time working toward a degree that will give him authoritative recognition in his field, the question of the Ph.D. degree versus the M.D. degree assumes considerable significance and brings up the main reason for focusing attention on this problem at the moment.

An increasing number of specialty areas closely allied to medicine and requiring the equivalent of Ph.D. training are either seeking or have already sought some form of recognition or endorsement through the development of independent American boards or subspecialty boards in their fields. Suggestions have been made in regard to the establishment of a new American Board of Microbiology and an American Board of Medical Microbiology in recent years. In the course of these efforts, certain problems have been encountered in regard to the possible relationship of such boards with medicine. The problem now confronting us is whether a mutually satisfactory solution to this situation can be developed that might well serve as a pattern of possible future developments in specialty areas requiring a similar high standard of training for eligibility as a specialist.

Using the microbiologists as an example again, it should be pointed out that if a microbiologist devotes adequate time to his basic training in this field so that he can qualify as a specialist in medical microbiology, the time spent in completing the requirements for a Ph.D. degree is essentially the equivalent of that required in obtaining an M.D. degree. Although there are certain obvious advantages for a medical microbiologist to have a full M.D. background in addition to his Ph.D. training, the question may be raised as to whether in the area of diagnosis which he covers the former degree in itself is or is not essential to the task he must assume. Actually, much of the time spent in certain phases of preparatory work qualifying for the degree of M.D. would be essentially wasted time for the individual who specifically plans to be a medical microbiologist. The same problem confronts those who might be primarily concerned with areas such as biochemistry. In view of the increasing time demands for training in all areas today, there seems to be a very real need for recognition of the possibilities of conservation of time in preparation for activities in various special fields.

The biochemist, the psychologist, the biophysicist, the health educator, and others requiring Ph.D.-type training, and who are to become part of the over-all team approach to medicine today, fall into a category somewhat similar to that of the microbiologist, as has already been indicated.

It is of paramount importance that in the diagnosis and care of patients the physician constantly remain the pivotal figure and that these various areas of activity allied to medical diagnosis, prevention, and therapy be as closely coordinated with medicine as possible. If such coordination is to be effectively accomplished there must be mutual understanding of the obligations of the various individuals representing these allied specialty fields to each other and to the patient. Such close cooperation can best be obtained through recognition of the responsibilities lying in the various areas of activity and through setting standards of the type that will render the best possible over-all end results from the standpoint of the welfare of the patients. The question may be raised, therefore, as to whether in light of the contributions which these qualified specialists in the areas associated with medicine make today in prevention, diagnosis, and therapy in cooperation with practitioners of medicine, they should or should not have some form of recognition or endorsement through recognized specialty or subspecialty boards, if their training and experience so indicates and providing they possess either an M.D. or Ph.D. degree or both. It is fairly obvious from the current trend of events that some of these groups have been seriously endeavoring to obtain endorsement for the development of such specialty or subspecialty boards during recent years. At the present time it is apparent that some will proceed to develop their own organizations in the relatively near future, with or without the sanction of the medical profession. The question can be raised as to whether it is more desirable to have these organizations proceed entirely independently or whether there might be certain mutual advantages through having close liaison with such groups and with medicine in general.

Actually, the questions that are presented in this situation seem to be relatively simple, but are deserving of very serious consideration at this time when there are constantly increasing efforts being made to set up boards in these various fields related to medical activities. Among these questions are the following:

1. In view of the importance of these specialties in other areas in the prevention, diagnosis, and treatment of disease, do you believe that the medical profession has a responsibility in assisting in developing the standards to be maintained by them?
2. If the medical profession has a responsibility in this regard, how can it best be assumed?
3. Should the Council on Medical Education and Hospitals of

the American Medical Association and/or certain other interested groups endeavor to assist in the development of certifying boards or agencies which would establish and maintain standards mutually acceptable to the Council and the specialty group?

4. What in your opinion is the best form of cooperative or liaison relationship between the medical profession and these various specialized groups?

Your cooperation in giving consideration to this problem and in sharing your views with the Council on Medical Education and Hospitals will be of great value in helping arrive at a solution in the best interest of all concerned.

EDWARD L. TURNER, M.D.

COMMITTEE ON CLINICAL CHEMISTRY

The Committee on Clinical Chemistry of the American Chemical Society met at the Netherlands Plaza Hotel, Cincinnati, Ohio, on April 1 and 2, 1955. The main topics under discussion dealt with legislation as it pertains to clinical chemistry. John G. Reinhold, past president of the Association, was present as Chairman of the committee.

NEW EDITOR OF *STANDARD METHODS*

Dr. David Seligson, director of the Division of Biochemistry, The Graduate Hospital, University of Pennsylvania, was appointed editor-in-chief of *Standard Methods for Clinical Chemistry*, a laboratory manual sponsored by the Association and published by the Academic Press, New York. The first volume appeared in 1953, and Volume II is now in preparation. Dr. Seligson's appointment on March 15, 1955, is for a five-year period.

NEW SECTIONS

Greater Kansas City

The Executive Committee of the American Association of Clinical Chemists has approved a Greater Kansas City Section. The charter date for this section was February 16, 1955.

Texas

The Executive Committee of the American Association of Clinical Chemists has approved a Texas Section. Temporary officers appointed at the organizational meeting were: *President pro tem*, Major J. A. Rivera of Fort Sam Houston; *Secretary pro tem*, Dr. J. W. Goldzieher of San Antonio. The charter date for this section was April 8, 1955, and is the ninth local section to be established.

REPORTS FROM THE SECTIONS

Metropolitan New York

A. Saifer

A symposium on bone and calcium metabolism was held on Tuesday, April 26, 1955, at Blumenthal Auditorium of the Mount Sinai Hospital. Franklin C. McLean of the University of Chicago spoke on "Homeostatic Regulation of Calcium Ion Concentration in Blood." Daniel Laszlo, Montefiore Hospital, presented "New Tools for the Study of Mineral Metabolism in Man." Albert E. Sobel, Jewish Hospital of Brooklyn, was symposium chairman. A general discussion followed the formal presentations.

The following slate of officers was elected for the year 1955: *Chairman*, Julius Carr, The Mount Sinai Hospital; *Vice-Chairman*, Harry Goldenberg, Hillside Hospital; and *Secretary-Treasurer*, Abraham Saifer, Jewish Chronic Disease Hospital. Members of the *Executive Committee* are Charles L. Fox, Jr., I. J. Greenblatt, Alexander I. Greenstein, Bernard Klein, Mary H. McKenna, and Kurt G. Stern.

Washington-Baltimore-Richmond

Marian E. Webster

One of the largest exhibits devoted exclusively to medical research instruments in this country was held at the National Institutes of Health, Bethesda, Md., May 2–5, 1955, under the sponsorship of the manufacturers whose products were exhibited.

A symposium on "Recent Developments in Research Methods and Instrumentation," sponsored by the Washington-Baltimore-Richmond Section of the Association, the Washington Section of the American Chemical Society, the Instrument Society of America, and the Society of American Bacteriologists was held concurrently.

Topics scheduled for the symposium sessions included "Electrophoresis and Chromatography," "Fluorescence Determination," "Optical Methods in Biochemistry," "Selection of Electronic Components for Medical Research," and "Instrumentation for Cytochemical and Microbiological Research."

There was an interesting demonstration of new apparatus, with many of the exhibited instruments in actual operation. The exhibit, which has been an annual event for the past five years, attracted a wide representation of research workers and other personnel from medical installations, pharmaceutical houses, universities, and hospitals in various parts of the country, as well as visitors from the many research installations in the Washington area.

The third meeting of the 1954–55 year was held on March 3, 1955, at the National Institutes of Health. A symposium on recent advances in hematologic technics was presented by Lt. Col. Joseph H. Akeroyd, who discussed the development and recent advances in the Coomb's test; Dr. William H. Crosby, Jr., who commented on the difficulties encountered in the standardization of methods for clinical hemoglobinometry and suggested the use of the Drabkin technic; Naomi Benjamin, who discussed the methods, errors, and reason for determination of red cell indices; and Dr. William A. O'Brien, who reported on the various technics for the determination of blood volumes.

Code of Ethics of the American Association of Clinical Chemists, Inc.

Approved and Passed by the National Executive Committee, September, 1953

ARTICLE I: DEFINITIONS AND GENERAL CONSIDERATIONS

What Constitutes Clinical Chemistry

Section 1

Clinical chemistry is that branch of chemistry which deals with the composition of the secretions, excretions, concretions and fluids of the human body in health and disease, and the chemical composition and metabolism of cells and tissues. Also the search for the presence of substances (or their derivatives) given for diagnostic or therapeutic reasons and the search for poisons (or their derivatives) are properly included in the field of clinical chemistry.

What Constitutes a Clinical Chemist

Section 2

Any individual equipped by education and experience to engage in the practice of clinical chemistry as defined above shall be considered a clinical chemist.

Responsibility of the Clinical Chemist

Section 3

The profession of clinical chemistry, as an adjunct to the profession of medicine, has as its ultimate responsibility the welfare of the public. The clinical chemist shall use to the best of his ability his scientific skills and knowledge to the benefit of all men without regard for racial or religious origin.

Education and Experience

Section 4

The clinical chemist shall have as his goal the acquisition of the best available education and experience in chemistry. He shall strive to constantly enlarge and improve his knowledge.

Relationship to the Medical Profession

Section 5

The clinical chemist shall deal with the medical profession at all times at the highest professional level. The compensation by the patient for chemical services shall include no rebates or commissions to any persons for solicitation or referral of analyses.

Relationship to the Patient

Section 6

The clinical chemist shall perform no services to the patient except on advice or prescription from any licensed practitioner of the medical arts. All reports and discussion of chemical findings shall be only between the chemist and the physician in charge.

ARTICLE II: PUBLICATION, PATENTS, AND ADVERTISING

Dissemination of Scientific Information

Section 1

The clinical chemist shall freely discuss with his fellow chemists and with scientists in related fields, advances in the science of clinical chemistry. To withhold information for personal gain shall be considered unethical. This Section shall not apply to information classified by a government agency for reasons of national security.

Publication of Research Findings

Section 2

An obligation to publish, after critical evaluations, new knowledge pertaining to the science of clinical chemistry obtained through research or other observations, shall be acknowledged.

Advertising and Publicity

Section 3

The clinical chemist shall not use, or allow his name to be used, in advertising directed to the public. Professional announcements shall be brief, dignified and consistent with accepted customs in medical and allied fields. The clinical chemist shall not seek publicity, yet he shall recognize the right of the public to have access to information concerning the public health and welfare. Publication of a scientific article or book shall precede the release of such material to the lay press. Because of the danger of misinterpretation, he must use restraint and great caution in releasing information having diagnostic or therapeutic implications.

Patents and Commissions

Section 4

The application of discoveries and developments in clinical chemistry, directly effecting public health and welfare, should not be limited by unreasonable restrictions for personal gains to the clinical chemist.

ARTICLE III: OBLIGATIONS AS A CHEMIST

Accuracy of Chemical Analyses

Section 1

The clinical chemist shall have as his goal the attainment of the highest precision and specificity that existing procedures permit.

Reporting of Significant Figures

Section 2

The analyst shall not report figures or decimal places that lack significance.

Critical Survey of Methods

Section 3

It shall be considered inadequate practice for a clinical chemist to use any procedure that has not been adequately studied in his own laboratory.

Replicates and Recoveries

Section 4

The systematic use of controlled procedures, such as replicates and recoveries, shall be considered indispensable to good practice.

Results of Uncertain Magnitude

Section 5

The clinical chemist shall not report any result of uncertain magnitude of error, unless this uncertainty is clearly made known to the recipient of the report.

ARTICLE IV: INTERPRETATION OF RESULTS

Relationship to the Physician

Section 1

The clinical chemist shall, at the request of the physician in charge of the patient, outline to the physician the significance of any chemical findings, and suggest further determinations that would aid the physician in making a diagnosis or prognosis. The clinical chemist shall under no circumstance transmit to the patient either the results or the interpretation of the results. The clinical chemist shall receive no compensation from the patient for interpretation of results to the physician.

ARTICLE V: THE CLINICAL CHEMIST AS AN INDIVIDUAL

A Scientist at All Times

Section 1

The clinical chemist shall conduct himself as a scientist at all times.

High Regard for Medical Profession

Section 2

The clinical chemist shall hold in high esteem the profession of medicine, to which he is an adjunct.

Relationship with Analysts

Section 3

The clinical chemist shall carefully supervise the analysts working in his laboratory. He shall train these workers to the best of his ability, encourage them to attain the highest professional competence, and teach them by word and example to adhere to the ethical standards herein outlined.

Publications and Collaborators

Section 4

The clinical chemist shall contribute as much as possible to research and advancement of his specialty. He shall encourage those working in his laboratory to do likewise. He shall accept as collaborators whenever possible the junior members of his staff and encourage these members to contribute to the science of clinical chemistry. He shall to the best of his ability assist physicians and other scientists by fully collaborating in their efforts to advance medical science.

ARTICLE VI: CONCLUSION

The ethics of the clinical chemist shall at no time be inferior to the standards long prevailing in the medical profession. The outline here presented can act only as a general guide, and shall be periodically reviewed and revised. It is for the individual to judge his professional conduct in the light of his obligation as a scientist to serve mankind.

ABSTRACTS

Editor: Ellenmae Viergiver. *Contributors:* Joseph A. Annino, Gladys J. Downey, Clyde A. Dubbs, Alex Kaplan, Margaret M. Kaser, Miriam Reiner, Herbert Thompson

Determination of ethylenediaminetetraacetic acid (EDTA) as the chromium complex. P. J. Cherney, B. Crafts, H. H. Hagermoser, A. J. Boule, R. Harbin, and B. Zak. (*Wayne University, Detroit, Mich.*)

A simple, rapid and reliable determination of EDTA is presented which depends on measuring the light absorbence of its purple Cr^{III} complex. The high stability of this complex prevents interference from other ions, since Cr^{III} is in excess.

Two ml. of urine are pipetted into a cuvette. Two ml. of Na_2CrO_4 solution (5 Gm./l.) and 2 ml. of 0.2N H_3AsO_3 solution are added (9.89 Gm. H_3AsO_3 + 7 Gm. NaOH in 300 ml. of water, neutralize with glac. $HC_2H_3O_2$, + 400 ml. excess, and dilute 1:1). The solution is heated in a boiling water bath 5 minutes, cooled, and read at 560 mμ.

Considerable data on favorable recovery are given. The nature, formation, and stability of the EDTA-Cr^{III} complex are discussed. Complete spectrophotometric data are included.—*Anal. Chem.* **26,** 1806 (1954).

C. D.

Some errors in the determination of calcium in aged blood serum eliminated by flame photometry. P. S. Chen, Jr., and T. Y. Toribara (*University of Rochester School of Medicine and Dentistry, Rochester, N. Y.*)

The calcium of aged (cloudy or partially denatured) serum, unlike that of fresh serum, cannot be quantitatively precipitated by oxalate, except after preliminary deproteinization with CCl_3COOH. Errors involved in the determination of Ca as CaC_2O_4 can be eliminated by direct Ca determination using the flame photometer. Very brief data are given.—*Anal. Chem.* **26,** 1967 (1954).

C. D.

Direct ethylenediamine tetraacetate (EDTA) titration methods for magnesium and calcium. C. W. Gehrke, H. E. Affsprung, and Y. C. Lee. (*Missouri Agricultural Experimental Station, Columbia, Mo.*)

An EDTA direct titration method, eliminating phosphate interference, has been used for 2 years for routine Ca determination in plant materials, milk, urine, serum, rations, grains, and other biologic materials.

A 10 Gm. sample of plant material is dry ashed at 550°, digested 2–3 hours with HCl-HNO_3, and diluted to 250 ml. Phosphate is removed by passing a neutralized 25 ml. aliquot containing 10–15 mg. of Ca through a column (23 × 2 cm. diameter) containing a 9 cm. zone of anion exchange resin, Amberlite IR-4B, Cl form, at a rate of 2–3 ml. per minute. The Ca is titrated in the combined eluate and washings with EDTA, using murexide indicator.

Considerable data indicate good Ca recoveries despite wide variations in phosphate concentration, and good agreement with and better precision than parallel results using the oxalate-permanganate method. Experience is necessary to detect the elusive purple end point. Magnesium determination is given for limestone only.—*Anal. Chem.* **26,** 1944 (1954).

C. D.

Rapid estimation of free and total cholesterol. B. Zak, R. C. Dickenman, E. G. White, H. Burnett, and P. J. Cherney. (*Detroit Receiving Hospital and Detroit Memorial Hospital, Detroit, Mich.*)

Simple and rapid procedures for total and free cholesterol determination in 1 ml. of serum are described. One milliliter of serum is placed in a 25 ml. volumetric flask containing about 10 ml. of acetone-alcohol (1:1) with swirling, after which the contents are heated to boiling in a water bath. After cooling, acetone-alcohol is added to 25 ml. and the contents are filtered. For total cholesterol, 2.5 ml. of filtrate in a 30 ml. test tube is evaporated to dryness. The residue is dissolved in 3 ml. of glac. $HC_2H_3O_2$ with heat. Two milliliters of color reagent [1 ml. of stock (2.5 Gm. $FeCl_3 \cdot 6H_2O$ in 25 ml. of glac. $HC_2H_3O_2$, stored in the refrigerator) in 100 ml. of conc. H_2SO_4] is added and the contents are mixed thoroughly. After cooling, the color is measured at 560 mμ. For free cholesterol, 2.5 ml. of filtrate in a 15 ml. conical centrifuge tube is evaporated to 0.5 to 1.0 ml. and 1 ml. of 1% digitonin in 50% ethanol is added. After 10 minutes, the tube is centrifuged for 10 minutes at 3500 rpm. and the supernatant liquid is removed by decanting. The precipitate is washed with 4 ml. of acetone and centrifuged. The acetone is decanted and the tube drained by inversion for several minutes on absorbent paper. The precipitate is dissolved in 3 ml. of glac. $HC_2H_3O_2$ with heat, 2 ml. of color reagent is added, and the color intensity measured as for total cholesterol.

A standard curve is prepared by subjecting 0.1, 0.2, and 0.3 ml. aliquots of a cholesterol standard (1 mg./ml. in glac. $HC_2H_3O_2$) to the color reagent.

Recovery experiments are shown as well as simultaneous analyses by the Kingsley-Schaffert procedure for total cholesterol [*J. Biol. Chem.* **180,** 315 (1949)] and by a modified procedure involving the Liebermann-Burchard reaction. Recoveries and correlations with the procedures mentioned are good. The sensitivity of this procedure is given as approximately 5 times that of the Schoenheimer-Sperry.

The abstracter concurs with the authors' conclusion that the simplicity, speed, accuracy, and reproducibility of the method may well recommend it for routine use.—*Am. J. Clin. Pathol.* **24,** 1307 (1954).

H. E. T.

Effect of rest and activity on the serum protein fractions. T. P. Whitehead, A. P. Prior, and D. F. Barrowcliff (*South Warwickshire Hospital Group (14), Warwick, England*)

Total serum protein, albumin, alpha, beta, and gamma globulin, hemoglobin, and hematocrit were determined on 15 normal persons after several hours of rest and after a similar period of normal activity. After activity there is a significant and consistent rise in total serum protein, with a mean increase of 0.47 Gm. per 100 ml., due almost entirely to an increase in the albumin fraction. No significant changes in average globulin, hemoglobin, and hematocrit were observed.—*Am. J. Clin. Pathol.* **24,** 1265 (1954).

H. E. T.

Coagulation studies in abruptio placentae complicated by hypofibrinogenemia. T. J. Greewalt and D. C. Triantaphyllopoulos. (*Milwaukee Blood Center, Milwaukee, Wisc.*)

Low fibrinogen levels and hemorrhagic manifestations may occur in abruptio placentae, amniotic fluid embolism, or with prolonged intrauterine retention of a dead fetus. The escape of thromboplastin-rich material causing in vivo defibrinogenemia within the maternal circulation may be the pathogenesis common to all these syndromes, although activation of fibrinolytic systems has been a suggested mechanism [Weiner *et al., Am. J. Obst. & Gynec.* **66,** 475 (1953)]. Levels of fibrinogen and labile factor (Ac-globulin) and prothrombin consumption and thromboplastinogen activity time were determined on 4 patients with premature separation of the placenta. All patients had fibrinogenopenia with fibrinogen below 0.2 mg./100 ml., and prolonged prothrombin times by the one-stage method, which were shown to be due to a deficiency of labile factor. Studies of prothrombin consumption and thromboplastinogen activity offer some suggestion of the presence of platelet factor deficiency and perhaps low thromboplastinogen levels also.—*Am. J. Clin. Pathol.* **24,** 1246 (1954).

H. E. T.

Studies on the excretion of chloride by man with and without congestive heart failure, using long-life radiochloride, Cl^{36}. C. T. Ray, S. A. Threefoot, G. E. Burch. (*Tulane University School of Medicine, New Orleans, La.*)

Daily excretion patterns of Cl^{36} in urine and stool were studied for prolonged periods after a single intravenous administration of 50 μc. of the tracer. The concentrations of Cl^{36}, Na, and K were determined in serum, urine, and other body fluids. Stools were assayed for Cl^{36} only. The method of Schales and Schales was used for Cl determination. From the fact that subjects with congestive heart failure are not able to excrete administered NaCl as readily as control subjects and the noted observation of the relationship of the immediate excretion of Cl^{36} and body weight, it is suggested that electrolyte excretory function tests might be developed as indicators of cardiorenal function in congestive heart failure.—*J. Lab. Clin. Med.* **44,** 663 (1954).

G. J. D.

The estimation of Darstine 1-(3-hydroxy-5-methyl-4-phenylhexyl)-1-methylpiperidinium bromide and its tertiary analog, 5-methyl-4-phenyl-1-(1-piperidyl)-3-hexanol hydrochloride in plasma and urine. E. K. Tillson, S. F. Paulson, and K. H. Beyer. (*Merck & Co., Inc., West Point, Pa.*)

The method described depends on the fact that the drugs can be extracted into ethylene dichloride from an alkaline aqueous medium. The solvent layer is shaken with an aqueous solution of methyl orange and the colored salt formed at the interface, which is soluble in ethylene dichloride, is acidified and read colorimetrically. A method for differentiating the two drugs depends on the fact that chloroform extracts the tertiary compound but not Darstine from an aqueous solution.—*J. Lab. Clin. Med.* **44,** 880 (1954).

G. J. D.

A new method for analysis of plasma fibrinogen utilizing a cationic detergent. R. F. Jacox. (*University of Rochester School of Medicine, Rochester, N. Y.*)

A turbidimetric technic for analysis of fibrinogen utilizes the property of fibrinogen to react with a cationic detergent, octadecyl dimethyl benzyl ammonium chloride (Octab), at a low *p*H and a high NaCl concentration. Fibrinogen is precipitated from a 1 ml. sample with sat. $(NH_4)_2SO_4$ and redissolved to a volume of 5 ml. with 1% NaCl. To 0.1 ml. of this solution is added 8.9 ml. of phosphate-NaCl buffer (0.1M Na_2HPO_4: 0.1 M NaH_2PO_4 with 0.4M NaCl; *p*H 5.1) and 1 ml. of Octab, 1% aqueous. At 15 minutes optical density is read with a 440 mμ filter against standard human fibrinogen. The accuracy of the procedure is ±6 per cent. Values by this method are high compared with a clotting method of fibrinogen assay, due to the fact that lysed fibrin as well as unaltered fibrinogen reacts with the reagent.—*J. Lab. Clin. Med.* **44,** 885 (1954).

G. J. D.

Separation of the bile pigments of serum, bile and urine. P. G. Cole, G. H. Lathe, and B. H. Billing (*University of London, London, England*)

The pigments of serum and urine of jaundiced patients and of bile were isolated by a combination of extraction procedures and reverse phase chromatography.

The absorption curves of the isolated pigments before and after diazotization were obtained in the ultraviolet and visible range. The nonpolar bile pigment that predominates in the serum of patients with hemolytic jaundice was bilirubin. The serum of patients with obstructive jaundice contained two pigments that reacted "directly" in the van den Bergh test. The visible absorption curves of the azo compounds of these three pigments are indistinguishable.—*Biochem. J.* **57,** 514 (1954).

A. K.

Quantitative estimation of glucose by paper partition chromatography. S. Baar. (*Birmingham Accident Hospital, Birmingham, England*)

Paper chromatograms were prepared of solutions containiug 50–200 μg. of glucose, using a *n*-propanol-ethyl acetate-water system. The glucose was stained by drawing the dried chromatogram through a solution consisting of isopropanol, phthalic acid, and aniline. After drying, the stained areas were cut out, eluted with glac. $HC_2H_3O_2$, and the glucose estimated quantitatively by measuring the light absorption of the eluate at 480 mμ. The recovery of glucose varied from 97.0 to 102.0%.—*Biochem. J.* **58,** 175 (1954).

A. K.

A colorimetric estimation of sugars using benzidine. J. K. N. Jones and J. B. Pridham. (*The University, Bristol, England*)

A new colorimetric method for the determination of aldopentoses, aldohexoses' hexuronic acids, methylated sugars, and disaccharides is described. The sugar solution is heated at 100° for prescribed periods of time, depending upon the sugar, with a solution of benzidine in glac. $HC_2H_3O_2$. The resulting color is read at 425 mμ. From 20 to 600 μg. of aldopentoses and aldohexoses may be determined with an accuracy of ±3 per cent.—*Biochem. J.* **58,** 288 (1954).

A. K.

The determination of *N*-methyl-2-pyridone-5-carboxamide in human urine. J. M. Price. (*University of Wisconsin, Madison, Wisc.*)

N-methyl-2-pyridone-5-carboxamide (pyridone) appears in urine as a metabolite of nicotinamide. Interfering substances are removed by passing the urine through cation and anion exchange resins. The effluent is then analyzed directly for pyridone by measuring its ultraviolet absorbence in a spectrophotometer. Recoveries are within 95 to 100.1%. Of 16 closely allied substances tested, only *N*-methyl-2-pyridone-3-carboxamide was found to interfere.—*J. Biol. Chem.* **211,** 117 (1954).

J. S. A.

The quantitative determination of fructose with skatole and hydrochloric acid. B. M. Pogell. (*Brooke Army Medical Center, Fort Sam Houston, Texas*)

To equal volumes of sample and 0.04% skatole in a colorimeter tube are added 8 ml. of ice-cold 30% HCl. The tube is heated for exactly 40 minutes at 37° and the optical density of the purple color formed is read at 510 mμ against a water blank. The method follows Beer's law closely and has a precision of ±1%. —*J. Biol. Chem.* **211,** 143 (1954).

J. S. A.

Studies on uric acid and related compounds: 1. Quantitative determination of uric acid in biological fluids. F. Bergmann and S. Dikstein. (*Hebrew University Hadassah Medical School, Jerusalem, Israel*)

Uric acid may be determined in urine or plasma by deproteinization with $HClO_4$, precipitation of the uric acid with $Hg(C_2H_3O_2)_2$, redissolving the uric acid in an NaCl solution and measuring absorbency at 290 mμ. The method requires at least 2.5 ml. of plasma. It is specific even in the presence of xanthines and substituted uric acids.—*J. Biol. Chem.* **211,** 149 (1954).

J. S. A.

Formazan formation compared to phosphatase activity in human serum. A. L. Waldo, R. E. Zipf, and P. Burton. (*Miami Valley Hospital, Dayton, Ohio*)

Two milliliters of 2,3,5-triphenyl-2-H-tetrazolium chloride (Eastman) in phosphate buffer, *p*H 7.2, were incubated with 0.2 ml. of serum in the dark at 38° for 24 hours. The tubes were cooled in an ice bath, 8.0 ml. of acetone were added, and the tubes shaken. The formazan formed was determined by measuring the color intensity at 485 mμ with the Beckman Model B spectrophotometer. Alkaline and acid phosphatase activities were determined by the methods of Bodansky and Gutman. Similar values were obtained for patients with cirrhosis, Cushing's syndrome, renal rickets, hypo- and hyperparathyroidism, and neoplasms. The greatest color intensities were found in cancer of the prostate and osteogenic sarcoma. Further investigation disclosed a marked correlation between serum phosphatase activity and formazan formation.

The authors were unable to confirm the report of Straus *et al.* [*Science* **108,** 113 (1948)] and of Black *et al.* [*Am. J. Path.* **26,** 1097 (1949)] that malignant tissues stain more deeply with tetrazolium salts than do normal tissues.—*Proc. Soc. Exp. Biol. Med.* **87,** 19 (1954).

M. M. K.

Blood, urine and tissue amylase in depancreatized rats. J. H. Roe, Jr., B. W. Smith, and C. R. Treadwell. (*George Washington University School of Medicine, Washington, D. C.*)

Eight adult rats were depancreatized by a technic previously described [*Proc. Soc. Exper. Biol. & Med.* **86,** 878 (1954)]. Twenty-four-hour urine specimens and tail blood samples were collected at intervals up to 30 days after pancreatectomy. No differences in blood or urinary amylase levels as determined by the method of Smith and Roe [*J. Biol. Chem.* **179,** 53 (1949)] were found between the depancreatectomized rats and a comparable group of unoperated animals. Analyses of the various organs showed amylase to be present in similar amounts in all organs except the small intestine and the liver. The lower values for the intestine after operation can be explained by the absence of pancreatic secretions. The decrease in liver amylase may have been due to the development of fatty livers in the operated rats. The data suggest that some organ or organs other than the pancreas is the source of blood, urinary, and tissue amylase in normal rats.—*Proc. Soc. Exp. Biol. Med.* **87,** 79 (1954).

M. M. K.

Vitamin B_{12} serum levels and diabetic retinopathy. B. F. Chow, D. A. Rosen, and C. A. Lang. (*John Hopkins Hospital, Baltimore, Md.*)

Serum vitamin B_{12} was determined by the method of Okuda, Wood, Lang, and Chow [*Fed. Proc.* **13,** 1546 (1954)]. Previous work has shown that following the intramuscular administration of a test dose of vitamin B_{12}, diabetics with retinopathy excreted significantly more of the vitamin than nondiabetics, and diabetics without retinopathy excreted less than nondiabetics.

In the present study there were 18 diabetics without and 16 diabetics with retinopathy. The mean serum vitamin B_{12} level of the group without retinopathy was 162 ± 18 μμg. per ml., and for the retinopathic group 292 ± 24. With the exception of one subject in the non-retinopathic group the two groups could be separated by a dividing line at 200 μμg./ml. The difference between the two groups was statistically significant, with $p < 0.001$.

These data suggest that vitamin B_{12} is intimately involved not only in the metabolism of carbohydrate but also plays a fundamental role in the development of retinopathy.—*Proc. Soc. Exp. Biol. Med.* **87,** 38 (1954).

M. M. K.

Response of serum inorganic phosphate to insulin in normal and diabetic subjects. F. De Venanzi, M. Roche, and J. Vera. (*Instituto de Investigaciones Médicas, Fundación Luis Roche, Caracas, Venezuela*)

Twenty diabetic patients were divided into two groups on the basis of the response of serum phosphate to the intravenous administration of 1 ml. per kg. of body weight of 50% glucose. At 45 minutes Group I (12 subjects) had a phosphate fall of less than 0.30 mg. per 100 ml., and Group II had a decrease of more than 0.30 mg. per 100 ml. Insulin in a dosage of 0.1 unit per kg. of body weight was given intravenously to 42 normal young adults and to the diabetic subjects, all of whom were fasting and kept at rest for one half hour before and during the test. Venous blood samples collected before and 12, 30, 45 and 60 minutes after the injection of insulin were analyzed for glucose by the Nelson method and for serum inorganic phosphate by the procedure of Fiske and Subba-Row. The mean decreases in blood sugar of the normal subjects were 39 mg. per 100 ml. at 15 min., 43 at 30 min., 32 at 45 min., and 18 at 60 min. The corresponding decreases for all the diabetics were 24, 39, 53, and 53 mg. per 100 ml.

All the differences between the normal and diabetic subjects were statistically significant, and only the initial blood sugar levels of 196 and 154 mg. per 100 ml. for Group I and Group II, respectively, of the diabetic subjects differed significantly.

The mean fall in serum inorganic phosphorus in the normal subjects was 0.53 mg. per 100 ml. at 15 min., 0.95 at 30 min., 0.99 at 45 min., and 0.75 at 60 min. For the diabetics these values were 0.29, 0.39, 0.51, and 0.33 mg. per 100 ml. All the differences between the normal and diabetic subjects were significant, and there was no significant difference between the two groups of diabetics.

The data indicate an inhibition of the response of phosphate to insulin in diabetes and that diabetics who differ in their serum-phosphate fall after glucose may be alike in the response of phosphate to insulin. It is believed that the phosphate fall after glucose reflects, at least in part, the ability of the pancreas to secrete insulin and that experimental data thus far available do not permit relating it to "peripheral utilization" of carbohydrate.—*Proc. Soc. Exp. Biol. Med.* **87,** 16 (1954).

M. M. K.

Determination of melanocyte-stimulating hormone in urine and blood.
K. Shizume and A. B. Lerner. (*University of Oregon Medical School, Portland, Ore.*)

A procedure is described for the extraction of melanocyte-stimulating hormone (MSH) from urine and from blood. The concentration is assayed by determining the darkening of isolated frog skin with a reflection meter. Recovery studies showed that approximately 20 per cent of MSH is recovered from urine and approximately 60 per cent from blood.

The concentration of MSH in urine and blood is the same for normal males and females. The 24-hour urinary excretion values range from 7.5 to 47.5 units, with an average of 27.7 units. In blood the range is 0.4–2.2 units/ml., with an average value of 1.3 units. During pregnancy, MSH excretion becomes elevated at the end of the second month and continues to increase until term. Following delivery, there is a return to normal within a few days. Seven of 12 patients with Addison's disease and 4 out of 8 patients who had bilateral adrenalectomies excreted increased quantities of MSH. Some of these patients may have excreted normal amounts because they were receiving cortisone. The MSH excretion was elevated in 1 patient each with one the following conditions: new lentigines, alopecia areata totalis, and retinitis pigmentosa. Negroes, albinos, and patients with vitiligo showed normal MSH excretion values. Two of 8 patients with decreased pituitary function excreted decreased amounts of MSH. Administration of cortisone to a patient with high levels of MSH in blood and urine reduced the hormone concentration to normal. Following adrenalectomy the blood MSH level increased markedly in a dog and returned to normal when cortisone was administered.—*J. Clin. Endocrinol. & Metab.* **14,** 1491 (1954).

M. R.

Renal function and I^{131} clearance in hyperthyroidism and myxedema. C. J. Hlad and N. S. Bricker. (*Fitzsimons Army Hospital, Denver, Colo.*)

Renal function studies have been performed on 4 patients with hyperthyroidism, 5 with primary myxedema, and 2 with panhypopituitarism and probably secondary hypothyroidism. Glomerular filtration rate, renal plasma flow, and TmPAH (maximum capacity of the tubules to transport *p*-amino hippurate) values were elevated in the hyperthyroid group and depressed in the myxedematous group. Following therapy in 1 hyperthyroid patient, renal functions were reversed toward normal. Following long-term therapy in 1 myxedematous patient, the glomerular filtration rate increased despite a fall in renal plasma flow. Triiodothyronine administered intravenously to an untreated myxedematous patient for a period of 6 days induced a striking increase in renal glomerular filtration rate and renal plasma flow.

It has been concluded that the state of thyroid activity exerts a definite effect on renal hemodynamics and tubular function. The clearance of I^{131} in hyperthyroid and myxedematous patients has been found to be a linear function of the glomerular filtration. The state of thyroid activity seems to influence the renal excretion of iodide indirectly through a filtration-rate effect, but not at the tubular level.—*J. Clin. Endocrinol. & Metab.* **14,** 1539 (1954).

M. R.

The diagnostic use of I^{132}. E. M. Hanbury, J. Heslin, L. G. Stang, W. D. Tucker, and J. E. Rall. (*Sloan-Kettering Institute, New York, N. Y.*)

The application of I^{132}, with a half-life of 2.33 hours, to previously designed tracer technics is presented. Clinical data on 11 patients studied with I^{132} include 1-hour thyroidal uptake determinations and 30-minute thyroidal clearance rates. $Iodine^{132}$ would seem to find its chief merit in tracer experiments in which minimal radiation is desired and in experiments in which frequent measurements of iodine uptake is desired.—*J. Clin. Endocrinol. & Metab.* **14,** 1530 (1954).

M. R.

The mechanism of endocrine control of melanin pigmentation. A. B. Lerner, K. Shizume, and I. Bunding. (*University of Oregon Medical School, Portland, Ore.*)

The melanocyte-stimulating hormone (MSH) from the pituitary gland causes darkening of human skin and nevi and formation of new nevi. When large doses of MSH were given to 1 patient, increased pigmentation was observed within a few hours. When MSH was given intramuscularly, from 1 to 4 per cent was excreted in the urine. After intravenous administration approximately twice as much was excreted.

The action of other hormones is related to that of MSH. Hydrocortisone and cortisone probably inhibit the release of MSH from the pituitary gland. Noradrenaline and adrenaline can block the local action of MSH on melanocytes, the pigment cells. The first factor is of clinical significance because cortisone and hydrocortisone can prevent the development of hyperpigmentation in patients who have undergone bilateral adrenalectomy and in patients who have Addison's disease. It can also decrease pigment already present in Addison's disease. The action of adrenaline and noradrenaline, although potent in vitro, has not yet proved to be of clinical significance. In addition, progesterone, which causes darkening of frog melanocytes, may have an effect on human melanocytes. Melanocyte-stimulating hormone seems to be a distinct pituitary hormone. Pigmentation associated with the clinical administration of ACTH is probably due to MSH contamination.—*J. Clin. Endocrinol. & Metab.* **14,** 1463 (1954).

M. R.

Effect of caloric restriction on cholesterol atherogenesis in the rabbit. M. G. Goldner, L. Loewe, R. Lasses, and I. Stern. (*Jewish Hospital, Brooklyn, N. Y.*)

Adult male rabbits were fed a diet of commercial rabbit pellets supplemented with raw carrots. For Experiment A, 18 animals were given 1 Gm. of cholesterol daily; 9 of these received a ration of pellets approximately half the average daily consumption of the 9 controls, which were fed *ad libitum.* In Experiment B, 22 animals were used. The food consumption of the 11 in the experimental group was decreased to one third that of the 11 controls, and the dose of cholesterol was increased to 2 Gm. daily for both controls and experimental animals. The durations of the two experiments were 12 and 8 weeks, respectively.

At intervals the following analyses were done: total blood cholesterol by the method of Abell *et al.* [*J. Biol. Chem.* **195,** 357 (1952)]; blood fatty acids by the method of Stern and Shapiro [*Brit. J. Clin. Path.* **6,** 158 (1953)]; lipid phosphorus by the procedure of Youngburg and Youngburg [*J. Lab. and Clin. Med.* **16,** 158 (1930)]; and lipoproteins according to Gofman *et al.* [*Circulation* **2,** 161 (1950)]. The two experiments gave similar results, with the experimental animals showing a loss of weight and a much more marked elevation of the blood lipid fractions than the controls. Arteriosclerotic changes with advanced lesions were present in the aortas of both groups and appeared to be more pronounced in the underfed rabbits. It is concluded that severe caloric restriction does not offer protection, but rather enhances the development of cholesterol-induced atherosclerosis in rabbits.—*Proc. Soc. Exp. Biol. Med.* **87,** 105 (1954).

M.M.K.

BOOK REVIEWS

Practical Clinical Biochemistry

HAROLD VARLEY. New York, Interscience Publishers, Inc., 1954, 558 pp., $6.50.

The author describes in 28 chapters procedures for all analyses required from a clinical chemistry laboratory, including clinical microscopy and the determination of the basal metabolic rate (Chapters VII and XX). The text contains 70 graphs and illustrations, almost all of very instructive character, also numerous tables and structural formulas in a little more than 500 pages of text. By painstaking compilation, the author has achieved a comprehensive description of technics, which include most of the more modern methods. In addition to the more commonly performed procedures, a large number, not usually found in routine manuals, are included, such as inulin and thiosulfate clearance tests, paper electrophoresis of serum proteins, choline esterase, serum copper, and pyruvic acid. Several alternatives for the analysis of a substance are frequently presented with the author's indications as to their individual usefulness.

The arrangement of the chapters is logical rather than systematic, as some chapters deal with groups of chemical entities, such as "The Plasma Proteins," "Chlorides, Sodium and Potassium," "Vitamins," "Hormones," while others deal with disease or dysfunction, for example, "Chemical Tests in Kidney Disease" and "Tests in Liver and Biliary Tract Disease." The same lack of pedantry is apparent in the organization of the subtitles. The description of every method is regularly followed by a few paragraphs with the author's extremely sound *interpretations* of the results. Each chapter concludes with a judiciously selected bibliography.

The prothrombin method described in Chapter XIV yields normal values of around 30 seconds rather than the usual figure of about 14 seconds, possibly owing to the selection of human brain rather than rabbit or horse liver as source for the thromboplastin. The instruments described for exemplification of photoelectric colorimetry and flame photometry (Chapters I and XVIII) are of British make. Besides such differences due to regional usage there are several points where this writer disagrees with statements and evaluations and where he misses some recent accessions to the armamentarium of clinical chemistry. This is of course to be expected in such a rapidly developing discipline, and Varley's book is altogether a most useful volume. Its strongest features are undoubtedly its comprehensiveness and the clear, unambiguous style in which technics and calculations are described.

The book will form an excellent basis for instruction in laboratory courses in routine chemistry for technicians and medical students. It is more than the usual phrase of approval by a reviewer when we say that no clinical laboratory should be without it, although the text may be a little too much for junior technicians working without chemical direction, say, in a physician's office.

Mt. Sinai Hospital, N. Y. HARRY SOBOTKA

The Lipids: Their Chemistry and Biochemistry

Volume II.: Biochemistry (Digestion, Absorption, Transport and Storage)

HARRY J. DEUEL, JR. New York, Interscience Publishers, Inc., 1955, 919 pp., $25.00.

Dr. Deuel's work of the past eight years started out to encompass two volumes. Volume I, dealing with the chemistry of the lipids, is the most comprehensive work on the subject to date. Volume II, which was to include the biochemical data, had to be divided into two volumes as the past few years has seen a tremendous increase in investigations and published data in this fertile field of study. This first volume on the biochemistry of lipids discusses four topics, Digestion, Absorption, Transport, and Storage. The next volume will include Biosynthesis, Metabolism, Oxidation, and Nutritional Value.

Once again, as in the first volume, the author has done an excellent work in the organization of the subject. The chapter heads are broken down into a multitude of subheads and further divisions that bring the data into sharp focus for the reader. This interesting approach can be seen from the following example: Chapter II, *The Digestion and Absorption of Fats in the Gastrointestinal Tract*, is divided into 9 major heads. Heading 2, *Enzymes Concerned with the Digestion of Lipids*, has 3 subheads, Lipases, Esterases, and Other Lipid-hydrolyzing Enzymes. These subheads are further divided into the specific points of discussion so that there is a definite portion of the discussion devoted to a specific topic, as Cholinesterases in Blood, Cholinesterases in Brain and Nervous Tissue, etc. It is by strict adherence to this excellent outline of the subject that Dr. Deuel has provided a source book that does not scatter the subject and makes for ready rapid reference.

Under the author's presentation of blood lipids is found a most complete discussion of lipid alterations in disease and organ dysfunction. Animal experimentation studies as well as data from clinical medicine are presented. Parts of this discussion are carried further under another heading, Lipid Storage under Abnormal Conditions.

Lipid Distribution in Specific Tissues also discusses data from investigations concerned with animal material used as food, such as eggs and milk.

What has been said of Dr. Deuel's first volume can be repeated for Volume II. The book is well written. When one views the amount of material contained in its 919 pages, one realizes that the author has presented the subject matter without being verbose, yet has kept good continuity and reader interest. This work will greatly influence research in the field because in even casual reading one can feel the author's ability to indicate to the reader just which parts of the data need further investigation and just where there is a definite lack of data, so that knowledge of a particular topic is sparse.

This book will save the researcher a tremendous amount of library work as the bibliography is most complete. The volume also contains a rather complete author, as well as subject index. There also is a listing of plant and animal sources of lipids.

Metropolitan Hospital, N. Y. H. D. APPLETON

Seromucoid in Hepatobiliary Disease

Emanuel E. Mandel, Thomas L. Gorsuch, and Gerald E. Cooper

With the technical assistance of *Florence L. Jones*

An increase in circulating carbohydrate-rich proteins has been known for some time to occur in diseases associated with neoplastic or inflammatory processes. These substances have been variously termed polypeptides (1–4), proteoses (5), mucoid-like material (6), seromucoid (7–10), and mucoprotein (11–15). It was only recently that the occurrence of a pathologic depression of the seromucoid (SM) level* was discovered, observed principally in hepatic disease (16–19). Thus, the incidence of a low SM level among 180 patients with either viral hepatitis or portal cirrhosis was about 80 per cent and compared favorably in diagnostic efficiency with the usual flocculation and other hepatic tests. On the other hand, only 2 per cent of 125 cases of obstructive jaundice showed a subnormal level, while 50 per cent had an increase (18, 19).

Since the test, in addition to its reputed diagnostic utility in such conditions as rheumatic fever and renal disease (20, 21), promised to be a useful means of distinguishing between "medical" and "surgical" jaundice (22)—an ever-present clinical problem—it was being considered by the authors for adoption in the routine hospital laboratory. As a necessary preliminary step, an attempt was made to reappraise the clinical significance of the test. The results of this study, which, in part, were in discord with the cited published findings, are reported here.

MATERIAL AND METHODS

Patients afflicted with various types of jaundice or hepatomegaly (other than that usually observed in congestive heart failure), or both,

---

From The Communicable Disease Center, Public Health Service, U. S. Department of Health, Education and Welfare; Emory University School of Medicine, Atlanta, Georgia; and The Chicago Medical School, Chicago, Illinois.

Presented in part at the Annual Meeting of the USPHS Clinical Society, New Orleans, La., April 1–3, 1954.

The assistance of Myron J. Willis, M.A., Statistics Section, Communicable Disease Center, in the statistical calculations is gratefully acknowledged.

Received for publication January 20, 1955.

* This term is adopted in accordance with Meyer's recent classification (10).

were studied. Only those patients were included in this report whose diagnosis appeared established by autopsy, biopsy, surgical operation, or prolonged clinical observation. "Normal" controls were recruited from the hospital* and Public Health Service staffs; "hospital" controls included patients with such localized lesions as were unlikely to exert a significant systemic effect and to influence the SM level, such as healing fracture, cataract, or peptic ulcer.

Blood specimens for SM analysis were usually secured in the morning from subjects in the preprandial state, except for experiments designed to determine the effect of food intake on the SM concentration (see below). Serum was separated promptly upon adequate clot retraction and stored at $-10°$ to $-15°$, if not analyzed the same day. Results of the usual hepatic tests, including serum bilirubin (23), cephalin cholesterol flocculation (24), thymol turbidity (24), and alkaline phosphatase (25), were used for correlation with SM values only if the interval between respective blood collections was no greater than three days.

For the purpose of adequate comparison with Greenspan's data (18), his method of analysis—originally described by Simkin and coworkers (16)—was adopted, although some of its shortcomings were recognized early in the study (26). Serum (usually 4 ml., never less than 2 ml.) was treated with twice the volume of 0.6M perchloric acid. After exactly 10 minutes of standing and subsequent filtering through Whatman #5 paper, filtrate and 5% phosphotungstic acid (in 2N HCl) were, in a volume ratio of 3:1, placed in a 15 ml. centrifuge tube, gently mixed, and spun 15 minutes later at about 500 G. for 10 minutes. The seromucoid precipitate was washed once with the phosphotungstic acid solution and, after thorough drainage, dissolved in 3 ml. of 0.2N NaOH and 0.6 ml. of biuret reagent. After one hour's standing in a dark cabinet, the samples were read in a Beckman Model DU spectrophotometer at 540 $m\mu$. Calculation of the SM content was made by reference to a standard curve obtained by means of solutions of 50 to 200 mg. of casein per 100 ml. of 0.2N NaOH, treated with biuret as indicated above.

RESULTS

Analysis of SM values determined among the normal controls revealed no striking difference between the fasting and nonfasting groups, if one discounts the low upper extreme in the nonfasting female group because of the small number of observations (Table 1). In individual cases, however, food intake did seem to influence the SM level, contrary to Green-

* Grady Memorial Hospital, Veterans Administration Hospital, and Emory University Hospital, Atlanta, Ga.

Table 1. NORMAL RANGE OF SEROMUCOID

Authors	Number of observations	Sex	Food intake before analysis	Seromucoid level (mg./100 ml.) Extreme values	Means	Standard deviation	Approximate 95% limits	Approximate 65% limits
Greenspan *et al.*	105	M	Not stated	38.9–78.7	59.2	7.3	48–75[a]	..
	80	F	Not stated	36.7–74.6	52.9	7.6	40–70[a]	..
Present authors	23	M	No	35.4–94.1	62.4	17.6	27–98	45–80[a]
	26	F	No	17.5–77.8	47.6	17.2	13–82	30–65[a]
	22	M	Yes	36.2–102.6	61.7	19.9	22–102	42–82
	11	F	Yes	27.6–55.5	38.8	9.2	20–57	30–48
	16[b]	M	No	31.2–98.8	70.3	20.3	30–111	50–91
	13[b]	F	No	23.4–93.3	51.9	18.7	15–89	33–71

[a] Range employed in diagnosis.
[b] Hospital controls.

span's experience (18), though not in a consistent manner (Fig. 1). Consequently, emphasis was placed on collecting blood for SM analysis from fasting subjects only. The range of values in the group of hospital controls was somewhat higher than among the "normals." In accordance with the findings of Greenspan and his associates (18), the range for females was distinctly lower than that for males in each control group. For each sex, however, the span of extreme values was considerably wider in this study than in the former authors' series, even though the latter included nearly four times as many observations. The lowest values in

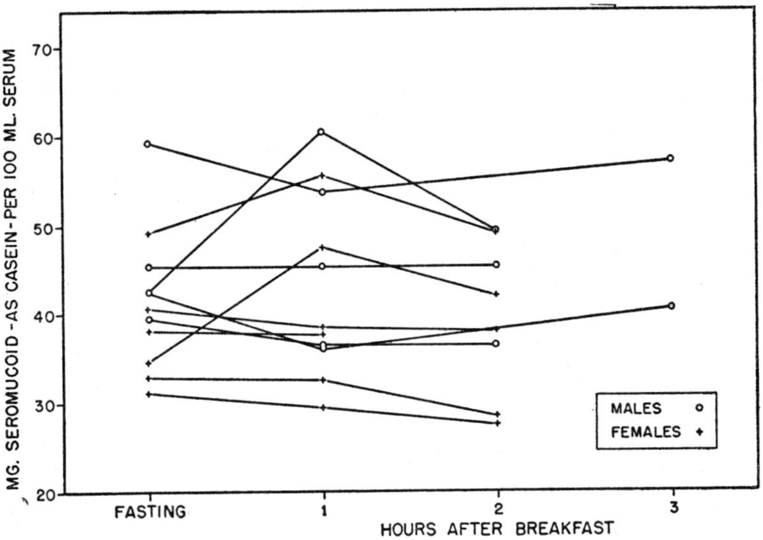

Fig. 1. Influence of food intake upon seromucoid level.

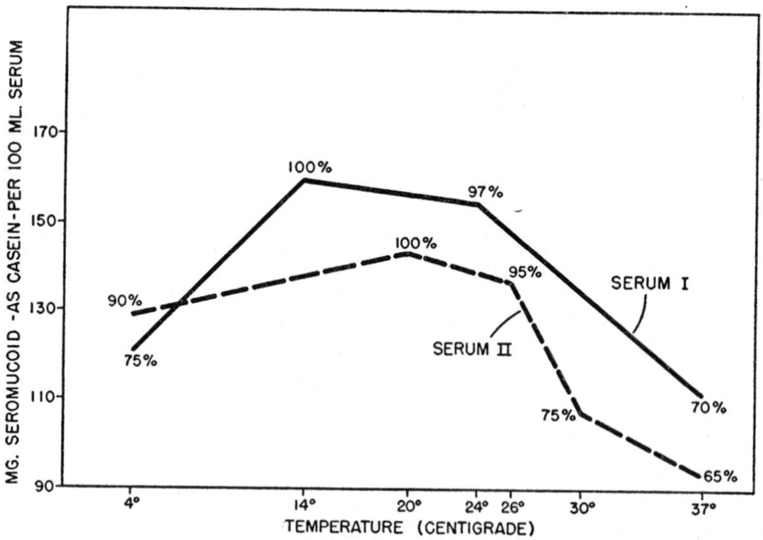

Fig. 2. Influence of temperature of perchloric-acid–serum mixture upon seromucoid yield.

the present control group were found in young and slender but obviously healthy nurses and medical technologists.

To a limited extent, these discrepancies can be explained by the difficulties encountered in analysis. The coefficient of variation (27) of duplicate determinations on 65 unselected consecutive sera was as high as 6.1 per cent.* In other words, the SM values that may be expected from a single serum range ±12% from the "ideal" or "true" value. If the latter were 50 mg./100 ml., 95% of the replicate determinations would fall between 44 and 56 mg. per 100 ml. The experimental error among values obtained from aliquots of a single serum analyzed several days apart was even greater, the coefficient of variation among aliquots of 10 such sera approaching 10 per cent. Among the factors (subsequently discovered) that may be responsible for this variation are differences in temperatures prevailing on different days of analysis (Fig. 2), as well as inadvertent changes in the procedure of pipetting and mixing serum and perchloric acid (26). The chief problem of precision is apparently inherent in this initial step in analysis, designed to separate the seromucoid from the other serum proteins. Analysis (in triplicates) upon 10 different perchloric acid filtrates yielded a coefficient of variation of 1%, and upon 30 different casein solutions, of 0.8% only.

In view of these limitations and the relatively small number of "nor-

* Winzler's method (11) yielded a coefficient of variation of 5 per cent.

mal" subjects studied, the 65 per cent confidence limits (27) were chosen to designate the normal range, which therefore constituted 45–80 mg./100 ml. for males and 30–65 mg./100 ml. for females. These extremes are in fairly close agreement with the 95 per cent confidence limits which represented the normal range of SM in Greenspan's series.

Among 44 cases of viral hepatitis (including 13 instances of presumed virus B infection), 17, or 39 per cent, showed a subnormal SM upon initial examination (Table 2). This percentage increased to 49 in the 29 cases in whom subsequent SM determinations could be secured. Nine of the above 44 patients were found to have complicating conditions (recent

Table 2. Seromucoid Levels in 165 Patients with Hepatobiliary Disease

Diagnosis	*No. of patients with:*		
	Increased values	*Normal values*	*Decreased values*
Acute hepatitis			
A or B virus	6(4)[a]	21(5)	17
Mononucleosis	1		
Leptospiral	1	1	
Amoebic	1		
Septic	1		
Toxic		1	
Chronic liver disease			
Fatty metamorphosis	1(1)	1	
Alcoholic cirrhosis	18(16)	17(11)	6(1)
Postnecrotic cirrhosis			3
Cardiac cirrhosis		1	1
Hemochromatosis	1		
Sarcoidosis	2		1
Biliary obstruction			
Benign			
Acute cholecystitis	4		
Chronic cholecystopathy	7		
Common duct stone	6	2	
Common duct stricture	1	1	
Congenital duct stenosis	1	1	
Malignant			
Carcinoma[b]	22	4	
Hepatoma	2	2	
Lymphoma	2		
Hemolytic jaundice			
Congenital spherocytosis	3(2)		
Sickle cell anemia	2(1)	1	
Transfusion reaction	1		
Malaria		1	

[a] Parentheses denote complicating illness (in hepatitis and hemolytic jaundice groups).

[b] Carcinoma of gastrointestinal tract (4 cases), pancreas (12), biliary tract (2), kidney (1), and of unknown origin (7), causing jaundice and/or metastatic hepatomegaly.

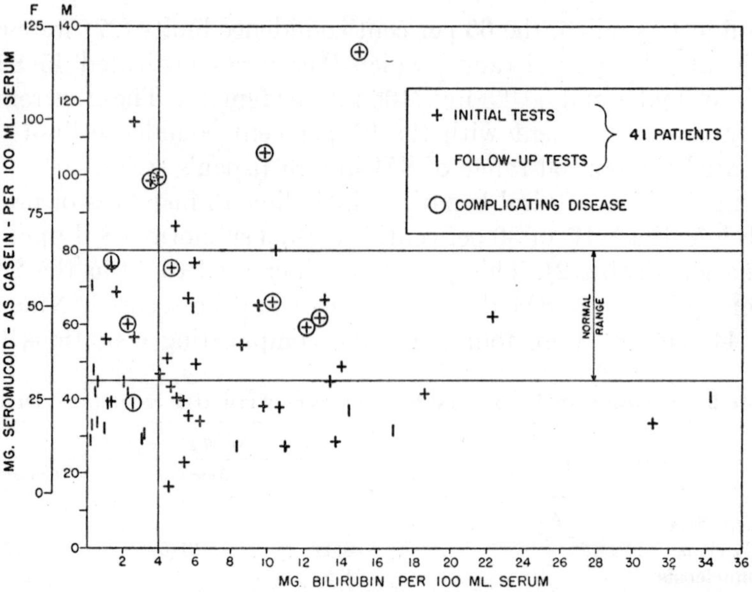

Fig. 3. Relation of seromucoid to severity of viral hepatitis as denoted by serum bilirubin. In all but 9 patients, the serum bilirubin was above 4 mg./100 ml. on initial examination. Most of the corresponding seromucoid values were either normal or low. χ^2 test (27) failed to suggest correlation between seromucoid and bilirubin.

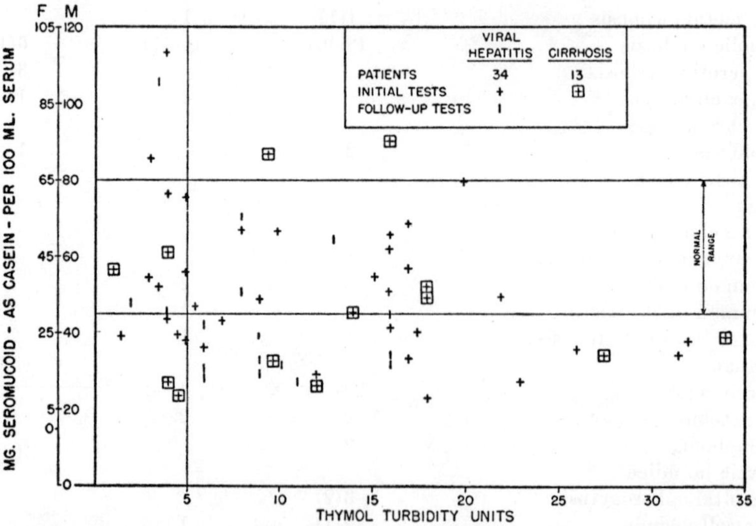

Fig. 4. Relation of seromucoid to thymol turbidity in uncomplicated hepatic disease. Less than one third of the cases showed, upon initial testing, a normal thymol turbidity (below 5 units) while more than one half had a normal or elevated (negative) seromucoid. In 6 instances, seromucoid was positive and thymol negative; in 9, both tests failed to indicate hepatic disease. χ^2 test (27) failed to suggest correlation between seromucoid and thymol turbidity.

surgical operations, pneumonia, pyelonephritis, mastitis, pregnancy), to which the failure of SM depression could be ascribed. Even if these cases were eliminated, reducing the group to 35 cases, there was still about one half of these which yielded a normal or, in 2 instances, elevated SM without evidence of an extrahepatic "SM-raising" process. While some of these patients had suffered a mild attack or were already in the recovery stage, as indicated by the low serum bilirubin level (Fig. 3), about one half of them showed considerable jaundice, malaise, and associated laboratory evidence of hepatic damage (Fig. 4) at the time of the SM test.

Absence of SM depression appeared to characterize a group of 6 patients presenting an acute hepatitis syndrome secondary to certain systemic disorders: infectious mononucleosis, leptospirosis (two), amoebiasis, acute bacterial endocarditis, and intoxication with bootleg whiskey.

Since complications likely to augment the SM level (chronic pyelonephritis, pneumonia, subphrenic abscess, lymphopathia venereum, urticaria, and delirium tremens) occurred in the majority of the 41 patients with alcoholic cirrhosis, it was not surprising that only 6 (15 per cent) showed a subnormal SM level. In 2 instances, a high initial SM was associated with prolonged fever and leukocytosis, attributed to enterogenous bacteremia; subsidence of these signs of inflammation weeks later was accompanied by SM depression. Of the 14 patients in this group who showed no evidence of complications, there were still 2 with an increased and only 6 (43 per cent) with a low SM. The latter finding was also encountered in the 3 cases of postnecrotic cirrhosis, in 1 of the 2 cases of cardiac cirrhosis, and in 1 of 3 cases of sarcoidosis. SM was elevated in a patient with hemochromatosis but apparently not affected by fatty infiltration of the liver.

Thus, the incidence of significantly reduced SM levels in the group of

Table 3. Efficiency of Seromucoid and of Three Other Serum Tests in the Diagnosis of Hepatobiliary Disease

Diagnosis	*Seromucoid* Above normal (%)		Below normal (%)	*Cephalin flocculation* Above 2+ (%)		0–2+ (%)	*Thymol turbidity* Above 5 units (%)		Below 5 units (%)	*Alkaline phosphatase* 4–10 units (%)		Above 10 units (%)
Viral hepatitis	14	(44)[a]	39	82	(39)		77	(39)		27	(22)	5
Cirrhosis	40	(47)	21	62	(39)		63	(38)		32	(19)	16
Benign obstruction	83	(23)	0		(20)	80		(22)	82	43	(14)	43
Malignant obstruction	81	(32)	0		(24)	79		(26)	81	55	(22)	27

[a] Parentheses denote number of patients in whom test was performed.

"primary" hepatic diseases was only 28 per cent, far below expectations based on Greenspan's reports (17, 18). This disappointment was enhanced upon comparison with some of the usual hepatic tests, performed concomitantly with the SM test. The cephalin flocculation and thymol turbidity tests were positive approximately twice as often in viral hepatitis and nearly three times as often in cirrhosis (Table 3). Even after exclusion of cases with extrahepatic complications, the incidence of diagnostic SM levels was still below 50 per cent. These findings are strikingly different from Greenspan's, who reported the incidence of a subnormal SM in hepatitis and cirrhosis as being 88 per cent and 70 per cent, respectively, while the cephalin flocculation and thymol turbidity tests gave less frequent positive results: 48 and 68 per cent, respectively, in hepatitis, and 41 and 39 per cent in cirrhosis.

With regard to the serum alkaline phosphatase, experiences of the authors correspond more closely with those of Greenspan's in that this test yielded a positive result less often than the SM test (results of the two series are not directly comparable because of the differences in critical enzyme levels used).

On the other hand, in 55 cases of biliary obstruction (Table 2; Fig. 3) not a single instance of a subnormal SM was encountered while the two routine flocculation tests gave 20 per cent of "false" positive reactions (Table 3); the alkaline phosphatase failed in 27 to 43 per cent of the cases to show a marked elevation. In nearly three times as many cases of obstructive jaundice, Greenspan and his associates found the incidence of a subnormal SM level to be less than 3 per cent (19).

Hence, a subnormal SM level in the presence of jaundice is almost specific for a primary parenchymal disease, a statement that cannot be made for any of the commonly used hepatic tests. The SM test may therefore be most valuable in problems involving the differentiation of "medical" from "surgical" jaundice when the usual clinical and laboratory technics give equivocal results: a subnormal level weighs heavily in favor of "medical" jaundice. The utility of the test was clearly enhanced by the use of follow-up determinations (17, 21); not infrequently, when the first test gave a normal or borderline SM value, examination a few days later revealed a distinct tendency of the SM level to rise or fall, suggesting obstructive or parenchymal disease, respectively. A single normal or increased SM concentration per se was of little help in ruling out parenchymal disease, even in the absence of extrahepatic complication. However, when such a diagnosis appeared to be well established, the finding of an elevated SM suggested the possibility—and, in several cases, initiated the discovery—of either an extrahepatic (inflammatory or neoplastic) complicating illness or an icterogenic agent other than the hepatitis virus (mononucleosis, leptospirosis, etc.). With about 80 per cent of both benign and malignant forms of biliary obstruction yielding high SM levels, the test could not be utilized to render a preoperative differentiation of the nature of the obstructive lesion.

DISCUSSION

Analysis of the data presented permits one to attribute a definite diagnostic value only to the finding of a subnormal SM level. Such a finding, in association with jaundice or hepatomegaly, or both, and in the absence of a nephrotic syndrome (20), of excessive hyperglobulinemia, and, perhaps, of certain endocrinopathies (19), is almost pathognomonic of hepatocellular disease. Normal or elevated levels are of very limited value and only occasionally make a decisive diagnostic contribution. In particular, high levels do not spell neoplastic disease, an observation which has been made in the past by Henry and coworkers (13) and, most recently, by Rhees and his associates (15). Although these investigators disregarded the existing sex difference in the normal SM concentration (Table 1) (17), their conclusions conform to Greenspan's (19) and the authors' experiences.

Recognition of abnormal (high or low) levels is obviously dependent

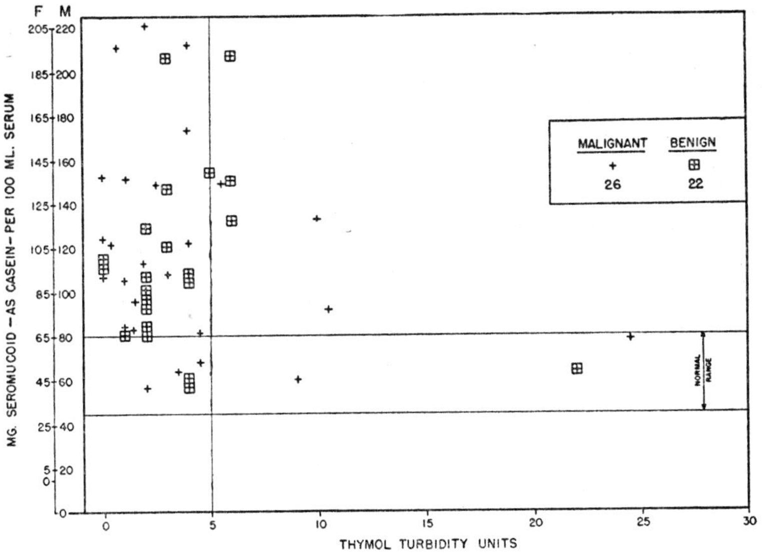

Fig. 5. Relation of seromucoid to thymol turbidity in biliary obstruction. The seromucoid test gave no false-positive (subnormal) result but the thymol turbidity was increased in 9 cases.

upon the definition of the "normal range," which in the present study was quite arbitrarily established as the 65 per cent confidence limits of all normal values encountered. Had the 95 per cent limits been used (Table 1), which would be more acceptable from a statistical point of view, the incidence of subnormal values would have been far lower than above recorded, whereas the number of high levels would have decreased but slightly (Figs. 3–5). The absence of any apparent false-positive results furnished by the values herein designated as subnormal lends some justification to the choice of the normal range as presented; additional support stems from the close similarity to the normal extremes employed by Greenspan and coworkers (17).

However, these, as well as other problems of a more technical nature mentioned initially, throw a suspicious light on the reliability of the analytic method and on the biologic significance of the results. Seromucoid obviously does not represent a single substance but rather a serum fraction whose separation from the other serum proteins by means of perchloric acid or other reagents (sulfosalicylic acid, trichloracetic acid [5, 11]) is quite arbitrary. This fact is evident from the marked changes in SM values that can be produced by relatively small alterations in the concentration of either acid or serum proteins or in the proportion of acid to serum (11, 26, 28). Increases in serum globulin such as are observed in sarcoidosis or multiple myeloma apparently tend to reduce the SM level (18), presumably through physicochemical action.

Electrophoretic analysis of perchloric-acid–serum filtrates revealed the presence of at least 3 peaks (MP-1, MP-2, and MP-3) (11, 29). Chemically, carbohydrate (galactose-mannose), hexosamine and protein (measured as tyrosine) constituted, aside from lipids, the chief components, in a ratio of 15.1:11.9:4.2 (by weight, on a moisture-free basis). Since the carbohydrate:protein (tyrosine) ratio was apparently maintained when the SM (tyrosine) level was markedly elevated in patients with cancer or pneumonia, it was concluded that the material responsible for the increase was chemically similar (but not necessarily identical!) to that isolated from normal serum (12). However, subnormal SM values (expressed as casein) encountered in liver disease were associated with increased carbohydrate:protein ratios (17).

With the use of ammonium sulfate fractionation, an electrophoretically and ultracentrifugally homogeneous plasma mucoid (M-1, corresponding to MP-1) was prepared by Winzler and his associates (30, 31). This had a molecular weight of 44,100, the mobility of α_1-globulin, and an isoelectric point of *p*H 1.8 at a buffer *p*H of 8.6; it contained approximately 26 per cent of carbohydrate (including hexosamine) and 10 per cent of "sialic acid" (32). The substance was finally isolated in crystallized form by Schmid from Cohn's fraction VI (33). Variations of this "acid glycoprotein" due to disease have, in the absence of a practical clinical method, not been reported.

It is thus obvious that seromucoid, as determined in perchloric acid filtrates, does not represent a chemical or biologic entity. There is much question as to whether increases or decreases of certain of its constituents —protein, hexosamine, hexose polysaccharide, or others—necessarily reflect equivalent fluctuations of the whole complex. Consequently, any speculation about the mechanism responsible for changes in SM concentration found in various disease states are bound to be superficial and fraught with error.

It has been suggested that serum glycoproteins originate from the depolymerization of ground substance of connective tissue (34, 35). This process, normally under enzymatic and hormonal control, may be augmented by certain alterations in tissue metabolism, particularly those associated with destruction or proliferation, causing an excess of soluble, lower-molecular substances to diffuse into the circulation (34–38) and be excreted in the urine (39). These substances are only in part represented by seromucoid which is devoid of hexuronic acids (10, 11, 30, 32, 33), the regular constituents of tissue glycoprotein (40). Hexuronic acids (41, 42), as well as polysaccharides other than those contained in seromucoid, are normally present in serum (37) and may be pathologically increased. The decrease in the concentration of seromucoid (but not of those carbohydrate derivatives) occurring in liver disease suggests that the liver may act either as another source of SM or as an organ capable of removing it from the blood stream. The former possibility, implying inadequate synthesis by the diseased liver (18), is suggested by Werner's observations on the serum hexosamine response of rabbits subjected to blood loss; the usual increase failed to occur when liver damage was produced by means of phosphorus or chlorobenzene (43). On the other hand, total protein-bound hexose polysaccharides have been found in normal or increased serum concentrations in viral hepatitis (17). The role of the liver as a source of SM is also suggested by the finding of reduced α_1-globulin in viral hepatitis (44, 45) and by the observation, based on C^{14} isotope studies, that most of the major serum protein fractions stem from the liver, except for γ-globulin and minute amounts of β- and α-globulins (46, 47).

As a working hypothesis, connective tissue and the hepatic parenchyma may be regarded as two independent sources of seromucoid, each source having a different type of response to physiologic stimulation or injury:

the former chiefly in the form of an increase, the latter by way of a decrease. The SM level, as analyzed at any given time, constitutes the sum of these responses. Thus, only marked preponderance of the response of one source over that of the other will result in a distinctly abnormal and diagnostically useful level. The combination of two severe responses, i.e., pneumonia and viral hepatitis, is liable to yield a normal level.

This theory leaves open the question of endocrine factors influencing the SM level (48–51) and, indeed, the distinct possibility that there may be many different sites of origin of SM and of different glycoproteins and their individual constituents, with different degrees or types of response to certain pathologic processes. Further clinical or physiologic studies of seromucoid would seem to be of little avail without the attainment of far greater precision in chemical identification and in analytic measurement of the substances involved. Any attempt at classification of diseases by seromucoid levels (19) must therefore be regarded as preliminary and subject to future revision.

SUMMARY AND CONCLUSIONS

Seromucoid was determined in 165 patients with jaundice or hepatomegaly, or both. Subnormal seromucoid concentrations were found in 39 per cent of 44 cases of viral hepatitis and in 15 per cent of 41 cases of alcoholic cirrhosis. This incidence increased to 50 and 43 per cent, respectively, when patients with complicating extrahepatic disease processes were excluded. No subnormal values were encountered in 55 cases of benign and malignant biliary obstruction which, however, yielded about 80 per cent of elevated values.

The empirical data point to the lower limit of the normal seromucoid range as providing a useful dividing line between obstructive and parenchymal jaundice: the finding of a subnormal level is strongly indicative of the latter. Normal or elevated levels may only occasionally be expected to make a decisive diagnostic contribution.

A more definitive evaluation of the clinical utility of this type of test must await improvements in analytic standardization, based on a more detailed knowledge of the chemical and physiologic identity of the compound than is available at present.

REFERENCES

1. Hahn, A., *Biochem. Z.* **121,** 262 (1921).
2. Wolff, E., *Ann. méd.* **10,** 185 (1909).
3. Cristol, P., and Puech, A., *Bull mém soc. méd. hôp. Paris* **50,** 1826 (1926).
4. Goiffen, R., and Spaey, J., *Bull. Soc. chim. biol.* **16,** 1675 (1934).

5. Winzler, R. J., and Burk, D., *J. Nat. Cancer Inst.* **4**, 417 (1944).
6. Mayer, K., *Z. physiol. Chem.* **275**, 16 (1942).
7. Zannetti, C. U., *Gazz. chim. ital.* **33**, 160 (1903).
8. Bywaters, H. W., *Biochem. Z.* **15**, 322 (1909).
9. Rimington, C., *Biochem. J.* **34**, 931 (1940).
10. Meyer, K., Rutgers Univ. Press, New Brunswick (1953).
11. Winzler, R. J., Devor, A. W., Mehl, J. W., and Smyth, I. M., *J. Clin. Invest.* **27**, 609 (1948).
12. Winzler, R. J., and Smyth, I. M., *J. Clin. Invest.* **27**, 617 (1948).
13. Henry, R. J., Berkman, S., Little, M. S., and Winzler, R. J., *J.A.M.A.* **147**, 37 (1951).
14. Winzler, R. J., *Advances in Cancer Research* **1**, 503 (1953).
15. Rhees, M. C., Ellerbrook, L. D., and Lippincott, S. W., *Am. J. Clin. Pathol.* **24**, 774 (1954).
16. Simkin, B., Bergman, H. C., and Prinzmetal, M., *Am. J. Med.* **6**, 734 (1949).
17. Greenspan, E. M., Tepper, B., Terry, L. L., and Schoenbach, E. B., *J. Lab. Clin. Med.* **39**, 44 (1952).
18. Greenspan, E. M., and Dreiling, D., *A.M.A. Arch. Internal Med.* **91**, 474 (1953).
19. Greenspan, E. M., *A.M.A. Arch. Internal Med.* **93**, 863 (1954).
20. Kelley, V. C., Good, R. A., Glick, D., and Ochs, M. J., *J. Clin. Invest.* **29**, 1500 (1950).
21. Kelley, V. C., Adams, F. H., and Good, A., *Pediatrics* **12**, 607 (1953).
22. Popper, M., and Steigmann, F., *Ann. Internal Med.* **29**, 496 (1948).
23. Malloy, M. T., and Evelyn, K. A., *J. Biol. Chem.* **119**, 491 (1937).
24. Neefe, J. R., Gambescia, J. M., Gardner, H. T., and Knowlton, M., *Am. J. Med.* **24**, 600 (1950).
25. Bodansky, A., and Jaffe, M. L., *Proc. Soc. Exp. Biol. Med.* **31**, 107 (1933).
26. Mandel, E. E., Jones, F. L., and Gorsuch, T. L., *Federation Proc.* **13**, 258 (1954).
27. Mainland, D., *Elementary Medical Statistics*, Philadelphia, Saunders, 1952.
28. Weimer, H. E., and Moshin, J. R., *Am. Rev. Tuberc.* **68**, 594 (1953).
29. Mehl, J. W., Humphrey, J., and Winzler, R. J., *Proc. Soc. Exp. Biol. Med.* **72**, 106 (1949).
30. Weimer, H. E., Mehl, J. W., and Winzler, R. J., *J. Biol. Chem.* **185**, 561 (1950).
31. Smith, E. L., Brown, D. M., Weimer, H. E., and Winzler, R. J., *J. Biol. Chem.* **185**, 569 (1950).
32. Odin, L., and Werner, I., *Acta Soc. Med. Upsaliensis* **57**, 227 (1952).
33. Schmid, K., *J. Am. Chem. Soc.* **75**, 60 (1953).
34. Gersh, I., and Catchpole, H. R., *Am. J. Anat.* **85**, 457 (1949).
35. Catchpole, H. R., *Proc. Soc. Exp. Biol. Med.* **75**, 221 (1950).
36. Engel, M. B., *Arch. Path.* **53**, 339 (1952).
37. Shetlar, M. R., Payne, R. W., Bullock, J. A., Patrick, D. R., Hellbaum, A. A., and Ishmael, W. K., *J. Clin. Invest.* **32**, 1208 (1953).
38. Maddock, C. L., *Proc. Soc. Exp. Biol. Med.* **85**, 598 (1954).
39. Engel, M. B., and Catchpole, H. R., *Proc. Soc. Exp. Biol. Med.* **84**, 336 (1953).
40. Cantarow, A., and Schepartz, B., *Biochemistry*, Philadelphia, Saunders, 1954.
41. Stary, Z., and Yuvanidis, M., *Biochem. Z.* **324**, 206 (1953).
42. Saltzman, A., Caraway, W. T., and Beck, I. A., Metabolism, *Clin. and Exp.* **3**, 11 (1954).
43. Werner, I., in *Acta Physiol. Scand.* **19**, 27 (1949) (abstr.).
44. Brante, G., *Scand. J. Clin. & Lab. Invest.* **4**, 293 (1952).
45. Mandel, E. E., and Cooper, G. R., Unpublished observations.
46. Miller, L. L., and Bale, W. F., *J. Exp. Med.* **99**, 125 (1954).
47. Miller, L. L., Bly, C. G., and Bale, W. F., *J. Exp. Med.* **99**, 133 (1954).
48. Boas, N. F., and Soffer, L. J., *J. Clin. Endocrinol.* **11**, 39 (1951).
49. Mancini, J. C., and Garberi, J. C., *J. Clin. Endocrinol.* **12**, 965 (1952).
50. Kelley, V. C., Kirschvink, J. F., and Ely, R. S., *Am. J. Physiol.* **171**, 738 (1952).
51. Weimer, H. E., and Redlich-Moshin, J., *Proc. Soc. Exp. Biol. Med.* **84**, 34 (1953).

Estimation of Hydrocortisone Secretion

Method of Calculation from Urinary-Excretion Data

Robert H. Silber

In 1938, Anderson, Haymaker, and Joseph (1) reported the finding of increased concentrations of cortin in the blood and urine of patients with Cushing's syndrome. Since then, as methods for the determination of cortical steroids have been improved, they have been applied to the urine and plasma of patients as a measure of adrenocortical activity. The reaction of 17,21-dihydroxy-20-ketosteroids with phenylhydrazine (2) has been applied to the analysis of plasma (3) and of urine (4) in Addison's disease and in Cushing's syndrome. In general, hyperactivity or hypoactivity of the adrenal cortex is reflected by increased or decreased plasma concentrations and excretion of 17,21-dihydroxy-20-ketosteroids. However, there may be conditions in which the output of the adrenal cortex is altered without demonstrable changes in the corticosteroid content of blood or urine. Therefore, it seemed desirable to devise a procedure which could be used clinically to estimate the adrenal output of hydrocortisone.

THEORETICAL CONSIDERATIONS

If a mathematical relationship between total (endogenous plus exogenous) hydrocortisone in the body and the fraction found in the urine can be established after administration of graded doses of hydrocortisone, it should be possible to extrapolate back to zero exogenous hydrocortisone and thereby determine the fraction of the endogenous hydrocortisone that is excreted. The calculation of endogenous production would then follow directly, after measurement of the basal steroid excretion in a given period of time. In theory, to accomplish this, the exogenous hydro-

---

From the Merck Institute for Therapeutic Research, Rahway, N. J.
Received for publication April 18, 1955.

cortisone should be administered slowly into the adrenal vein to mix intimately with the endogenous steroid and to share its metabolic fate in the body. This mode of administration is obviously impractical and due to the required manipulation of the subject would not necessarily reflect the normal output of the adrenal cortex. Oral administration has been found to yield surprisingly satisfactory results, with a constant fraction of the exogenous steroid detected in the urine by the procedure of Silber and Porter (5) over the dosage range studied.

MATERIAL AND METHOD

Since, by the analytic procedure employed, we find that the increase in excretion of 17,21-dihydroxy-20-ketosteroids after oral administration of hydrocortisone is essentially complete within 8 hours, this period appeared to be satisfactory for the experimental demonstration of the method. In practice a 24-hour period has also been used and may be preferred.

On 4 consecutive days 5 male laboratory workers consumed a light breakfast at 7:00 A.M., voided at 8:30 A.M., ingested 0, 10, 25 or 50 mg. of hydrocortisone (free alcohol) with about 200 ml. of water, and collected all urine until 4:30 P.M. The subjects were permitted to have lunch at 11:30 A.M. Creatinine determinations were performed on all urines to check the adequacy of the collections. Phenol was added as preservative and samples of urine were frozen until all could be treated with glucuronidase[1] and assayed simultaneously.

Effects of Drugs

One subject (No. 2) ingested additional doses of 75 and 100 mg. (Table 1). This subject was studied again several weeks later and in subsequent weeks was used to determine the effect of several drugs on adrenocortical activity. During one series of collections, 2.7 Gm. of aspirin were ingested daily in 3 equal portions at 0 time, 2½ hours, and 5 hours; in a second, 300 mg. of ascorbic acid were taken, again in 3 equal portions; in a third, 100 mg. of Pyribenzamine, in 2 equal portions, were ingested; and in a fourth, 40 units of ACTH (Armour H. P. ACTHAR Gel) was administered daily by intramuscular injection (Table 2).

---

[1] Due to possible changes in the enzyme preparation, we now check each lot before use and usually find that 5–10 times as much enzyme as indicated in the published method (5) is needed.

RESULTS

Four of the subjects (see Table 1) excreted 24–32 per cent of the oral hydrocortisone as 17,21-dihydroxy-20-ketosteroids. The fifth subject excreted only 13.6 per cent. By applying these percentages to the 8-hour basal excretion values the secretion of hydrocortisone by the adrenals of these subjects in 8 hours may be estimated in milligrams. However, it may be more desirable to employ an extrapolated basal value for this calculation because analytic errors are minimized after administration of the steroid. In most instances the extrapolated value and the actual basal excretion were not significantly different.

The adrenal output of these subjects averaged 13.8 mg. of hydrocortisone in the 8-hour period. When the above approach was applied to a group of 20 males (21–35 years of age) studied with Dr. Bacon Chow

Table 1. Urinary Excretion of 17,21-Dihydroxy-20-ketosteroids by Human Subjects
Milligrams Free plus Conjugated in 8 Hours

Hydrocortisone dose (mg.)	*Subject 1*	*Subject 2*[a]	*Subject 3*	*Subject 4*	*Subject 5*
0	5.3 (4.7)	3.8 (2.7)	2.9 (2.8)	3.0	2.95
10	7.9	5.73	5.15	5.35	4.2
25	12.6	10.3	9.3	9.0	6.2
50	20.6	18.0	15.9	15.4	10.6
% excreted	31.8	30.4	25.2	24.0	13.6
Adrenal output (mg./8 hr.)	14.8	8.9	11.1	12.5	21.7

Parenthetical figures are extrapolated basal excretion values which were used in the calculations.

[a] After 75-mg. dose, 25.6 mg. excreted; after 100 mg. dose, 32.1 mg.

Table 2. Effect of Several Drugs on Adrenal Output of Subject 2
Milligrams free plus conjugated in 8 hours

Hydrocortisone dose (mg.)	*Control (first)*	*Aspirin (2.7 Gm.)*	*Ascorbic acid (300 mg.)*	*Pyribenzamine (100 mg.)*	*ACTH (40 units)*	*Control (second)*
0	2.94 (2.9)	4.0	4.15 (4.0)	4.2	11.5	3.65
10	5.6	6.63	6.4	7.07	16.9	5.7
20	8.2	9.25	9.3	9.2	22.6	9.05
30	11.2	..	11.9	12.7	..	11.05
% excreted	27.1	26.3	25.6	27.3	54.8	24.1
Adrenal output (mg./8 hr.)	10.7	15.2	15.6	15.4	21.0	15.1

Parenthetical figures are extrapolated basal excretion values which were used in the calculations.

of Johns Hopkins (6), 24-hour urine collections were made and the adrenal output was calculated to be 21.9 ± 8.2 mg. (s.d.) per 24 hours. In this study (6) only 2 urine collections were made—one before and one after administration of 40 mg. of hydrocortisone.

Calculations

For purposes of illustration, the data obtained on subject No. 2 (see Table 2) during the first control period are shown below:

$$\frac{\text{mg. excreted after test dose} - \text{basal excretion in mg.}}{\text{test dose in mg.}} = \text{fraction excreted}$$

$$\frac{5.6 - 2.9}{10} = .27$$

$$\frac{8.2 - 2.9}{20} = .265$$

$$\frac{11.2 - 2.9}{30} = .277$$

$$\text{Av.} = \overline{.271} \text{ of dose excreted}$$

Then, $\frac{\text{basal excretion in mg.}}{\text{fraction excreted}} = \text{adrenal output (mg. in 8 hours)}$

$$\frac{2.9}{0.271} = 10.7 \text{ mg.}$$

It is also possible to determine the fraction excreted by the application of simultaneous equations. (In dogs we find this procedure necessary.)

a = exogenous hydrocortisone, mg. (known)
b = a constant
x = fraction excreted
y = steroid excreted

$$(a + b)x = y$$
$$(10 + b)x = 5.6$$
$$(20 + b)x = 8.2$$

Then, subtracting the first from the second,

$$10x = 2.6$$
$$x = 0.26 \text{ or } 26\%$$

This fraction is then applied to the analytically determined basal excretion value (as in dogs), or, if desired, to the extrapolated basal value (as in man).

DISCUSSION

The quantity of hydrocortisone secreted by the adrenal glands of human subjects has been the subject of a great deal of speculation, but relatively little pertinent data have been published. Weichselbaum (7) has found that administration of approximately 40 mg. of hydrocortisone to adrenalectomized subjects in a 24-hour period brings their plasma concentrations into the normal range. This value compares favorably with the average values reported in this paper, 13.8 mg. in the 8-hour period, or 21.9 mg. in 24 hours (6).

Comparative Evaluation of Procedures

In the dog the urinary analyses are less accurate, due in part to the low excretion of 17,21-dihydroxy-20-ketosteroids (basal about 0.2–0.3 mg. per day) but application of the procedure herein described indicates that the adrenals of a 10–12-Kg. dog secrete about 1–2 mg. per day, and after 80 units of ACTHAR daily intramuscularly this increases to 5–6 mg. Since it has been found in our laboratory that the 24-hour excretion of 17-hydroxycorticoids by adrenalectomized dogs was increased from zero to the normal range of 0.2–0.3 mg. after administration of 1 or 2 mg. of hydrocortisone, it appears that the procedure is valid and can yield satisfactory results in the dog. Analysis of blood from the adrenal vein of intact 14–20-Kg. dogs by Hume and Nelson (8) revealed an adrenal output of 0.6–2.0 μg. per minute. A dog secreting a total of 2 mg. in a 24-hour period would have an average secretion of 1.4 μg. per minute from the 2 adrenals, so the results of the direct and indirect procedures are in reasonably satisfactory agreement.

Pharmacologic Influences

The data on the effect of aspirin, ascorbic acid, and Pyribenzamine are presented here more to illustrate the method than to determine whether these materials influence adrenal output, but it does appear that these substances did not significantly influence adrenal activity. ACTH, as expected, increased adrenal output to 21 mg. in 8 hours (and 30 mg. in 12 hours). The shift of the fraction of steroid excreted from 25 or 30 per cent to 55 per cent during ACTH treatment is very interesting and suggests that ACTH may not only stimulate secretion by the adrenal cortex but may also influence hydrocortisone metabolism. When sufficient data are obtained on patients it may be found that the fraction excreted in the urine has diagnostic significance.

Absorption and Metabolism

Oral administration of the steroid appears to be justified. The normal urinary excretion of 17,21-dihydroxy-20-ketosteroids in man as measured here is about 6.6 mg. per 24 hours, with only about 5 per cent in chloroform-soluble form—that is, not conjugated (5). After oral administration of hydrocortisone the proportion of free to conjugated steroid is relatively unchanged. Furthermore, after oral or intravenous administration of 25 or 100 mg. to dogs (9), the excretion of total (free plus conjugated) 17,21-dihydroxy-20-ketosteroids is essentially the same. Peterson (10) has reported similar findings in men given hydrocortisone orally or intravenously. Therefore, it is reasonable to conclude that not only is the hydrocortisone practically quantitatively absorbed from the intestinal tract but also its metabolism is similar to that of the endogenous steroid.

CONCLUSIONS

Although one may have reservations regarding the absolute validity of results obtained with the procedure described, it nevertheless appears adequate to reveal changes in adrenal output.

The experimental approach used in this study may be applied to the study of other substances, provided certain conditions are fulfilled. Thus, if one can exclude the substance in question from the diet for several days, if an excretion product can be accurately determined in the urine, if the subject is in a reasonably steady state, and if the substance can be administered in graded doses, it may be possible to estimate the formation or synthesis of that substance in the body.

SUMMARY

A method has been described for the estimation of the secretion of hydrocortisone by the adrenals of man, based exclusively upon urinary-excretion data. In an 8-hour period (8:30 A.M.–4:30 P.M.) 5 subjects secreted an average of 13.8 mg. of hydrocortisone. In 1 subject ACTH was found to increase the adrenal output whereas aspirin, ascorbic acid, and Pyribenzamine had little, if any, effect.

The possible application of the approach to the measurement of the formation of other substances in the body has been noted.

REFERENCES

1. Anderson, E., Haymaker, W., and Joseph, M., *Endocrinol.* **23**, 398 (1938).
2. Porter, C. C., and Silber, R. H., *J. Biol. Chem.* **185**, 201 (1950).
3. Perkoff, G. T., Sandberg, A. A., Nelson, D. H., and Tyler, F. H., *A.M.A. Arch. Int. Med.* **92**, 1 (1954).

4. Liddle, G. W., Island, D., Renfret, A. P., and Forsham, P. H., *J. Clin. Endocrinol. and Metabolism* **14,** 839 (1954).
5. Silber, R. H., and Porter, C. C., *J. Biol. Chem.* **210,** 923 (1954).
6. Silber, R. H., Yamamoto, R., and Chow, B. F., to be published.
7. Eckert, C., Weichselbaum, T. E., *et al.*, personal communication, 1954.
8. Hume, D. M. and Nelson, D. H., *Fed. Proc.* **13,** 73 (1954).
9. Silber, R. H. and Morgan, E., to be published.
10. Peterson, R. E., and Wyngaarden, J. B., *Ann. N. Y. Acad. Sci.* **61,** 297 (1955).

Quantitative Identification of Urinary Calculi

Reid H. Leonard and Arthur J. Butt

THE USUAL METHODS of identification of urinary calculi are based upon qualitative chemical reactions (1, 2, 3). These methods are difficult to interpret and easily lead to erroneous conclusions. Other, more specific, methods are based upon mineralogic technics, x-ray patterns, and infrared absorption curves (4, 5) but are of limited use because of the infrequent availability of the required instrumentation.

Calculi may be identified by quantitative methods in regular clinical use. Most specimens may be identified by determination of calcium, phosphorus, and oxalic acid, while the less frequent types may require a determination of ammonia and soluble nitrogen. In addition to the quantitative determinations, 2 observations and 4 qualitative tests assure accuracy in identification of calculi.

The compounds found in calculi are well defined with the exception of the phosphates. Table 1 gives the analytical compositions of the compounds which are ordinarily found in calculi.

PROCEDURE

Preparation

The sample should be free of tissue, blood, lint, and such extraneous matter. It is dried in a vacuum for 15 minutes in fragments weighing not over 100 mg. placed in a tube immersed in boiling water. Small calculi may be weighed whole but larger ones should be ground to a powder before sampling. With large laminated calculi it is clinically important to separate the nucleus and portions of predominating layers and analyze them separately. About 10 mg. is sufficient for analysis, although with care as little as 1 mg. may be used.

The weighed specimen is placed in a tube and 1–2 ml. of 1:4 hydrochloric acid (HCl) is added. Solution takes place, sometimes slowly, at or near the boiling point. Observation of copious evolution of gas indi-

Received for publication April 25, 1955.

Table 1. Analytical Composition of Compounds Found in Calculi

Compound	*Calcium* (%)	*Phosphorus* (%)	*Oxalic acid* (%)	*Other*
Calcium oxalate hydrate	27.4	0.0	61.6	..
Calcium oxalate dihydrate	24.4	0.0	54.8	..
Dicalcium phosphate dihydrate	23.3	18.0	0.0	..
Carbonate-apatite	38.8	18.0	0.0	carbon dioxide
Hydroxy-apatite	39.3	18.3	0.0	..
Calcium carbonate	40.0	0.0	0.0	carbon dioxide
Magnesium ammonium phosphate hexahydrate	0.0	12.6	0.0	5.7% ammonia nitrogen 9.9% magnesium
Uric acid	0.0	0.0	130.[a]	33.3% alkali soluble nitrogen
Cystine	0.0	0.0	150.[a]	11.7% nitrogen, soluble in 1:4 HCl
Protein	0.0	0.0	0.0	16% insoluble nitrogen

[a] Calculated from the permanganate consumed.

cates carbonate and should be recorded. A second observation of the relative amount and apparent nature of the insoluble residue is made. Since uric acid and protein do not dissolve, they are removed by centrifugation at this point. The supernatant is analyzed as any acid-soluble specimen, while the residue (a) is dissolved in alkali (e.g., 5N potassium hydroxide [KOH] or 2.5N sodium hydroxide [NaOH]) if it is uric acid or it (b) may be digested and the nitrogen content of the digest determined. After the calculus is dissolved it is diluted to a definite volume in either a calibrated tube, cylinder, or flask. A final dilution to give approximately 1 mg. of calculus per 1 ml. solution is convenient.

Calcium Determination

An aliquot containing about 0.5 mg. of calculus is diluted to 5 ml. with water and isopropanol in such a way that the final solution is 40% alcohol. The calcium is read with appropriate alcoholic standards on a Model B Beckman flame photometer. On small specimens 0.1 mg. will suffice for this determination. Although use of the flame photometer is particularly expedient other methods may be applied. The calcium content for a 1 ml. aliquot (about 1 mg. of calculus) ranges from 0 to 4 times the calcium content of 1 ml. of serum.

Phosphorus Determination

An aliquot representing about 0.2 mg. of calculus is analyzed by the method of Fiske and SubbaRow (6).

Oxalic Acid Determination

An aliquot representing 1–5 mg. of calculus is acidified with 2 ml. of 2N sulfuric acid (H_2SO_4), a drop of 5% manganese sulfate ($MnSO_4$) is added, and after warming the mixture is titrated rapidly with 0.010N potassium permanganate ($KMnO_4$). Most samples give sharp endpoints; however, both uric acid and cystine react and give indefinite and fading endpoints. Uric acid calculi give a brown color. One milliliter of 0.010N $KMnO_4$ is equivalent to 0.45 mg. of oxalic acid, about 0.6 mg. of uric acid, and about 0.7 mg. of cystine. Consequently the presence or absence of uric acid and cystine must be determined by qualitative or quantitative reactions on every specimen which shows a significant permanganate consumption.

Auxiliary Determinations

A qualitative test for ammonia is made with Nessler's reagent added by drops to a small portion of the solution. If much ammonia is shown to be present then this constituent is analyzed quantitatively; however, the presence of calcium will require separation of the ammonia either by distillation or diffusion before it can be quantitatively determined. Magnesium ammonium phosphate usually can be determined by direct nesslerization. Insoluble residues, alkali-soluble calculi, and those not containing much calcium and phosphorus are digested with concentrated H_2SO_4 and potassium persulfate ($K_2S_2O_8$). After dilution of the digest a portion is used for the nitrogen determination. Magnesium is detectable by flame photometry or by the color reaction with *p*-nitrobenzene-azo-resorcinol. Uric acid is detected and determined by the method of Brown (7). Cystine is detected by the nitroprusside reaction (8).

Although this particular selection of procedures is used in our laboratory, the specimen solution may be analyzed by adaptation of methods routinely used for calcium, phosphorus, nitrogen, and uric acid.

INTERPRETATION OF RESULTS

For purposes of interpretation, urinary calculi have been placed in 4 groups: oxalate, phosphate, mixed oxalate-phosphate, and nitrogen-containing.

Oxalate Calculi

The oxalate calculi are the most common type and are simple to identify. Some representative analyses and interpretations are given in Table 2. Oxalate types do not evolve carbon dioxide upon solution in acid;

Table 2. Analysis of Oxalate-type Calculi

	Found			Computed			
						Calcium oxalate dihydrate	
#	Calcium (%)	Oxalic acid (%)	Phosphorus (%)	Calculated phosphate (%)	Corrected calcium (%)	on calcium (%)	on oxalic acid (%)
130	23.8	51.7	1.0	5.6	22.5	92	94
157	24.1	55.0	0.5	2.8	23.5	96	100
164	25.2	54.0	0.25	1.4	24.9	102	99
199	26.7	57.8	0.5	2.8	26.1	107	106
275	24.9	53.0	0.37	2.1	24.4	100	97
312	26.6	55.8	0.59	3.3	25.8	106	102
336	25.0	51.0	0.9	5.0	23.8	98	93
338	28.6	53.4	0.36	2.0	28.1	115	97
351	24.8	54.6	0.29	1.6	24.4	100	100
418	27.2	60.8	0.3	1.7	26.8	110	111
471	28.4	57.9	0.11	0.6	28.3	116	106

a trace of protein or material containing insoluble nitrogen is usually left after solution; a faint test for ammonia is usually found; uric acid and cystine are usually absent or present in trace amounts; and magnesium is absent. Small amounts of phosphorus are usually found.

In order to calculate the composition, it is first necessary to correct the total calcium figure for that which is combined with phosphorus. To do this, the percentage of phosphorus is multiplied by 1.29 and the result subtracted from the total calcium. The calculation of calculi components is made on the basis of the composition given in Table 1. Calcium oxalate as the di- or monohydrate form may then be calculated from both the corrected calcium and the oxalic acid. The examples given in Table 2 are all as the dihydrate form. The agreement between the two methods of calculation is good and serves as evidence of the validity of the oxalic acid determination. When calcium oxalate monohydrate is calculated as calcium oxalate dihydrate, a value of 112.5 per cent is obtained. Oxalate calculi which figure more than 100 per cent as the dihydrate probably contain much monohydrate material. Examples 418 and 471 are apparently almost entirely the monohydrate form. Example 338 shows a much higher result when based on the calcium content than when based on the oxalic acid. We have encountered other specimens which exhibited this high calcium content for an oxalate-type calculus. The nature of the binding anion in these cases is not known.

Phosphate Calculi

The phosphate calculi have been reported to contain several different calcium phosphate salts (4). The usual phosphate specimen contains

Table 3. Analysis of Phosphate-type Calculi

	Found				Computed			
							Computed from calcium	
#	Calcium (%)	Oxalic acid (%)	Phosphorus (%)	Carbon[a] dioxide	Calculated phosphate (%)	Calcium: phosphorus ratio	as apatites (%)	as dicalcium phosphate (%)
156	27.8	3.4	16.8	0	93	1.56	68	113
184	21.1	3.6	16.0	0	89	1.22	50	84
187	19.0	4.5	16.4	P	91	1.04	44	73
204	23.9	2.6	16.2	P	90	1.40	59	97
265	26.9	2.1	14.9	P	83	1.74	67	112
268*	25.4	3.2	19.0	P	105	1.26	62	103
299	33.5	8.3	15.6	P	87	1.91	77	128
335	25.6	5.2	13.3	P	74	1.75	60	100
354	29.2	4.8	16.3	0	91	1.66	70	116
364	22.1	2.2	13.1	P	73	1.61	54	91
436	26.0	2.1	13.3	P	74	1.89	65	108
458	19.1	2.1	14.4	P	80	1.26	47	78

[a] #268 is a calculus from prostate. P = present, 0 = absent.

some carbonate; traces of protein; no uric acid, cystine, or magnesium; and small amounts of oxalic acid. The total calcium may be corrected for calcium oxalate by deducting 0.45, the oxalic acid percentage. Table 1 shows the similar phosphorus contents of apatites and dicalcium phosphate. Examples of the phosphate-type calculi are given in Table 3. Since the apatites and dicalcium phosphate dihydrate calculate the same on the basis of phosphorus, this figure is given in Table 3 under the column heading "Calculated phosphate." The weight ratio of calcium to phosphorus has been useful as a guide to the nature of the calcium phosphate salts in calculi. The ratios for carbonate-apatite, hydroxy-apatite, and dicalcium phosphate are 2.15, 2.15, and 1.29, respectively. The ratios shown in Table 3 are made after the calcium has been corrected for oxalate. It is possible to calculate from the ratio any proportion of two out of the possible salts. However, for clinical purposes it is sufficient to know that a "calcium phosphate" is the calculus component, although for investigative purposes the nature of the calcium phosphate is important.

Infrared spectroscopy strongly suggests an apatite-like crystal structure even in those instances where the ratio of calcium to phosphorus is considerably below that required for an apatite (5). The ratios obtained show a composition that usually falls between dicalcium phosphate and the apatites. In order to more clearly demonstrate this, the apatite and dicalcium phosphate dihydrate contents based upon the calcium found are given in Table 3. The apatite values are uniformly low while the

Table 4. Analysis of Mixed Oxalate-Phosphate Calculi

	Found				*Computed*			
							Calcium in products as % of Ca found when based on	
#	*Calcium* (%)	*Oxalic acid* (%)	*Phosphorus* (%)	*Carbon dioxide*	*Calcium oxalate dihydrate* (%)	*Calculated phosphate* (%)	*Dicalcium phosphate* (%)	*Apatites* (%)
134	26.8	27.0	9.3	0	49	52	90	120
143	27.5	21.2	11.9	0	39	66	90	127
163	27.0	13.5	14.3	P	25	79	90	136
227	32.2	35.1	6.6	0	64	37	75	93
235	25.3	31.0	6.8	P	57	38	89	113
239	28.5	39.5	4.8	0	72	27	84	98
246	29.0	13.9	12.5	P	25	69	77	113
258	33.0	31.0	8.2	0	57	46	74	96
309	28.6	9.5	14.6	P	17	81	80	124
337	36.1	41.7	4.3	0	76	24	67	77

P = present; 0 = absent.

dicalcium phosphate values are frequently much too high. The large variability of the phosphate-type calculi precludes any simple but precise means of expressing their composition. It is not yet known how much significance can be attached to the calcium:phosphorus ratio.

Mixed Oxalate-Phosphate Calculi

The mixed oxalate-phosphate types are calculated on the basis of oxalic acid to calcium oxalate dihydrate and on the basis of phosphorus to "calculated phosphate." Examples are given in Table 4. The sum of the two calculated salts is within 5 per cent of a complete accounting of the calculi weights. However, when the calcium contents of the calculated salts are compared to the calcium determined by analysis there is poor correlation. Table 4 gives the calculated calcium sum or recovery as percentage of the calcium found. These recovery figures are consistently low when the composition is on the basis of dicalcium phosphate dihydrate and generally high when calculated on the basis of carbonate apatite. The results are adequate to classify the calculi for clinical significance.

Nitrogen-Containing Calculi

Examples of nitrogen-containing calculi are given in Table 5. When a high oxalic acid value but a low or absent calcium value is found then either uric acid or cystine should be suspected. A determination of soluble nitrogen, aided by qualitative tests, will establish which of the

Table 5. Analysis of Nitrogen-containing Calculi

	Found									Computed
#	*Calcium* (%)	*Oxalic acid* (%)	*Phosphorus* (%)	*Carbon dioxide*	*Soluble nitrogen* (%)	*Uric acid* (%)	*Ammonia nitrogen* (%)	*Cystine* (%)	*Magnesium* (%)	*Composition*
95	0.3	70	0.0	0	12.2	0	1.0	P	0	96% cystine
166	10.2	1.8	14.1	0	0	0	P	0	8	81% magnesium ammonium phosphate; 22% calcium phosphates
175	0.0	60	0.0	0	31.5	87.5	0	0	0	87% uric acid
182	0.6	129	0.0	0	12.0	0	0	P	0	103% cystine
183	0.0	73	0.0	0	30.6	P	0	0	0	92% uric acid
192	0.0	135	0.6	P	12.1	P	0	86	0	86% cystine
279	1.9	45	0.0	0	..	80	0	0	0	80% uric acid; 8% calcium oxalate ?
437	2.8	60	0.1	0	..	67	0	0	0	67% uric acid; 11% calcium oxalate ?
451	8.6	1.7	13.2	P	..	0	4.4	0	P	77% magnesium ammonium phosphate; 19% calcium phosphates
52	14.9	1.8	13.0	P	..	0	4.2	0	P	74% magnesium ammonium phosphate; 21% calcium phosphates; 17% calcium carbonate ?

P = present; 0 = absent.

two is present. Since uric acid is insoluble in 1:4 HCl, while cystine is soluble, the distinction between these two components is frequently known from the start. Quantitative determination of either uric acid or cystine is used in cases where there is still doubt as to the major component of the calculus. Magnesium ammonium phosphate can be identified by the determination of either ammonia nitrogen or of magnesium.

DISCUSSION

Determination of the major component of a calculus is usually adequate for clinical purposes but cases of mixed composition sometimes require the differentiation of components occurring to the extent of only about 10 per cent. It is frequently possible to remove a nucleus from a laminated calculus as well as samples from different layers. Calculi which exhibit marked lamination are apt to differ in composition. The nuclei and small embryonic specimens, of less than 20 mg., are of much diagnostic value since they frequently point to the underlying cause of the calculus formation. The procedure as outlined has been able to identify all specimens submitted, except for 1 prostatic calculus. In 2 instances inert material has been encountered in a portion of the specimen.

The distinction between the 2 hydrates of calcium oxalate is primarily theoretical and is thought to be related to the hydration of the patient. The calcium:phosphorus ratio is important from the etiologic viewpoint and may be helpful in treating some cases. The proportion of oxalate to phosphate is of theoretical and therapeutic importance.

Few specimens are apt to give deceptive results. These are clarified by performing the qualitative tests routinely with the quantitative determinations. Deceptive conditions are produced by the presence of calcium compounds with magnesium ammonium phosphate, calcium oxalate with uric acid, and calcium phosphate with cystine.

SUMMARY

Quantitative determination of calcium, phosphorus, and oxalic acid, assisted by occasional determination of ammonia nitrogen and insoluble nitrogen when indicated by qualitative tests, provides a means of computing the component substances of calculi. The determinations may be performed by slight modifications of the methods in use in the routine clinical chemistry laboratory, although flame photometry is particularly convenient for the determination of calcium.

2544 Escambia Ave.
Pensacola, Fla.

REFERENCES

1. Higgins, C. C., *Renal Lithiasis*, Springfield, Ill., Thomas (1944), p. 53.
2. Hawk, P. B., Oser, B. L., and Summerson, W. H., *Practical Physiological Chemistry*, (ed. 13) Philadelphia, Blakiston (1954), p. 854.
3. Hepler, O. E., *Manual of Clinical Laboratory Methods*, (ed. 4), Springfield, Ill., Thomas (1949), p. 16.
4. Prien, E. L., and Frondel, C., *J. Urol.* 57, 949 (1947).
5. Beischer, D. E., *J. Urol.* 73, 653 (1955).
6. Fiske, C. H., and SubbaRow, Y., *J. Biol. Chem.* 66, 375 (1925).
7. Brown, H., *J. Biol. Chem.* 158, 601 (1945).
8. Block, R. J., and Bolling, D., *Amino Acid Composition of Proteins and Foods* (ed. 1), Springfield, Ill., Thomas (1945), p. 164.

Calcium Determination in Biologic Material

Eugene Y. Berger

THE CLASSICAL PROCEDURE for the determination of calcium in biologic fluids involves the precipitation of calcium as the oxalate and titration of the oxalate with potassium permanganate. The permanganate titration has certain difficulties. The oxalate solution has to be heated during the titration (1) and the end point is unreliable in dilute solutions (2). The use of cerate oxidimetry avoids these circumstances. The principles of cerate oxidimetry have been well established in the chemical literature and there have been numerous applications to the determination of calcium (2–8). The present report defines conditions which proved to be most satisfactory for the determination of calcium in biologic material. The method has proved reliable through several years of use since 1940 in this and other laboratories. The accuracy is ±2 per cent as measured by the recovery of known amounts of calcium.

PRINCIPLE OF METHOD

Calcium is precipitated as the oxalate salt which is then oxidized by ammonium hexanitratocerate (9). The excess cerate is titrated with ferrous ion, using ortho-phenanthroline as an oxidation-reduction indicator.

REAGENTS

(1) 0.4% aqueous solution phenol red.
(2) 4N ammonium hydroxide.
(3) 10% glacial acetic acid.
(4) 4% ammonium oxalate.

From the Research Service, Third (New York University) Medical Division, Goldwater Memorial Hospital, Welfare Island, New York, N. Y.
Received for publication May 6, 1955.

(5) Wash solution (10): Equal parts of 95% ethanol, ethyl ether, and water containing 2% ammonium hydroxide. Prepare daily.
(6) 2N sulfuric acid.
(7) 0.014M ammonium hexanitratocerate in 2N sulfuric acid. 7.67 Gm. of ammonium hexanitratocerate is dissolved in liter of 2N H_2SO_4.
(8) 0.025M *o*-phenanthroline ferrous sulfate ("Ferroin").[1] Dilute with water to 0.005M for use.
(9) 0.1M ferrous ammonium sulfate stock solution. 19.6 Gm. of ferrous ammonium sulfate is dissolved in 500 ml. 0.36N H_2SO_4. Stock solution is diluted with water to 0.005M for use.
(10) Standard 0.01N sodium oxalate. To 0.6698 Gm. of sodium oxalate dissolved in distilled water is added 5 ml. of conc. H_2SO_4 and the solution diluted to 1 liter (11).
(11) 4N sulfuric acid.

METHODS

Serum or Heparinized Plasma

In a 15 ml. conical centrifuge tube 2 ml. of serum or heparinized plasma is mixed with 2 ml. of distilled water; 1 ml. of 4% ammonium oxalate is added. The mixture is allowed to stand about 12 hours or if more convenient, overnight.

The sample is centrifuged at 2500 rpm for 15 minutes and the supernatant fluid removed by aspiration, using a fine-tipped pipet. The precipitate is washed with 3 ml. of wash solution. To insure thorough removal of excess oxalate, the wash solution is added slowly along the side of the tube. The precipitate is stirred with a thin glass rod and the rod is washed with wash solution as it is removed from the sample. The sample is centrifuged for 10 minutes at 2500 rpm. The supernatant wash is carefully decanted and the tube allowed to drain for a few minutes while resting inverted on absorbent paper. The washing procedure is repeated.

The moist calcium oxalate precipitate is dried by placing the tube in a water bath at room temperature and bringing the bath slowly to a boil. To the dried oxalate 2 ml. of 2N H_2SO_4 is added and the tube is heated for 1 minute to bring all the precipitate into solution. The tube is cooled to room temperature and 1 ml. of 0.014M cerate is added. The sample is stirred and allowed to stand for 30 minutes, with the stirring rod left in the tube. Orthophenanthroline indicator, 0.02 ml. of 0.005M, is added and the excess cerate is titrated with 0.005M ferrous ammonium sulfate,

[1] This oxidation-reduction indicator is purchased as an 0.025M solution.

using a 5 ml. microburet. The color change is from yellow to colorless, to a faint blue, and then to salmon pink, which represents the end point. The end point is quite sharp and distinct. Only 0.002 ml. of 0.005M ferrous ammonium sulfate is needed to effect the color change.[2, 3]

Urine

One to three milliliters of urine is pipetted into a 15 ml. conical centrifuge tube. The *p*H is adjusted to 6.5 by adding 1 drop of phenol red indicator solution and 4N NH_4OH by drops until the solution is pink. Ten per cent glacial acetic acid is then added by drops until the solution turns yellow. The calcium is precipitated by adding 1 ml. of 4% ammonium oxalate.[4] The solution is mixed and allowed to stand. After precipitation of the calcium oxalate the procedure is followed as described for plasma.

Dried Tissues and Feces

A sample of about 1 Gm. is placed in a platinum crucible (about 10 ml. capacity) with enough concentrated sulfuric acid to cover the specimen. The sample is dried at 100° and then ashed in a muffle furnace at 700° for 12 hours. The white ash is dissolved in 1–3 ml. of concentrated hydrochloric acid and transferred to a 25 ml. volumetric flask with hot water. The sample is allowed to cool and then diluted to 25 ml. A sample containing about 10 microequivalents of calcium is placed in a 15 ml. conical centrifuge tube, and the *p*H is adjusted to 6.5 and the calcium precipitated following the procedure detailed for the determination of calcium in urine.

STANDARDIZATION

The ferrous ammonium sulfate is standardized against 0.01N sodium oxalate and the cerate is standardized against the iron. One milliliter of

---

[2] At the time the cerate is added to the oxalate, there should be sufficient excess cerate to impart some yellow color to the solution. If the solution turns colorless, indicating that there is more than 14 microequivalents of calcium present, more cerate is added so that some yellow color persists.

[3] Do not use Tygon tubing as part of the titration apparatus, as this tubing oxidizes the ferrous iron.

[4] The precipitate of 10 microequivalents of calcium oxalate just about covers the bottom of a 15 ml. conical centrifuge tube. Should the precipitate appear considerably smaller or larger than this after the addition of ammonium oxalate, it would be advisable to alter the amount of the sample. One ml. of 0.014N cerate will be sufficient to titrate 14 microequivalents of calcium. If there is more calcium present than 14 microequivalents, more cerate may be added at the time of titration, but it becomes inconvenient to add much more than 5 ml. of cerate to a 15 ml. centrifuge tube.

0.014M cerate is added to 1 ml. of 0.01N sodium oxalate plus 1 ml. of 4N sulfuric acid. The solution is allowed to stand for 30 minutes. Orthophenanthroline, 0.02 ml. of 0.005M, is added and the solution is titrated against the iron solution. One milliliter of cerate plus 2 ml. of 2N sulfuric acid are also titrated directly against the iron without the addition of oxalate. The titration difference between the cerate with oxalate and cerate without oxalate represents the amount of iron which is equivalent to 1 ml. of 0.01N oxalate, which in turn is equivalent to 0.2 mg. of calcium.

SUMMARY

A method has been described for the determination of calcium in plasma, urine, and tissue and feces. Calcium is precipitated as the oxalate salt and the oxalate is determined by cerate oxidimetry.

REFERENCES

1. Clark, E. P., and Collip, J. B., *J. Biol. Chem.* **63**, 461 (1925).
2. Kirk, P. L., and Tompkins, P. C., *Ind. Eng. Chem., Anal. Ed.* **13**, 277 (1941).
3. Katzman, E., and Jacobi, M., *J. Biol. Chem.* **118**, 539 (1937).
4. Ellis, G. H., *Ind. Eng. Chem., Anal. Ed.* **10**, 112 (1938).
5. Larson, C. E., and Greenberg, D. M., *J. Biol. Chem.* **123**, 199 (1938).
6. Kochakian, C. D., and Fox, R. P., *Ind. Eng. Chem., Anal. Ed.* **16**, 762 (1944).
7. Smith, W. R., *Analyst* **69**, 14 (1944).
8. Wheatly, V. R., *Analyst* **69**, 207 (1944).
9. Smith, G. F., Sullivan, V. R., and Frank, G., *Ind. Eng. Chem., Anal. Ed.* **8**, 449 (1936).
10. Wang, C. C., *J. Biol. Chem.* **111**, 443 (1935).
11. Hawk, P. B., and Bergeim, O., *Practical Physiological Chemistry* (ed. 11). Philadelphia, Blakiston, 1937, p. 469.

Serum Beta-Lipoproteins of Normal, Atherosclerotic, and Lipemic Individuals

Changes in Concentration, Stability, and Mobility upon Incubation at 6.5° and 37.5°, as Determined by Paper Electrophoresis

Sidney P. Gottfried, Russell H. Pope, Nathan H. Friedman, Irving B. Akerson, and Salvatore Di Mauro

IT HAS BEEN OBSERVED by many investigators that the serum lipoproteins tend to decrease when allowed to stand for any length of time at room temperature or at refrigerator temperature. The latter, together with the observations of Horlick (1) who reported that the serum lipoproteins of a person with atherosclerosis were less stable when incubated with *Clostridium welchii* lecithinase than the serum lipoproteins of a normal individual, prompted us to study any changes in the concentration and stability of the serum of normal, lipemic, and atherosclerotic individuals upon incubation at 6.5° and 37.5°.

Hoch and Chanutin (2) reported that in serum stored at room temperature, a portion of the β-globulin, as measured by a Tiselius electrophoretic apparatus, increased its mobility within 36 hours of storage. Since the β-lipoproteins appear to be associated with the β-globulin fraction as far as mobility is concerned, it was decided to determine whether β-lipoproteins of normal, lipemic, and atherosclerotic sera would show a similar change in mobility on standing.

METHODS

Clotted blood was obtained from 8 normal, 8 lipemic, and 7 atherosclerotic individuals. The serum was separated as quickly as possible,

From the Biochemistry, Pathology, and Medical Departments of Bridgeport Hospital Bridgeport, Conn.
This study was aided by a grant from the Bridgeport Heart Association.
Received for publication, February 4, 1955.

and a lipoprotein pattern was run. The sera were allowed to stand for 24, 48, and 72 hours in a refrigerator at 6.5° and in a water bath at 37°. The appearance of a turbidity in the serum was noted, and lipoprotein patterns were obtained every 24 hours. In some cases, serum protein patterns were run along with the lipoproteins.

Lipoprotein and protein curves were obtained by a method previously described (3). This consisted in streaking filter paper with 0.04 ml. and 0.01 ml. serum, for a lipoprotein and protein separation respectively, and running for 24 hours in an Ivan Sorvall apparatus at 360 V. (4–6 ma.) in a barbiturate buffer at a *p*H of 8.55. The lipids were visualized by staining with Sudan III and the proteins by Amido Black B. The density of the stains was obtained by means of a Photovolt densitometer using no filter. The curves were plotted and the position of the peaks noted in inches from the origin. The concentration of the beta lipoproteins was expressed as square inches of area under the respective curves as measured by a planimeter.

A normal individual was defined as any person under 55 years of age who had no organic disturbances at the time, whose serum lipids were between 350 and 800 mg./100 ml. and whose serum cholesterol was between 150 and 300 mg./100 ml. Serum lipids were determined gravimetrically by a modification of the method of Bloor (4, 5) while the serum cholesterol was determined by the method of Kaye (6). A lipemic individual was one under 55 years of age who had no previous history of coronary involvement, but whose serum lipids were either greater than 800 mg./100 ml. or whose serum cholesterol was more than 300 mg./100 ml. Atherosclerotic individuals were chosen according to criteria set forth in a previous publication (7).

RESULTS AND DISCUSSION

In Tables 1, 2, and 3 are listed the concentration and mobility of the β-lipoproteins of normal, atherosclerotic, and lipemic serum freshly drawn and after incubating at either 6.5° or 37° for 24, 48, and 72 hours. An asterisk denotes the appearance of a visible turbidity in the serum upon incubation. In such cases, a repeat study was performed. Generally, the concentration of the β-lipoproteins tended to decrease upon standing, the decrease being practically the same for normal, atherosclerotic, or lipemic serum, and being independent of the temperatures at which the serum was incubated.

The average results denote that at either 6.5° or 37°, standing for 24 hours resulted in a decrease in the β-lipoproteins of about 10 per cent,

Table 1. β-LIPOPROTEIN STUDIES ON NORMAL SERUM

Patient	Total cholesterol (mg./100 ml.)	Total lipids (mg./100 ml.)	Concentration of β-lipoprotein (in.²/0.04 ml.)							Mobility of β-lipoprotein peak (inches from origin)						
			Fresh serum	24-Hour incubation		48-Hour incubation		72-Hour incubation		Fresh serum	24-Hour incubation		48-Hour incubation		72-Hour incubation	
				6.5°	37°	6.5°	37°	6.5°	37°		6.5°	37°	6.5°	37°	6.5°	37°
1	197	578	2.64	2.23	2.34	1.85	2.13	1.51	1.64	2.38	1.75	2.38	1.88	2.36	1.88	2.25
2	208	510	2.54	2.17	2.68	1.76	1.64	1.74	1.23	2.38	1.63	2.13	2.00	2.38	1.75	2.38
3	165	605	2.43	1.99	2.14	1.58	2.11	1.73	1.72	2.13	1.63	2.38	1.00	2.25	1.25	2.50
4	230	700	2.36	2.07	2.23	2.07	1.88	2.14	1.82*	1.88	1.13	2.25	1.00	2.25	0.75	0.38*
	235	747	2.24	1.95	1.93	1.83	1.85	1.95	1.92	1.88	2.25	2.75	1.63	2.50	2.00	..
5	193	580	2.29	2.03	1.76	1.97	1.92	1.94	2.07*	1.88	1.25	1.50	1.63	2.25	1.25	0.50*
	..	..	2.09	1.92	1.78	1.71	1.58*	1.65	1.81*	2.13	1.50	2.13	2.38	2.00*	1.75	0.0*
6	157	570	1.94	1.74	1.64	1.43	1.30	1.45	1.03	1.88	1.88	2.63	2.50	2.38	2.13	1.38
7	153	700	2.67	2.68	2.56	2.20	2.12	2.23	2.56	1.75	2.00	2.38	1.88	..	1.38	..
8	188	587	1.94	1.74	1.63*	1.80	1.63*	1.67	1.43*	2.13	1.88	1.00*	1.88	0.25*	1.00	0.0*
AVERAGE	..	..	2.31	2.05	2.07	1.82	1.82	1.80	1.72	..	..	..	..	..	..	..

* Denotes a turbid serum.

Table 2. β-Lipoprotein Studies on Atherosclerotic Serum

Patient	Total cholesterol (mg./100 ml.)	Total lipids (mg./100 ml.)	Concentration of β-lipoprotein (in.²/0.04 ml.)							Mobility of β-lipoprotein peak (inches from origin)						
			Fresh serum	24-Hour incubation		48-Hour incubation		72-Hour incubation		Fresh serum	24-Hour incubation		48-Hour incubation		72-Hour incubation	
				6.5°	37°	6.5°	37°	6.5°	37°		6.5°	37°	6.5°	37°	6.5°	37°
1	267	980	2.37	2.36	2.34	2.13	2.33	1.43	1.76	2.25	2.25	2.75	2.00	2.38	2.13	3.00
2	295	900	2.40	2.20	2.10	2.08	1.97*	2.01	2.03*	2.50	2.25	2.50	2.00	0*	2.00	0*
	357	973	2.44	2.33	2.21	2.23	2.01	1.78	1.82	1.80	1.13	2.38	2.00	2.63	2.13	2.88
3	237	950	2.57	2.12	2.06	2.21	1.80*	2.01	1.65*	2.63	2.00	2.75	2.25	0.38*	2.38	0*
	254	847	2.63	2.42	2.30	2.20	2.12*	2.29	2.22*	2.00	2.00	2.75	1.88	1.13*	1.63	0.25*
4	256	880	1.95	1.66	1.86*	..	2.08*	1.65	1.64*	2.50	1.75	0.25*	..	0*	2.13	0*
	245	963	2.23	2.09	2.02	1.90	1.58*	1.86	1.64*	1.63	1.75	1.75	1.50	1.13*	2.00	0*
5	267	933	2.62	2.17	2.22	2.08	1.77*	1.57	1.41*	2.38	1.88	2.75	1.88	0.38*	1.88	0.38*
	228	933	2.43	2.29	2.24	1.91	2.03	1.84	1.81*	2.00	1.88	2.75	2.25	2.63	1.63	1.50*
6	290	1062	1.90	1.61	2.02	1.90	2.03	1.43	1.72	2.00	2.13	2.75	2.00	2.25	2.25	2.87
7	292	850	2.73	2.14	2.32	1.97	1.99	1.72	1.96	1.80	1.25	2.25	1.75	2.50	1.88	2.50
8	284	950	2.19	1.97	2.00	1.85	2.11	1.63	..	1.88	1.88	2.25	1.63	2.38	2.00	..
Average	..	..	2.37	2.11	2.14	2.04	1.98	1.77	1.79	..	..	..	..	..	..	..

*Denotes a turbid serum.

Table 3. β-Lipoprotein Studies on Lipemic Serum

Patient	Total cholesterol (mg./100 ml.)	Total lipids (mg./100 ml.)	*Concentration of β-lipoprotein* (in.²/0.04 ml.)							*Mobility of β-lipoprotein peak* (inches from origin)						
			Fresh serum	24-Hour incubation		48-Hour incubation		72-Hour incubation		Fresh serum	24-Hour incubation		48-Hour incubation		72-Hour incubation	
				6.5°	37°	6.5°	37°	6.5°	37°		6.5°	37°	6.5°	37°	6.5°	37°
1	273	935	2.75	2.01	1.84	2.21	1.76	1.60	1.63	1.88	2.00	2.38	2.00	2.88	2.00	2.88
2	312	938	2.51	2.18	2.27	2.09	2.22	1.89	2.16	2.50	1.88	2.50	1.88	2.13	2.13	2.75
3	256	843	2.49	2.31	2.14	1.79	2.17	1.78	2.05	2.25	2.00	2.38	1.88	2.38	1.13	2.75
4	280	873	2.50	2.28	2.38	2.18	1.92*	2.09	1.87*	2.25	2.25	2.63	1.75	1.13*	2.13	0.63*
	278	910	2.21	1.96	2.06*	1.83	2.02*	..	..	2.25	1.87	1.25*	1.75	0.25*	..	..
5	249	920	2.69	2.44	2.54	2.50	2.63*	2.37	2.05*	2.50	2.00	2.75	2.25	2.13*	1.75	0*
	..	..	2.40	2.34	2.41	2.27	2.37	2.21	2.19	1.75	2.25	3.00	2.75	3.50	2.00	2.87
6	280	1273	2.91	2.76	2.70	2.69	2.71	2.34	2.60	2.13	1.13	2.13	1.88	2.38	1.75	2.50
7	220	1050	2.23	2.18	2.18	2.30	1.98	..	..	1.88	1.88	2.38	1.88	2.38	..	..
Average	..	..	2.53	2.27	2.28	2.21	2.20	2.04	2.08	..	..	..	..	..	..	..

* Denotes a turbid serum.

after 48 hours the decrease was 20 per cent, and after 72 hours, 25 per cent.

If the average results for the β-lipoprotein concentrations in fresh serum are examined, it will be noticed that the results are the same for both normal and atherosclerotic individuals, 2.31 and 2.37 respectively. The atherosclerotic patients studied in this report were all ambulatory, and more or less had returned to their normal routine which had been interrupted by the immobilizing myocardial infarct. The above results are in agreement with those reported by the authors in a recent publication (8). The latter stated that in many cases, soon after an immobilizing infarct, the β-lipoproteins were elevated but tended to become normal as the time from the infarct increased. Table 3, however, shows that the β-lipoproteins in fresh lipemic sera run slightly higher than in fresh normal or atherosclerotic sera, averaging 2.53. None of these lipemic sera showed any marked initial turbidity.

Attention is drawn to the very close agreement between the average results of the β-lipoprotein concentrations of sera incubated at 6.5° and at 37°. The greatest difference is 4.5 per cent.

When the figures for the mobility of the β-lipoprotein peaks are examined before and after incubation, the following observations can be made. If the position of the β-lipoprotein peak of freshly drawn serum is used as a reference point, it will be observed that in practically all cases of normal, atherosclerotic, and lipemic serum incubated at 37° the peak becomes more mobile and migrates further from the origin. This change in mobility is somewhat accentuated as the time of incubation is increased from 24 to 72 hours. However, this phenomena does not occur when the serum becomes turbid. In such cases, the peak becomes less mobile, migrating toward the origin.

If the position of the peaks obtained by incubating at 6.5° are noted, a decrease in the mobility of the β-lipoproteins will be found to occur in most cases, the peak of the freshly drawn serum again being used as the reference. This decrease in mobility does not always become greater as the period of incubation is increased. In many cases it becomes less, and in a few cases the decrease in mobility turns into an increase after incubating 48 or 72 hours. This irregularity in results may be due to an inability to obtain a reproducible peak for the β-lipoproteins. If the tables are examined, it will be noted that the peak of the β-lipoproteins of freshly drawn serum varies from 1.63 to 2.63 inches from the origin. This large spread in the position of the β-lipoprotein peak indicates that the increase in mobility of the β-lipoproteins, which has been reported to occur after incubating at 37°, might not be real. Those cases which report an increase in mobility of less than 1.00 inch lie within the above reported spread, and cannot be considered significant.

However, since the mobilities of a serum incubated at 6.5 and 37° were always determined in a simultaneous run, the observation that the mobility of the β-lipoprotein peak after incubating at 37° is always greater than the peak obtained after incubating at 6.5° must be considered significant. This holds for either normal, atherosclerotic, or lipemic serum. The only exceptions that occur are upon the appearance of a visible turbidity in the serum. This takes place only upon incubating at 37°, never at 6.5°. In most cases, the turbidity appeared after 48 hours. In only 1 case did it appear as early as after 24 hours. When repeat determinations were performed on those sera in which a turbidity did occur, in 5 of 8 cases a turbidity reoccurred. Although the total number of cases is not large enough, it does appear from Tables 1, 2, and 3 that atherosclerotic serum has the greatest tendency to become turbid upon incubating at 37°.

In order to study more fully the variations in the β-lipoprotein pattern after incubation, serum protein as well as lipoprotein patterns were obtained on 12 normal, atherosclerotic, and lipemic sera according to the procedure already described. Two types of curves were obtained, one in which no turbidity occurred, the other in which a turbidity did occur. Figure 1, *A–E*, is typical of a case in which no turbidity occurred after incubation. They represent the protein and lipoprotein curves in an atherosclerotic serum before and after incubation at 6.5° and 37° for 24 and 48 hours.

The curves reveal that the mobility of the protein fractions remain constant whether incubated at 6.5° or at 37°. Likewise, the β-lipoproteins incubated at 6.5° do not show any change in mobility, the peak lying between the β- and γ-globulins. However, the β-lipoproteins incubated at 37° do reveal an increase in mobility after 24 hours, the peak shifting to between the β- and α_2-globulins. This increase in mobility is somewhat accentuated after incubating for 48 hours. Therefore, it is evident that these curves corroborate the inference from figures reported in Tables 1, 2, and 3—that the mobility of the β-lipoproteins incubated at 37° is greater than the mobility of the β-lipoproteins incubated at 6.5°. In addition, Fig. 1, *A–E,* denotes that incubating at 6.5° probably does not cause a decrease in the mobility of the β-lipoproteins.

Although the mobility of the β-lipoproteins increases upon incubating at 37°, no increase was observed in the mobility of the β-globulins. This

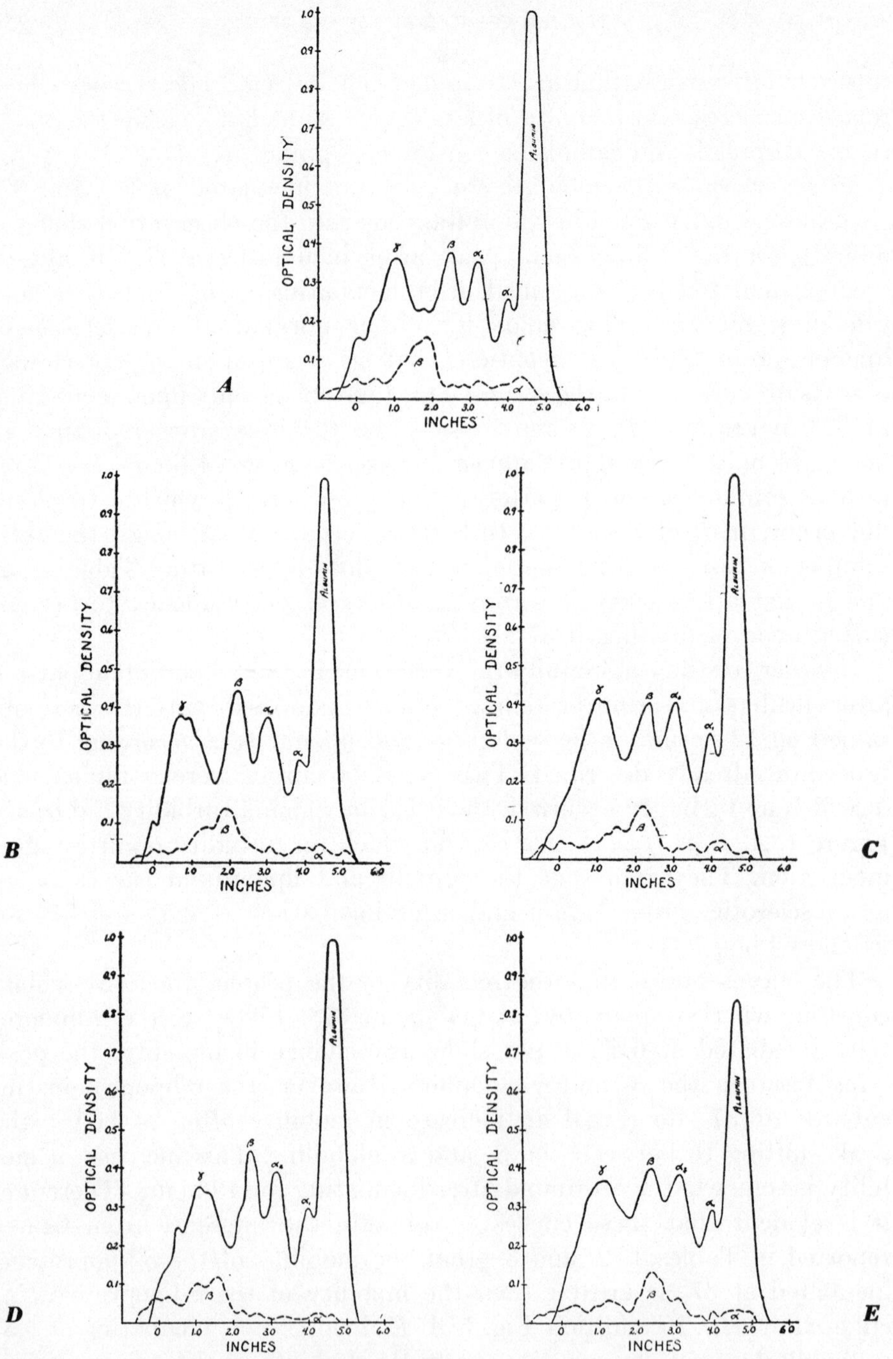

Fig. 1*A*. Protein and lipoprotein fractionation curves of fresh serum in a case of atherosclerosis. Solid lines represent the protein; broken lines the lipid profiles. ***B.*** After 24 hour incubation at 6.5°. ***C.*** After 24 hour incubation at 37.5°. ***D.*** After 48 hour incubation at 6.5°. ***E.*** After 48 hour incubation at 37.5°.

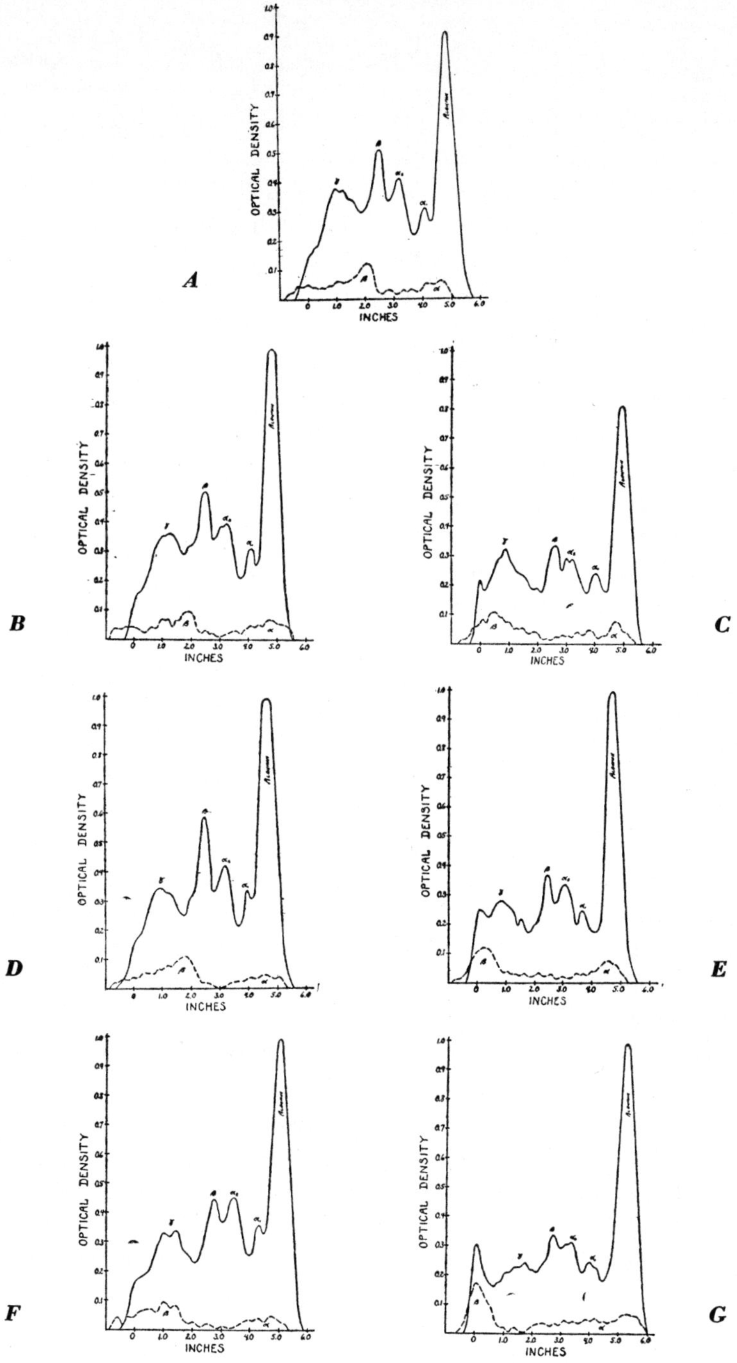

Fig. 2*A*. Protein and lipoprotein fractionation curves of fresh serum from a normal adult. Solid lines represent the protein; broken lines the lipid profiles. ***B*.** After 24 hour incubation at 6.5°. ***C*.** After 24 hour incubation at 37.5°. ***D*.** After 48 hour incubation at 6.5°. ***E*.** After 48 hour incubation at 37.5°. ***F*.** After 72 hour incubation at 6.5°. ***G*.** After 72 hour incubation at 37.5°.

is at variance with the observations of Hoch and Chanutin (2), who stated that using the Tiselius electrophoresis technic, an increase was obtained in the mobility of the β-globulins of stored serum.

Figure 2, *A–G*, is typical of a case in which a turbidity occurred after incubation. They represent the protein and lipoprotein curves in a normal serum before and after incubation at 6.5° and 37° for 24, 48, and 72 hours. It is noticed that at 37° after a period of 24 hours the appearance of a turbidity in the serum is accompanied by a decrease in the mobility of the β-lipoproteins, the peak shifting toward the origin. After 48 hours, when an increase in the turbidity of the serum is evident, it is noticed that the β-lipoprotein peak has moved closer to the origin. At the end of 72 hours, practically the entire β-lipoprotein fraction has concentrated at the origin, denoting an almost complete loss of mobility.

Along with the appearance of a turbidity in the serum is the formation of a sixth protein fraction less mobile than the γ-globulins. As the turbidity increases after incubating for 48 hours, this sixth protein fraction increases at the expense of the β- and γ-globulins, and moves closer to the origin. At 72 hours this new protein fraction has increased even more, and has shifted to such an extent that the peak is located directly at the origin, coinciding with the peak of the β-lipoproteins. The β- and γ-globulins have continued to decrease, and at this point the α-globulins also have begun to decrease.

In the case presented above, the turbidity appeared after only a 24-hour incubation, and was considerable. In other cases where the turbidity does not appear until after 48 or 72 hours and is not marked, this sixth protein fraction is small, and little or no decrease in the other globulins occurs.

The sixth protein fraction is probably "denatured" protein as evidenced by the concomitant decrease in solubility (increase in serum turbidity) and decrease in mobility. Likewise, the β-lipoproteins are probably "denatured" after incubating at 37°, since with increasing turbidity the mobility of the β-lipoproteins decrease considerably.

Two questions arise: first, why the proteins and lipoproteins of some sera should change upon incubation at 37° and some not; second, why a turbidity appears in one serum specimen but not in another, when obtained from the same individual at a later date. These questions may possibly have some bearing upon the pathogenesis of atherosclerosis.

Nothing has been stated concerning the α-lipoproteins, since no marked change in the concentration, stability, and mobility of this fraction after incubation at 6.5° or 37° has been noted, employing the separation and staining technic described in this paper.

SUMMARY

1. Serum lipids, cholesterol, and lipoproteins were determined on 8 normal, 7 atherosclerotic, and 8 lipemic individuals in the fasting state. Serum lipids and cholesterol were determined chemically, the lipoproteins by paper electrophoresis. Serum lipoproteins were also performed after incubating at 6.5° and 37° for 24, 48, and 72 hours, and changes in the physical appearance of the serum, and in the concentration and mobility of the β-lipoproteins were observed. In 12 of the above cases, serum protein patterns were noted with the lipoprotein patterns.

2. In many cases a visible turbidity appeared upon incubating at 37°, never upon incubating at 6.5°. In most cases this turbidity appeared after incubating for 48 hours, and tended to occur more frequently in atherosclerotic sera than in normal sera.

3. The concentration of β-lipoproteins decreased upon incubating either at 6.5° or at 37°, the decrease being of the same order of magnitude for normal, atherosclerotic, or lipemic sera.

4. Incubating at 37° increased the mobility of the β-lipoproteins (except when a turbidity appeared), the peak shifting from between the β- and γ-globulins to between the β- and α_2-globulins. Incubating at 6.5° had no effect on the mobility of the β-lipoproteins.

5. When a turbidity appeared upon incubating at 37°, the mobility of the β-lipoproteins decreased, the peak shifting toward the origin. As the turbidity became marked, a sixth protein fraction appeared, of slower mobility than the γ-globulin. This protein fraction first appeared to form at the expense of the β- and γ-globulins and then at the expense of the α-globulins, all of which decreased. It is considered that the turbidity is due to the formation of "denatured" proteins and lipoproteins which are characterized by a decrease in mobility.

6. No consistent changes were noted in the concentration, stability and mobility of the α-lipoproteins upon incubating at either 6.5° or 37°.

REFERENCES

1. Horlick, L., *Circulation* **10**, 30 (1954).
2. Hoch, H., and Chanutin, A., *J. Biol. Chem.* **209**, 661 (1954).
3. Gottfried, S. P., Pope, R. H., Friedman, N. H., and Di Mauro, S., *J. Lab. Clin. Med.* **44**, 651 (1954).
4. Bloor, W. R., *J. Biol. Chem.* **17**, 377 (1914).
5. Bloor, W. R., *J. Biol. Chem.* **77**, 53 (1928).
6. Kaye, I. A., *J. Lab. Clin. Med.* **25**, 966 (1940).
7. Gottfried, S. P., Friedman, N. H., Pope, R. H., Akerson, I. B., and Di Mauro, S., *Circulation* **10**, 271 (1954).
8. Gottfried, S. P., Pope, R. H., Friedman, N. H., Akerson, I. B., and Di Mauro, S. *Am. J. Med. Sci.* **229**, 34 (1955).

A Note on Quantitative Urobilinogen Determinations

Bernard Balikov

The Watson method for the quantitative estimation of urobilinogen in urine and feces in the evaluation of hepatic and hemolytic diseases (1–4) has become widely accepted as a useful tool in clinical practice. The optimum acidity for extraction of urobilinogen from the ferrous hydroxide filtrate, however, has been dealt with vaguely in the literature. Studies on this step of the procedure show it to have a marked influence upon the result.

MATERIAL AND METHOD

The urine specimens were selected from patients under observation for various forms of liver disease and the stool specimens from those received in the laboratory for routine parasitologic or bacteriologic examinations.

The method of Schwartz, Sborov and Watson (1) was employed for the urobilinogen determinations except for the establishment of the standard curve using pontacyl dyes which is described by Watson and Hawkinson (4). Readings were made at 565 mμ on the Coleman Junior Spectrophotometer Model 6A.

The critical aspect of this study is concerned with the concentration of acetic acid in urine or fecal samples after the addition of fresh ferrous sulfate and 10% sodium hydroxide which yields final concentrations of 2.5% sodium hydroxide in urine samples and 2.0% in fecal specimens. At this point varying amounts of water and glacial acetic acid were

From the Percy Jones Army Hospital, Battle Creek, Mich.

Present address: Chemistry Section, The Surgical Research Unit, Brooke Army Medical Center, Fort Sam Houston, Texas.

Reprinted essentially unchanged from *The Clinical Chemist* 5, 89 (1954).

added to the ferrous hydroxide filtrate to make final acid concentrations ranging from 0.1% to 50%. Extraction with petroleum benzine was then carried out in the usual fashion.

RESULTS

Urine

Identical aliquots of ferrous hydroxide filtrate were pipetted into each of several separatory funnels. Water and glacial acetic acid were added to make the final volume 50 ml. and extraction with petroleum benzine, and so on, was carried out in the usual fashion. Results of a series of experiments are shown in Fig. 1. It is apparent that the most complete extraction is realized with a glacial acetic acid concentration of 2%. That this extraction actually is complete was checked by a second extraction made immediately after the first, in which a negligible amount of urobilinogen was recovered (99% transmittance). Similar results were obtained using either 5 or 10 ml. of filtrate for extraction, indicating complete extraction of at least 10 ml. of filtrate.

Determinations of *p*H over the critical range of 0.5 to 4.0% glacial

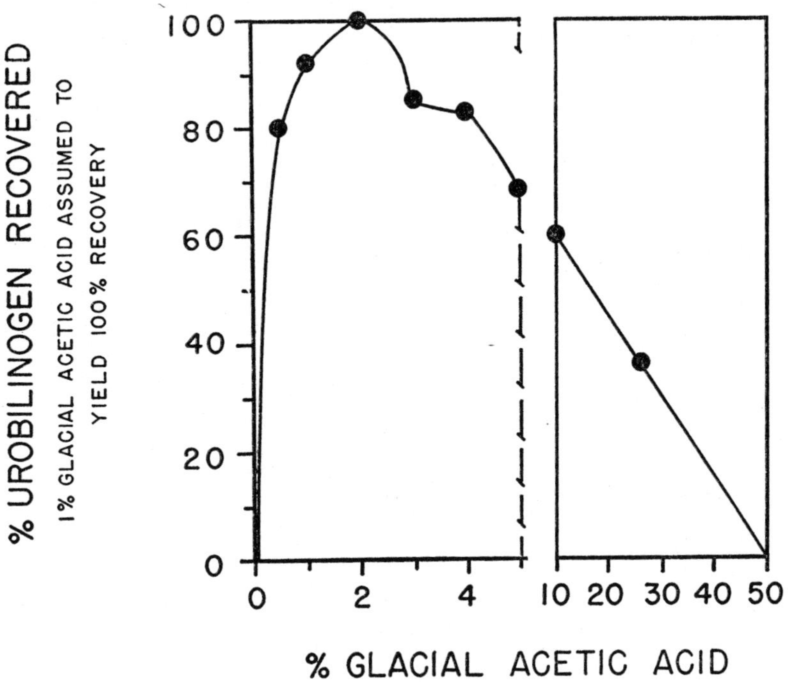

Fig. 1. Recovery of urine urobilinogen from varying glacial acetic acid concentrations.

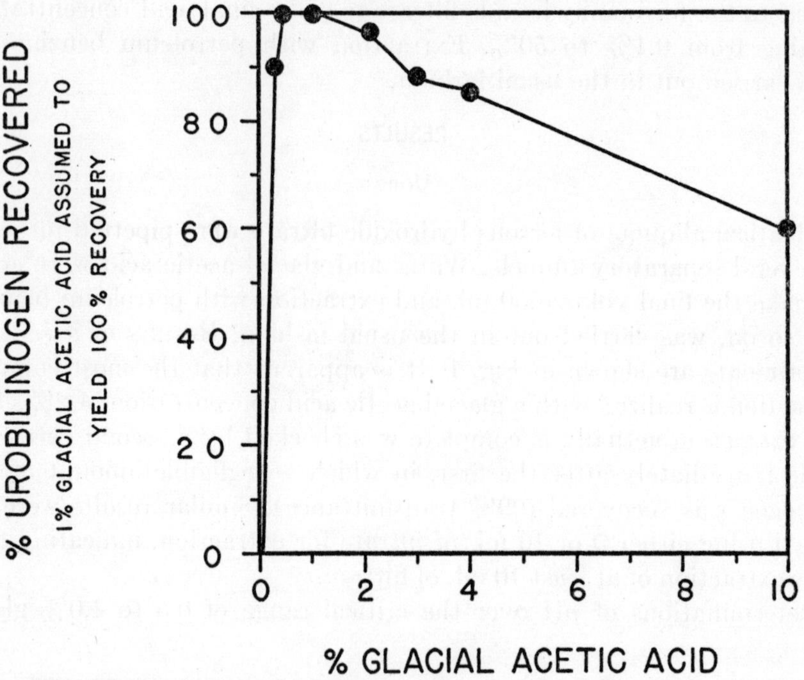

Fig. 2. Recovery of fecal urobilinogen from varying glacial acetic acid concentrations.

Table 1. Relation between Concentration of Acetic Acid and *p*H of Ferrous Hydroxide Filtrate

Glacial acetic acid concentration (%)	*p*H	
	5 ml. of filtrate	*10 ml. of filtrate*
	URINE	
0.5	4.4	4.9
1.0	4.0	4.3
2.0	3.7	3.9
3.0	3.5	3.8
4.0	3.3	3.6
	FECES	
0.1	6.1	11.6
0.5	4.0	4.4
1.0	3.7	3.9
2.0	3.3	3.6
3.0	3.2	3.4

acetic acid are shown in Table 1. A Beckman *p*H Meter Model G was used for all *p*H measurements.

Feces

Identical experiments were carried out on feces as described for urine, above. Glacial acetic acid concentrations ranged from 0.1 to 10%. From Fig. 2, it can be seen that the optimum concentration of glacial acetic acid is between 0.5% and approximately 1.5%. Here also similar results were obtained using 5 or 10 ml. of filtrate for extraction.

Determination of *p*H over the critical range of 0.1 to 3.0% glacial acetic acid are shown in Table 1.

The experiments were repeated on 5 separate samples of both urine and feces and yielded identical results in each instance.

DISCUSSION

Various references (2, 3) to the methods for extraction of urobilinogen from urine and feces are somewhat vague as to the specific degree of acidification optimum in the procedure. The importance of this aspect of the method has been a matter of some speculation in this laboratory. We were gratified, therefore, to note that optimum extractions were obtained uniformly when acidification of urine filtrates were held rigidly at the end concentrations of 2.0% glacial acetic acid, and the fecal filtrates at 1%. We have, therefore, instituted the following modifications of the standard Watson method referred to above.

Urine

Either 5 or 10 ml. of ferrous hydroxide filtrate is transferred to a separatory funnel. Water is added to bring the volume to 49 ml. One ml. of c.p. glacial acetic acid is added and the solution is mixed. Petroleum benzine is added and the analysis is continued as outlined by Watson and co-workers (1, 4).

Feces

The ferrous hydroxide filtrate is treated precisely as is urine except that water is added to bring the volume to 49.5 ml. and 0.5 ml. of C.P. glacial acetic acid is added.

The above findings have suggested that additional study of urobilinogen at various *p*H levels and its possible solubility in organic acids would be of value. Such a study will be undertaken shortly.

It is not surprising that the optimum acetic acid concentration is less for the fecal ferrous hydroxide filtrate than for the urine since the former is less alkaline than the urine.

The significance of the plateaus in Figs. 1 and 2 between acid concentrations of 3 and 4% is not known.

SUMMARY

A procedure has been discussed whereby the optimum extraction of urobilinogen from feces and urine can be accomplished by standardization of acidulation of the ferrous hydroxide filtrates in the Watson method.

REFERENCES

1. Schwartz, S., Sborov, V., and Watson, C. J., *Am. J. Clin. Path.* **14,** 598 (1944).
2. Watson, C. J., *Arch. Int. Med.* **47,** 698 (1931).
3. Watson, C. J., *Am. J. Clin. Path.* **6,** 458 (1936).
4. Watson, C. J., and Hawkinson, V., *Am. J. Clin. Path.* **17,** 108 (1947).

Cross-Contaminator Exclusion Test for Dry-Ashing Determination of Protein-Bound Iodine

Meyer Samson, Herman Brown, and Seymour Eichen

Oxidation of organic material as a preliminary to determination of iodine, whether by wet or dry methods, entails loss of iodine if insufficient organic matter is present during the reaction (1, 2, 3). In blood serum, the organic content suffices to prevent this loss when the amount of iodine in the specimen is in the range found in physiological or pathological sera, 0–30 μg./100 ml., as has been repeatedly shown in recovery experiments (4, 5, 6, 7). When the iodine content of serum exceeds 500 μg./100 ml., as is sometimes the case after administration of iodinated radiopaque media, or other contact with iodinated medication, iodine may be volatilized in the ashing stage of the analysis, to be reabsorbed in other tubes. Such cross-contamination invalidates the entire series of tests, with loss of analyst's time and delay of reports.

To avoid delays caused by the presence of such cross-contaminators, a simple method of screening them out in advance was desirable. In connection with the quantitative dry-ashing procedure in use in this laboratory (7), the cross-contaminator exclusion test described below has proven satisfactory. It requires only 1 drop of serum, and adds no more than 30 minutes of operating time to a series of 20–40 PBI determinations.

REAGENTS AND APPARATUS

* 4N Sodium carbonate in dropper bottle.

Approximately 4N hydrochloric acid in dropper bottle.

* Approximately 0.15N arsenious acid in dropper bottle.

From the Departments of Research and Clinical Chemistry, The Samson Laboratories, Philadelphia, Pa.

Received for publication April 12, 1955.

* These items are identical with those used in quantitative PBI procedure (7).

* Approximately 0.065N ceric ammonium sulfate in dropper bottle.
* Muffle furnace, with control for 600° ± 25°.

Automatic electric Time Switch.[1]

Twin infrared heater with reflectors.[2]

Stainless steel test tube rack, 6 rows of 15 x 14 mm. holes.[3]

Pyrex test tubes with lip, 75 x 12 mm.

PROCEDURE

1. Place 1 drop (0.05 ml.) of serum and 2 drops of 4N Na_2CO_3 into a test tube. Shake rack. Dry completely under infrared heater.

   The serum is dropped from the pipet used for the quantitative tests. Step 1 is set up simultaneously with the start of protein precipitation for the quantitative work. The Fisher Infra-rediator effects good drying in 2 hours if the lamps are adjusted about ½ in. from the tops of the tubes.

2. Put rack into muffle furnace preheated to 600°. Set automatic time switch to shut off at 2½ hours.

   Step 2 is started at about the same time that the material in the quantitative tests goes into the drying oven.

3. To the cold ash, add 2 drops 4N HCl plus 1 drop arsenious acid solution. Shake. Allow to stand ten minutes. Add 1 drop ceric ammonium sulfate solution. Shake. Allow to stand 5 minutes. Read colors over a white background immediately at the end of 5 minutes, looking downward through tubes. Decolorized tubes indicate potential cross-contaminators.[4]

   Step 3 is carried out the morning after Step 2. Reading of cross-contaminator exclusion tests is complete by the time the muffle is preheated to 600° for the quantitative determinations.

   To guard against reagent deterioration, a blank containing Na_2CO_3 only, as well as a normal serum and one to which inorganic iodide equivalent to 400 μg. of iodine per 100 ml. has been added, are included in the qualitative series. The first two should be clear yellow at 5 minutes, the last completely decolorized.

EXPERIMENTAL DATA

When the need for a test to exclude cross-contaminating artefactual sera from the muffle furnace stage of dry ashing PBI determinations

[1] Electric Hotpack Company, Inc., Philadelphia: #6080B Limitor.

[2] Fisher Scientific Company, Pittsburgh: Heater, Infra-rediator, #11-504-5.

[3] Drummond Scientific Company, Philadelphia.

[4] Specimens decolorizing in 5 minutes are withdrawn from the quantitative ashing procedure. The dried proteinate, however, is not discarded. Instead, it is ashed separately and run through the quantitative procedure as usual, as a verification of the qualitative test.

became apparent, a search was made for a simple qualitative procedure. Feigl's (10) spot plate test for iodine appeared most promising, since its reagents were similar to those used in most quantitative procedures for serum iodine. It was accordingly adapted to serum ash. Pyrex test tubes were found to be the best ashing containers, as in quantitative work, since iodine losses occurred during ashing in shallow platewells or micro-crucibles.

RESULTS

Typical results appear in Table 1. Decolorization of cerium within 5 minutes after its addition to the acidified and arsenized ash solution was regularly obtained at a level of 0.2 μg. I_2 per drop (0.05 ml.) of serum,

Table 1. DECOLORIZATION TIMES OF CERIC SOLUTIONS

Iodine (*μg./100 ml.*)	*I_2 plus reagents unmuffled* (*min.*)	*I_2 plus reagents muffled* (*min.*)	*I_2 plus serum and reagents muffled* (*min.*)
100	Y 10	Y 10	Y 10
200	D 3	D 4	D 7
400	D 1	D 3	D 4
800	D 0.75	D 1.5	D 3

Y = yellow; D = decolorized.

equivalent to 400 μg. I_2/100 ml. This finding was not affected by the source of the added iodine, whether inorganic, as thyroxin, or as artefactual serum with an unknown iodine compound content. To avoid occasional cross-contamination during the qualitative muffling by sera containing very large amounts of iodine ($>$9000 μg./100 ml.), the proportion of carbonate to serum was increased to double that in the quantitative procedure. The effectiveness of this measure has led to consideration of the possibility of improvement of quantitative dry-ashing procedures in the same direction, a matter now being studied in our laboratory.

DISCUSSION

Practical methods for the determination of iodine in the fractional microgram amounts present in small serum samples depend on the catalytic acceleration of the reduction of ceric salts by arsenite in acid solutions, first described by Kolthoff and Sandell (8). While with the aid of instrumental analysis (9), this reaction is capable of differentiating increments of inorganic iodide in pure aqueous solution as small as 0.02 μg./100 ml., its sensitivity in qualitative work, in which the distinction is between clearly visible yellow and colorlessness, is considerably lower. Feigl's (10) spot plate modification of the Kolthoff-Sandell reaction is read at 30 minutes, for which time an identification limit of 0.05 μg. KI per drop is given, equivalent to 75 μg. iodine per 100 ml. The sensitivity of the serum cross-contaminator exclusion test described above, for which a time limit of 5 minutes has been established for convenient inclusion in the quantitative procedure, and which contains much sodium chloride, is of the order of 400 μg. per 100 ml., or one twenty-thousandth that of increment differentiation under optimum conditions. It is nevertheless sufficient for the purpose. Concentrations of iodine below this level have not, in experience with the method in use in this laboratory, caused cross-contamination. If further analytical experience, or the advent of iodinated medications of cross-contaminating capacity at lower concentration, makes a more sensitive test desirable, one may be readily adapted from the experimental data set forth.

Not all artefactual sera have the same cross-contaminating potential. Some sera having iodine content upward of 5000 μg./100 ml. did not cross-contaminate known control sera included in the series. On the other hand, some artefactual sera with iodine content one tenth the above level have been implicated. It is evident that volatilization of iodine depends to a large extent on the nature of the compound present. Further study to evaluate the analytical characteristics of the various iodinated medications apt to be found in serum may prove valuable.

SUMMARY

A simple qualitative test for iodine in blood serum has been described. It is designed to detect sera which are potential cross-contaminators in dry-ashing PBI procedures. One drop of serum is used. Added operating time in a PBI series of 20–40 determinations is not over 30 minutes.

REFERENCES

1. Taurog, A., and Chaikoff, I. L., *J. Biol. Chem.* **163**, 313 (1946).
2. Barker, S. B., *J. Biol. Chem.*, **173**, 715 (1948).
3. Association of Official Agricultural Chemists, Washington, D. C., *Methods of Analysis*, "Iodine in Drugs-official", p. 597 (1950).
4. Decker, J. W., and Hayden, H. J. *Anal. Chem.* **23**, 798 (1951).
5. Barker, S. B., Humphrey, M. J., and Soley, M. H., *J. Clin. Invest.* **30**, 55 (1951).
6. Man, E. B., Kydd, D. M., and Peters, J. B., *J. Clin. Invest.* **30**, 531 (1951).
7. Brown, H., Reingold, A. M., and Samson, M., *J. Clin. Endocrinol. and Metabolism* **13**, 444 (1953).
8. Kolthoff, I. M., and Sandell, E. B., *J. Am. Chem. Soc.* **56**, 1426 (1934).
9. Chaney, A. L., *Anal. Chem.* **22**, 939 (1950).
10. Feigl, F., *Spot Tests*, Houston, Texas, Elsevier Press, 1954, Vol. I, p. 250.

the Clinical Chemist

EDITORIAL

AT THE TIME this is being written, a lawsuit is in process in Des Moines, Iowa, to determine whether hospitals are engaging in the practice of medicine when they own and operate laboratories and hire specialists to work in these laboratories. This suit was initiated by the Iowa Hospital Association and 34 member hospitals, and they have requested the court, with District Judge C. Edwin Moore presiding, to overrule the Iowa Attorney General's opinion, that hospitals owning and operating laboratories are practicing medicine illegally. Defendants in this action are the Attorney General's Office, the Iowa State Board of Medical Examiners, and the Iowa Association of Pathologists.

The clinical chemist is not a principal in this controversy, yet he obviously will be very directly affected in any decision as to what constitutes the practice of medicine as it relates to laboratory procedures. The American Association of Clinical Chemists has contended from the beginning that clinical chemistry is not the practice of medicine and the chemist is not engaged in the practice of medicine when he performs chemical determinations requested by a physician, or when he discusses these determinations with a physician who may seek information in the interest of his patient. These concepts are clearly stated in the Resolution on Legislation and in the Code of Ethics of the American Association of Clinical Chemists.

The Association does not of course take any official position in this Iowa controversy. The points of conflict are far-reaching and extend much beyond the chemistry laboratory. But the Association is prepared, however, to defend the rights of the clinical chemist at all times to practice his specialty at the highest professional and scientific level. This is in the public interest.

MAX M. FRIEDMAN
National Secretary

Following are accounts of the testimony that appeared in the Des Moines, Iowa, *Register* and *Tribune*, May 24 and 25, 1955. (Reprinted by permission of the publishers.)

Says Chemists Are Underpaid

By Walter Shotwell.

Clinical chemists associated with hospitals or universities generally are "miserably underpaid and overworked," Dr. John G. Reinhold, Glen Mills, Penn., testified Monday in Polk county district court.

But, he added, money is a "secondary consideration" because "a good scientist usually is a dedicated man."

Second Witness.

Senior consultant in biochemistry to the United States army's surgeon, Dr. Reinhold was the second witness called by the Iowa Hospital Association in a trial to determine whether Iowa hospitals may legally operate laboratories staffed with hired specialists.

Dr. Reinhold said in response to questions that never in his experience has a hospital administration interfered with his professional judgment.

He testified that he prefers employment with a hospital because he feels that employment by an individual pathologist would limit the "free relationship between physician and scientist" and the scope of scientific research.

He termed it "highly significant" that few laboratory techniques have been developed by medical doctors, explaining that "they haven't had the interest."

Still, Dr. Reinhold testified, "We (the U. S.) lead the world in clinical chemistry."

Under cross-examination, Dr. Reinhold testified that he regards his responsibility as providing information to the physician, who then makes appropriate decisions.

He said no relationship exists directly between the chemist and the patient and that the chemist receives no money from the patient. However, he said the chemist will occasionally view the patient's medical record during consultation with the physician.

Friedman Testifies.

Also testifying Tuesday afternoon was Dr. Max M. Friedman, Rego Park, N. Y., chemist of Lebanon Hospital in New York, N. Y.

Dr. Friedman testified as to contributions made by clinical chemists to medical advancements but said chemists "are not competent" to practice medicine as such.

He testified that if individual clinical chemists were required to work only for individual pathologists, it "would hamper the progress of biochemistry, discourage well-trained chemists" from entering the medical field and would force chemists to work with poor facilities.

Chemists also would have less time for research, Dr. Friedman testified. He said he "disagrees violently" with one leading chemist who predicted in a nationally-circulated journal that in the future chemists may actually treat patients.

Dr. Friedman also denied under cross-examination that "formidable warfare" exists between chemists and pathologists. However, he admitted that the chemists have been seeking legislation to grant them "recognition."

AACC ELECTIONS

President

Otto Schales, of the Alton Ochsner Clinic in New Orleans, La., was elected President of the American Association of Clinical Chemists to succeed Lt. Col. Monroe E. Freeman, whose term of office expired on June 30, 1955. Dr. Schales has served the Association in many capacities and was Vice-President for the past year. He is well known to his colleagues for his scientific and professional attainments. His term of office is to extend until June 30, 1956.

Officers

The other officers elected for the same period were Robert M. Hill, University of Colorado Medical School, Vice-President; Max M. Friedman, Lebanon Hospital, New York City, National Secretary; and Louis B. Dotti, St. Luke's Hospital, New York City, National Treasurer.

Executive Committee

The new Executive Committee will consist of the above officers in addition to the following members: Monroe E. Freeman, Medical Service Corps, Washington, D. C.; Joseph H. Gast, Baylor University School of Medicine; William H. Goldwater, U. S. Naval Radiological Defense Laboratory, San Francisco; Icie M. Hoobler, Children's Fund of Michigan, Detroit; and Samuel Natelson, Rockford Memorial Hospital, Rockford, Ill.

Nominating Committee

The new Nominating Committee elected by the membership will consist of John G. Reinhold, chairman; Miriam Reiner, District of Columbia General Hospital; Harry Sobotka, Mount Sinai Hospital, New York; Joseph I. Routh, University Hospitals, Iowa City; Arnold G. Ware, Los

Angeles County Hospital; Albert E. Sobel, Jewish Hospital of Brooklyn; and Warren M. Sperry, N. Y. State Psychiatric Institute, New York.

It will be the function of this Nominating Committee to propose a slate of officers and members for the 1956–57 Executive Committee.

The ballots were counted and the election certified by Julius J. Carr, Albert Hanok, and Andre C. Kibrick.

1955 ANNUAL MEETING OF THE AACC

The Annual Meeting of the American Association of Clinical Chemists will be held once again with the Fall National Meeting of The American Chemical Society in Minneapolis, Minn., sometime during the week of September 11–16, 1955. The exact dates are not yet available and since the next issue of CLINICAL CHEMISTRY will not appear until after the meeting it will be necessary for our members to obtain the meeting program from *Chemical and Engineering News*. The final program will appear in the August 8 issue of *Chemical and Engineering News*, in which all the Association events will be scheduled with the exception of the membership meeting. In the past this meeting was held immediately following the symposium with the Division of Biological Chemistry and preceding the Annual Dinner.

The social highlight of the year has been the annual dinner at which the Ernst Bischoff Award is presented. The success of these dinners can be best attested to by the fact that for the one held last year in New York it was necessary to set up tables in the alcoves to accommodate the overflow from the dining room.

SPANISH TRANSLATION OF *STANDARD METHODS*

Arrangements have been made with a publishing firm in Madrid for the translation of *Standard Methods in Clinical Chemistry* into the Spanish language. The Association will receive royalties for the translated edition as for the English edition.

ENZYME SYMPOSIUM

A three-day International Symposium on "Enzymes: Units of Biological Structure and Function," sponsored by the Henry Ford Hospital and The Edsel B. Ford Institute for Medical Research, will be held in the auditorium of Henry Ford Hospital, Detroit, Mich., November 1, 2, and 3, 1955.

Interrelationships between enzymology and other fields—notably genetics, physiology, biochemistry, and pharmacology—will constitute the general theme of the symposium. The specific topics for the six sessions will be: Origin of Enzymes, Status of the Gene-Enzyme Relationship, Enzymes and Cell Structure, Enzymatic Basis of Some Physiological Functions, Cellular Energy Sources, and Regulation of Enzyme Activity. More than thirty internationally known scientists have accepted invitations to participate.

A copy of the Preliminary Announcement may be obtained by writing to Dr. Clarence E. Rupe, Henry Ford Hospital, Detroit 2, Mich.

Invitations will be sent to as many as can be accommodated.

AAAS ANNUAL MEETING

The American Association of Clinical Chemists will participate in the 122nd meeting of the American Association for the Advancement of Science to be held in Atlanta, Ga., December 26–31, 1955. The preliminary program has already been published in *Science*, May 12, 1955, page 751. The Association, with Albert E. Sobel as program chairman, has arranged a symposium on "Recent Concepts in Clinical Chemistry" and a dinner on December 26. There will also be two sessions for contributed papers in clinical chemistry on December 27.

This is the first occasion for the Association to collaborate with the AAAS in their national meetings. It is to be hoped that our members will be well represented at these meetings and that this collaboration will become an annual event. The Association has been an affiliated society of the AAAS for several years.

AMERICAN BOARD OF CLINICAL CHEMISTRY

The American Board of Clinical Chemistry, Inc., held its annual meeting at the Henry Ford Hospital, Detroit, Mich., on May 20–21, 1955. Three clinical chemists who successfully passed examinations given by the board last October were certified: Sol I. Bulkin, Lawrence C. Kier, and Otto E. Loebstein. The total number of certified clinical chemists is now 241.

A complete *Directory of Certified Clinical Chemists* may be obtained by writing to the Secretary-Treasurer, Dr. O. H. Gaebler, Henry Ford Hospital, Detroit, Mich., and will be sent without charge to hospital departments or other laboratories which engage in clinical chemistry.

Clinical chemists interested in being certified should write for the *Instructions to Applicants for Certification*. In order to be considered for admission to the next regional examination, which will probably be held during October, 1955, candidates should file their applications immediately.

The Board elected the following officers for the coming year: Marschelle H. Power, *President*; Clarence W. Muehlberger, *Vice President*; and Oliver H. Gaebler, Secretary-Treasurer. The other members of the Board are: Joseph W. E. Harrisson, Arnold E. Osterberg, William A. Wolff, Warren M. Sperry, Harry Sobotka, Robert M. Hill, and Albert L. Chaney.

REPORTS FROM THE SECTIONS

Southern California

Clyde A. Dubbs

The third symposium of the season was held on February 1 at the Los Angeles County Hospital. Robert Stragnell and Gerard Lanchantin, both of the University of Southern California Medical School, discussed "Recent Advances in Blood Coagulation and Their Clinical Significance."

ABSTRACTS

Editor: Ellenmae Viergiver. *Contributors:* Joseph A. Annino, Gladys J. Downey, Clyde A. Dubbs, Alex Kaplan, Margaret M. Kaser, Miriam Reiner, Herbert Thompson

Effect of glucagon on peripheral utilization of glucose in man. T. B. van Itallie, M. C. Morgan, and L. B. Dotti (*St. Luke's Hospital, New York, N. Y.*).

Peripheral glucose uptake in normal human subjects during and after glucagon-induced hyperglycemia was compared with peripheral uptakes during and after similar hyperglycemias produced by intravenous infusion of glucose, and by ingestion of glucose following subcutaneous injection of epinephrine. Comparison of CV differences following glucagon administration with those following the infusion of glucose showed that peripheral utilization of glucose was not inhibited by glucagon and may have been enhanced. In contrast, epinephrine injection was followed by apparent inhibition. It is suggested that the description of glucagon as an "insulin antagonist" is misleading.—*J. Clin. Endocrinol. and Metabolism* **15,** 28, 1955. (M. R.)

Effect of long-term administration of desiccated thyroid on serum lipoprotein and cholesterol levels. B. Strisower, J. W. Gofman, E. Galioni, J. H. Rubinger, G. W. O'Brien, and A. Simon (*University of California, Berkeley, Calif.*).

In a series of 50 schizophrenic patients receiving a daily dosage of 3 gr. of desiccated thyroid, the concentrations of the mean Standard S_f0-12 and mean Standard S_f12-20 serum lipoproteins were significantly reduced within a period of 3 weeks, but by 24 weeks the Standard S_f0-12 concentration had returned to the prethyroid level. The magnitude of the drop in the Standard S_f0-12 concentration was directly related to the prethyroid value.—*J. Clin. Endocrinol. and Metabolism* **15,** 73, 1955. (M. R.)

The determination of sugar in blood and spinal fluid with anthrone reagent. J. H. Roe (*George Washington University, Washington, D. C.*).

Glucose in blood or spinal fluid is determined by first deproteinizing with trichloroacetic acid, tungstic acid, or barium hydroxide-zinc sulfate. Anthrone reagent is then added to the filtrate, the solution is heated in a boiling water bath, and the density of the resultant color is measured at 620 mμ. An anthrone reagent containing thiourea is described which is stable for two weeks. Comparisons of results with the standard copper reduction methods are in good agreement.—*J. Biol. Chem.* **212,** 335, 1955. (J. A.)

Progressive changes in renal phosphate and calcium excretion in rats following parathyroidectomy or parathyroid administration. R. V. Talmage and F. W. Kraintz (*Rice Institute, Houston, Texas*).

The urinary excretion of Ca^{45} or P^{32} was followed for 27 hours after their administration to adult rats 1 hour after parathyroidectomy or after the first injection of parathyroid extract, and serum calcium and phosphorus were determined in animals sacrificed at intervals during the experimental period. Parathyroidectomy caused an increase in the urinary excretion of calcium for at least 12 hours and an immediate drop in urinary phosphorus, but at 24–27 hours the rates of excretion of both ions had returned to normal. Throughout the experimental period the serum calcium fell and serum phosphorus rose. The results following parathyroid extract were in the opposite directions, but the rates were comparable. It is concluded that the control of the renal thresholds for both calcium and phosphate by parathyroid hormone is the cause of the altered serum levels observed, and that any changes in excretion occurring after 24 hours are due to extrarenal effects of parathyroid administration or deprivation.—*Proc. Soc. Exp. Biol. Med.* **87,** 263, 1954. (M. K.)

Simultaneous measurement of the iodide-concentrating and protein-binding capacities of the normal and hyperfunctioning human thyroid gland. S. H. Ingbar (*Walter Reed Army Medical Center, Washington, D. C.*).

It is possible in man to measure simultaneously the ability of the thyroid gland to concentrate inorganic iodide and to bind thyroidal iodide to protein as shown in a study of 29 normal individuals and 20 patients with untreated Graves' disease. The increased rate of hormone synthesis in the latter group was usually the result of increases in both the iodide-concentrating and protein-binding capacities of the thyroid gland. The method also makes possible the measurement of the rate of transfer of plasma iodide to hormonal iodine which can be applied to patients receiving large doses of antithyroid drugs.—*J. Clin. Endocrinol. and Metabolism* **15,** 238, 1955. (M. R.)

A rapid, simple method for the determination of reduced, dehydro-, and total ascorbic acid in biological material. R. R. Schaffert and J. R. Kingsley (*University of California, Los Angeles, Calif.*).

Total ascorbic acid is determined as follows: a protein-free filtrate is prepared using 6% trichloroacetic acid. The filtrate is treated with Norit (amorphous carbon) and filtered. To the filtrate is added 10% thiourea and 2,4-dinitrophenylhydrazine. The mixture is then heated in a water bath. After cooling, 85% H_2SO_4 is added and the resultant color density is measured at 515 mμ. When the procedure is carried out omitting the Norit, dehydroascorbic acid is measured. The L-ascorbic acid is the difference between the total and the dehydroascorbic acid.—*J. Biol. Chem.* **212,** 59, 1955. (J. A.)

Effects of intravenous hydrocortisone on electrolytes of serum and urine in man. R. P. Knight, D. S. Kornfeld, G. H. Glaser, and P. K. Bondy (*Yale University School of Medicine, New Haven, Conn.*).

When hydrocortisone was given in large amounts (50 or 100 mg.) intravenously over a period of 4 hours to 5 subjects, the blood eosinophil count fell, but urine and serum sodium and chloride levels failed to exhibit a consistent pattern of response. It was also possible to demonstrate a heretofore undescribed early increase in the serum potassium level concomitant with the expected rise in urine potassium. These increases in the serum potassium ranged from 0.6 to 1.1 mEq. in 4 of the 5 subjects over the 4 hours. This suggests that one of the major early effects of hydrocortisone on electrolyte metabolism is on the distribution of cations between intracellular and extracellular fluid since the increased urinary potassium excretion induced was insufficient to prevent a rise of the serum potassium.—*J. Clin. Endocrinol. and Metab.* **15,** 176, 1955. (M. R.)

Determination of estrogens in stored urines of pregnancy. R. M. Anker (*University of Colorado Medical School, Denver, Colo.*).

The Allen modification of the Kober colorimetric assay was investigated and improved. The uncertainty is estimated to be at most 300 μg. per 24-hour urine specimen, depending upon the colored impurities present in the urine. The specimens may be stored for 2 years at room temperature under a layer of *n*-butanol; the recovery is much better than when aqueous mineral acid is used as the means of clearing the conjugates.—*J. Clin. Endocrinol. and Metabolism* **15,** 210, 1955. (M. R.)

Quantitative determination of urine sodium by means of ion-exchange resins. J. S. Vanatta and C. C. Cox (*University of Texas, Dallas, Texas*).

A modification of a serum sodium technic previously published (*J. Biol. Chem.* **210,** 719, 1954) is described. Urine is passed through IR-112 which removes sodium. The sodium is eluted with $BaCl_2$ solution and the barium is precipitated as $BaSO_4$. The supernatant is then passed through IRA-400 to convert the NaCl to NaOH. Subsequently the NaOH is titrated with standard HCl using bromthymol blue as an indicator. Data are presented showing good agreement with the Butler and Tuthill method.—*J. Biol. Chem.* **212,** 599, 1955. (J. A.)

Estimation of plasma phosphatase by determination of hydrolysed phenol with amino-antipyrine. P. R. N. Kind and E. J. King (*Postgraduate Medical School, London, England*).

The method of Grifols-Lucas (*Brit. Med. J.* **2,** 295, 1951) has been modified by the present authors to yield results comparable to those obtained by the King-Armstrong procedure. The amount of phenol liberated by enzymatic hydrolysis is determined by reaction with 4-amino-antipyrine (AAP). A red-colored quinone is produced which can be measured colorimetrically. Proteins do not react with AAP and therefore need not be removed.—*J. Clin. Pathol.* **7,** 322, 1954.

(E. V.)

The endogenous creatinine clearance in normal subjects. M. H. Roscoe (*Manchester University, Manchester, England*).

The data presented in this paper show that the excretion of endogenous creatinine is very constant in spite of considerable variation in urine flow, decreasing only slightly at low urine volumes. The creatinine clearance was lower than the expected filtration rate as determined by the clearance of inulin. It is suggested that this discrepancy is probably due to overestimation of the plasma creatinine. If, as has been found by Roscoe (*J. Clin. Pathol.* **6,** 201, 1953), 20 per cent of the estimated chromogen is not creatinine, the differences in the clearances can be accounted for.—*J. Clin. Path.* **7,** 327, 1954. (E. V.)

Permanent color standards for determination of phosphate by molybdenum blue method. E. P. Parry and A. L. McClelland (*University of Connecticut, Storrs, Conn.*).

Stable color standards, having hue and absorption spectrum (400 to 700 mμ) similar to molybdenum blue, are prepared. A standard containing 4.98 mg. of copper sulphate and 0.920 mg. of bromophenol blue in 10 ml. of acetate buffer (*p*H 4.63) showed no absorption spectrum change when exposed for 24 days in the direct morning sunlight.—*Anal. Chem.* **27,** 140, 1955. (C. D.)

Silica gel microcolumn for chromatographic resolution of cortical steroids. M. L. Sweat (*University of Utah College of Medicine, Salt Lake City, Utah*).

As little as 0.25 μg. of a steroid can be chromatographically determined using a 40 $\times$ 5 mm. O.D. microcolumn containing 0.1 Gm. of silica gel. The column is suspended in a water-jacketed condenser having a stopcock outlet. Corticosterone and 17-hydroxycorticosterone can be determined in 2 ml. of plasma. A synthetic mixture was resolved, by elution with 100 ml. of alcohol-chloroform, into desoxycorticosterone, 17-hydroxy-11-desoxycorticosterone, corticosterone, cortisone, 17-hydroxycorticosterone, and 4-pregnene-11β, 17α, 20β, 21-tetrol-3-one in that order of elution. While some overlapping occurred, the relative specificities of the fluorescent and phenylhydrazine analytical methods permit satisfactory individual determinations in most cases. Applications to human, dog, and rat blood are described elsewhere.—*Anal. Chem.* **26,** 1964, 1954.

(C. D.)

Potassium and reducing substances in proximal tubule fluid of the rat kidney. H. Wirz and P. A. Bott (*Women's Medical College of Pennsylvania, Philadelphia, Pa.*).

The kidneys of rats were exposed, the middle third of the proximal tubule of a single nephron was isolated and punctured as described by Walker and Oliver (*Am. J. Physiol.* **134,** 562, 1941), and a ureter was cannulated. Potassium in plasma, tubule fluid, and urine was determined by means of an internal standard flame photometer and reducing substances by an ultramicro adaptation of the Sumner method as described by Walker and Reisinger (*J. Biol. Chem.* **101,** 223, 1933).

Lower concentrations of potassium in tubule fluid than in plasma, together with reabsorption of water in the proximal tubule of the rat kidney, demonstrate that considerable reabsorption of potassium takes place. This is also the site of active glucose reabsorption.—*Proc. Soc. Exp. Biol. Med.* **87,** 405, 1954.

(M. K.)

Effects of hormone administration on serum protein patterns. C. H. Ligeti and K. Irvine (*School of Medicine, University of Virginia, Charlottesville, Va.*).

Previous studies have revealed the occurrence of lowered serum albumin levels and increases in the α_1- and α_2-globulins after surgery. In these experiments large doses of cortisone increased the total serum protein concentration, but no other hormone tested had a significant effect. Serum albumin was decreased by pituitary adrenocorticotropic hormone and increased by testosterone, hydrocortone, and cortisone. Insulin increased α_1-globulin and estrogen increased the α_2-globulin. Serum γ-globulin was depressed by hydrocortone, but not by cortisone. The other pituitary and adrenal hormones, progesterone, and thyroid had no effect on serum protein patterns. *Proc. Soc. Exp. Biol. Med.* **87,** 324, 1954.

(M. K.)

Occurrence of glucose in combination with acetoacetate in normal urine. M. C. Nath and V. K. Sahu (*University Department of Biochemistry, Nagpur, India*).

Previously a metabolic relationship between glucose and acetoacetate in rabbits had been demonstrated by hypoglycemia followed by hyperglycemia after repeated injections of acetoacetate, the production of hyperglycemia by either glucose or acetoacetate but not by the two together, and the protection afforded by glucose and acetoacetate together or their condensation product (2-tetrahydroxy butyl, 5-methyl, 4-carbethoxy furan) against alloxan diabetes.

In the present experiments, urine from rats, rabbits, and normal and diabetic human subjects subjected to hydrolysis with HCl reduced Nylander's reagent and yielded glucosazone but did not do so before hydrolysis. Anthrone gave a marked color and tests for acetone were positive after hydrolysis. Unhydrolyzed urines gave a red-orange color with $FeCl_3$, as did the glucose-acetoacetate condensation product. Several urines from patients with glycosuria and acetonuria showed no increase in glucose or acetone with hydrolysis. The data indicate that glucose and acetoacetate occur in normal urine in a combined form, which is not present in diabetes.—*Proc. Soc. Exp. Biol. Med.* **87,** 287, 1954. (M. K.)

Conjugates of adrenal corticoids in human plasma. A. M. Bongiovanni, W. R. Eberlein, M. M. Grumbach, J. J. VanWyk, and G. Clayton (*Johns Hopkins School of Medicine, Baltimore, Md.*).

Concentrated chloroform extracts of plasma chromatographed on Florosil and treated with phenylhydrazine according to Nelson and Samuels (*J. Clin. Endocrinol. & Metabolism* **12,** 519, 1952) constituted the "free" corticoids. The remaining plasma was acidified to *p*H 5.5 with 40% H_2SO_4 and then to *p*H 4.5 with acetate buffer. Beta-glucuronidase (1000 units/ml. plasma) was added and the plasma incubated at 37° for 24 hrs. Dialysis was carried out at room temperature for 48 hr. against 12 volumes of 10% methanol in water, and the dialysate was extracted with chloroform. The extracts were treated as for the "free" fraction.

Normal values for free corticoids ranged from 2 to 10 μg./100 ml. and comparable values were found for the conjugated corticoids in 8 patients without adrenal disease. Both were increased in two subjects after acute injuries; the free fraction was elevated in a child with adrenocortical carcinoma with metastases; and the results in 2 patients with Cushing's disease were variable but the proportion of conjugated steroids was elevated. ACTH and Compound E acetate caused increases in both free and conjugated fractions, with the conjugated portion exceeding the free after about two hours. Disposition of excessive hormone involves conjugation, which was impaired in cirrhosis of the liver. Evidence is presented to support the belief that the material measured in the conjugated fraction consists of corticoids.—*Proc. Soc. Exp. Biol. Med.* **87,** 282, 1954. (M. K.)

Comparative value of the basal metabolic rate, chemical protein-bound iodine, and radioactive iodine excretion or uptake in the diagnosis of borderline hyperthyroidism when used individually or in combination. L. Zieve, B. Skanse and A. L. Schultz (*Veterans Administration Hospital and University of Minnesota, Minneapolis, Minn.*).

Considered individually, radioactive iodine uptake, or excretion, in 24 hours is the most valuable index for distinguishing between borderline euthyroid and borderline hyperthyroid patients. Protein-bound iodine is about 80 per cent as effective, and the basal metabolic rate about 20 per cent as effective. A weighted combination of protein-bound iodine and radioactive iodine uptake is better, although not greatly so, than either one alone. Both are needed for maximum diagnostic effectiveness.—*J. Lab. Clin. Med.* **45,** 281, 1955. (G. D.)

Correction for color differences between standards and urine extracts and their ketonic fractions in the Callow-Zimmerman reaction. H. P.

Schedl, W. B. Bean, B. M. Stevenson, and E. R. Schumacher (*State University of Iowa, Iowa City, Iowa*).

Following analysis of urine extracts for 17-ketosteroids, aliquots of the original ethanol solution were dried in vacuo. After Girard separation (Pincus and Pearlman, *Endocrinology* **29,** 413, 1941), both ketonic and nonketonic fractions were analyzed, all Zimmerman reactions being performed by the method of Callow (Callow, Callow, and Emmons, *Biochem. J.* **32,** 2, 1312, 1938). Since the Zimmerman reaction absorption spectra of ketonic substances in urine extracts are not the same as that of the standard, dehydroisoandrosterone acetate, and since destruction of chromogens occurs during the Girard procedure, uncorrected analyses on ketonic fractions may be misleading. Using measurements made at three wave lengths—425, 510, and 595 mμ—the authors propose that the 17-ketosteroid content of the sample be corrected by comparing the absorption peak of the unknown with that of the standard.—*J. Lab. Clin. Med.* **45,** 191, 1955. (G. D.)

Turbidimetric method of fibrinogen assay: Results with the Coleman Junior spectrophotometer. A. H. Fowell (*Cutler Laboratories, Berkeley, Calif.*).

The recent recognition of afibrinogenemia of pregnancy has emphasized the need for a rapid method of fibrinogen assay in blood. The method of Parfentjev, Johnson, and Clifton [*Arch. Biochem.* **46,** 470 (1953)] has been adapted for use with the Coleman Junior spectrophotometer, Model 6A. Five milliliters of blood are collected in a test tube containing 0.5 ml. of 4% sodium citrate dihydrate. Plasma is separated by centrifugation at 2500 rpm for 10 minutes. The blank is 1 ml. of plasma plus 9 ml. of normal saline; the sample is 1 ml. of plasma plus 9 ml. of Parfentjev reagent (133.33 Gm. of ammonium sulfate, 10.0 Gm. of sodium chloride, and 0.25 Gm. of Merthiolate in 1 liter of aqueous solution; *p*H is adjusted to 7.00 with 10M NaOH). The spectrophotometer is set to read 100% transmittance at 510 mμ with the blank. The optical density of the sample is measured at exactly 3 minutes after the addition of the reagent. If coagulation has occurred, the cuvette is given a vigorous shake just before reading. Fibrinogen concentration of the sample in grams per 100 ml. equals $\frac{\text{O.D.} + 0.019}{0.509}$. The lower levels of fibrinogen, 0.05 to 0.150 Gm./100 ml., where fibrinogen replacement therapy is required, will be clearly indicated by this method.—*Am. J. Clin. Pathol.* **25,** 340 (1955). (H. T.)

Determination of quinine in urine in "tubeless method" of gastric analysis. R. D. Lewis and A. G. Foord (*Huntington Memorial Hospital, Pasadena, Calif.*).

Modifications of the "tubeless method" of gastric analysis of Segal, Miller, and Morton [(*Proc. Soc. Exp. Biol. Med.* **74,** 218 (1950)] are described. The authors substituted chloroform for ether in the urine extraction because in their experience recoveries were poor with the gentle ether extraction. Ten milliliters samples of urine are transferred to 16 × 100 mm. tubes and 0.5 ml. of 0.1N NaOH is added, followed by 5 ml. of chloroform. The tubes are covered with the thumb protected by a clean rubber cot and vigorously shaken for 10 seconds. They are then centrifuged and the urine phase is removed by aspiration. The chloroform is washed with 5 ml. H_2O and recentrifuged. The water phase is removed. Ten milliliters of 0.1N H_2SO_4 is added to the chloroform extract and the tubes are again shaken. The sulfuric acid phase (upper layer) is removed and the fluorescence of the specimen is compared with standards in ultraviolet light. Recoveries with ether were found to be 38–60 per cent; when chloroform was used recoveries were 76–93 per cent.—*Am. J. Clin. Pathol.* **25,** 199 (1955).

(H. T.)

Ultramicro procedures in clinical chemistry. W. T. Caraway and H. Fanger (*Rhode Island Hospital, Providence, R. I.*)

This is a report of the authors' study of procedures for all the common clinical chemistry determinations on 0.01 ml. samples of serum. Nearly all the procedures described can be adapted to larger samples by multiplying all quantities by a factor of 10 or 100. Details concerning equipment and capillary blood collection are given and procedures are described in detail for the ultramicro determination of glucose, urea nitrogen, creatinine, total protein, albumin, sodium, potassium, calcium, chloride, carbon dioxide combining power, inorganic phosphorus, icterus index, bilirubin, cholesterol, thymol turbidity, cephalin flocculation, alkaline phosphatase, and amylase. Only a small working area is required for these ultramicroprocedures but this should be used exclusively for this work. The procedures are somewhat more time-consuming than are the standard methods and are less adaptable to a large volume of work. Data shown demonstrate that the precision of the ultramicromethods is in conformity with that of standard accepted macro procedures.—*Am. J. Clin. Pathol.* **25,** 317 (1955).

(H. T.)

Identification of urinary sugar. F. W. Fales (*Emory University, Atlanta, Ga.*)

The presence of reducing sugar in urine is determined by Benedict's qualitative reagent. If the concentration is low, the urine is concentrated to 1% sugar by evaporation. A fermentation test is made to establish the presence or absence of fermentable sugar. If fermentation is present, the sugar may be glucose or fructose; if absent, either galactose, lactose, or pentose is present. Final identification of the unknown sugar is obtained by paper chromatography, using known sugars as controls.—*Am. J. Clin. Pathol.* **25,** 336 (1955). (H. T.)

Counter-current distribution procedure for the quantitative-qualitative analysis of small amounts of urinary corticosteroids. N. B. Talbot, S.

Ulick, A. Koupreianow, and A. Zygmuntowicz (*Harvard Medical School, Boston, Mass.*)

A 24-hour urine specimen (adjusted to *p*H 6) is extracted 4 times with 1/7 volume of chloroform. The chloroform extract is separated by centrifugation and washed 3 times with 1/10 volume of 0.1N NaOH and 3 times with 1/10 volume of water. The residue from this extract is dissolved in the contents of the zero tube of the distribution apparatus, which is filled with equal volumes of pure upper and lower layer solvents (iso-octane and secondary butanol). The distribution is performed according to Craig; the apparatus is gently inverted for 45 seconds at each transfer and checked for the separation of the two layers by direct observation. After 1 hour the material in each tube is transferred to one of a series of bottles. The contents are dried in vacuo and the residue is dissolved in 5 ml. of ethanol. The optical density is determined at 302 mμ (Value A). A 3 ml. aliquot is then transferred to a 15 ml. glass-stoppered test tube and 0.5 ml. of thiocarbazide reagent is added. After 90 minutes at room temperature the optical density is determined at 302 mμ. This value is multiplied by a factor of 1.17 to correct for the dilution caused by the addition of reagent (Value B). The increase in optical density at 302 mμ (Value C) attributable to thiosemicarbazones is found by subtracting Value A from Value B.

Clinical studies indicate that the excretion pattern per square meter per day of healthy persons is quite steady. Gross qualitative as well as quantitative changes in the urinary corticosteroids have been observed in a small series of patients suffering either severe stress or definite adrenocortical disease.—*J. Clin. Endocrinol. and Metabolism* **15,** 301 (1955). (M. R.)

Simultaneous Determination of *p*H, CO_2 Content, and Cell Volume in 0.1 ml. Aliquots of Cutaneous Blood

A Modification of the Shock and Hastings Technic

Richard B. Singer, Jane Shohl, and Dolores B. Bluemle

In 1934 SHOCK AND HASTINGS (1) described the construction and use of a micropipet, by means of which blood in 0.1 ml. aliquots could be used for the simultaneous determination of *p*H, CO_2 content, and red cell volume. In this method the blood in two pipets was diluted to 2.0 ml. with saline-phenol red solution, centrifuged, and used first for the determination of hematocrit value, second for the colorimetric determination of *p*H by visual comparison with previously prepared standards, and last, for the determination of CO_2 content in whole blood in the manometric Van Slyke apparatus. One or two additional pipets were filled with blood and 0.9% NaCl to serve as color blanks. A sample size of 0.5 ml. or less is thus sufficient for the determination of all three factors in duplicate, and cutaneous blood may therefore be utilized as an easily obtainable substitute for arterial blood. The method is particularly useful for the study of acid-base balance in infants.

Although the original method is suitable for most clinical purposes, the

---

From The Departments of Research Medicine and Biochemistry, School of Medicine, University of Pennsylvania, Philadelphia, Pa.

This work was aided by grants from the Committee for the Advancement of Research and the C. Mahlon Kline Fund for Development in the Department of Medicine, the University of Pennsylvania, and the Life Insurance Medical Research Fund.

Present addresses: 501 Boylston Street, Boston, Mass. (R.B.S.) and 2010 Boxwood Drive, Broomall, Pa. (J.S.).

Received for publication May 11, 1955.

following modifications were found, after a thorough trial, to offer certain advantages in operation and improvements in accuracy. The need for the preparation and checking of a large set of bicolor standards has been eliminated by adapting the micropipet in such a way that the optical density of the unknown can be compared with the optical density of a phenol red solution in phosphate buffer of known *p*H, in a suitable filter photometer. A similar method of photometric estimation of *p*H in blood or plasma in standard colorimeter tubes has been described by Van Slyke, Weisiger, and Van Slyke (2). To obviate the difficulty of filling the stem of the micropipet with blood under oil, without accidental admixture of the latter, we utilized the method of collection and handling of blood proposed by Lilienthal and Riley (3). In our hands this resulted in a more accurate measurement of the 0.1 ml. aliquot of blood, a crucial factor in any microtechnic. Since the technic thus modified has proved its value in five years of use at the Hospital of the University of Pennsylvania, it has seemed worthwhile to describe the modifications in detail to encourage a wider clinical application of the technic. Evidence will also be presented to support the accuracy of the determinations and the validity of handling blood samples in a way that appears to violate traditional anaerobic methods.

RELATIONSHIP BETWEEN *p*H AND PHOTOMETRIC MEASUREMENT

The basic principles involved in the adaptation of a *p*H method utilizing indicators from a visual colorimetric to a photometric measurement have been reviewed by Van Slyke *et al.* (2). Phenol red behaves like a monovalent weak acid, so that the dissociated salt and undissociated acid components are related to the *p*H of the solution in the familiar Henderson-Hasselbalch equation:

$$\mathrm{p}H = \mathrm{p}K'_{PR} + \frac{(PR^-)}{(HPR)} \tag{1}$$

The total concentration of indicator, (PR), or the sum of (PR^-) and (HPR), is kept very much less than the final buffer concentration of the mixture of the indicator solution with a test solution, such as blood or phosphate. It is therefore possible for the salt-acid ratio of the indicator to adjust to the *p*H of the test solution virtually without alteration of the latter.

Indicators like phenol red have the further property in both the dissociated and undissociated forms of possessing distinctive colors in solution. The alkaline form, PR^-, of phenol red is a deep purple color, and the acid form, HPR, is yellow. Each form has a characteristic spectrophotometric absorption curve (4). In the *p*H range 6.7 to 8.6, mixture of the salt and acid forms gives a continuous series of intermediate colors, which can be analyzed visually by comparison with prepared standards or spectrophotometrically by making absorption curves or readings at two crucial wavelengths. The absorption curve for the alkaline phenol red has a maximum at $\lambda = 560$ mμ, and that for the acid form, a maximum at $\lambda = 430$ mμ, with virtually zero absorption at 560 mμ.

A reading of optical density or light extinction on a phenol red solution varies almost linearly with the concentration of alkaline phenol red, when a filter photometer with a green filter transmitting at about 540 to 560 mμ is used. The diameter of the colorimeter tubes and other parameters must be constant to maintain this relationship. In solutions in which the total phenol red concentration is known and constant, the photometer reading can therefore be related to *p*H through the concentration, (PR^-), and the factor pK'_{PR} in Equation 1. A series of phosphate buffer solutions containing the proper amount of phenol red is read in the photometer, and a calibration curve is prepared for optical density or extinction against the known values of *p*H (2). It is convenient to use a photometer such as the Klett-Summerson, in which the scale reading is proportional to optical density rather than to transmission.

APPARATUS

Micropipets of the Shock and Hastings design, with certain dimensions specified so that the pipets can be easily centrifuged and also placed in a uniform and suitable position in the photometer. Critical dimensions of the micropipets used originally in our work are shown in Fig. 1. This design required the drilling of a hole at the bottom of the cuvette or tube holder of the photometer, and insertion of a cork spacer on the inside of the bottom cover for the purpose of aligning the pipet bulb vertically with the light aperture of the holder (see Fig. 1). The hole does not interfere with the use of the ordinary photometer tubes in the holder. However, to avoid the need for this modification, the micropipet has been redesigned by the supplier. The model currently available fits directly into a metal adapter which can easily be inserted into or removed from the standard tube holder of the Klett-Summerson filter photometer.[1]

A filter photometer, capable of receiving the pipets and matching tubes of about 13 mm. outside diameter. A Klett-Summerson instrument was

[1] The adapter and micropipets made in accordance with such specifications are obtainable from Arthur H. Thomas Co., Philadelphia, Pa.

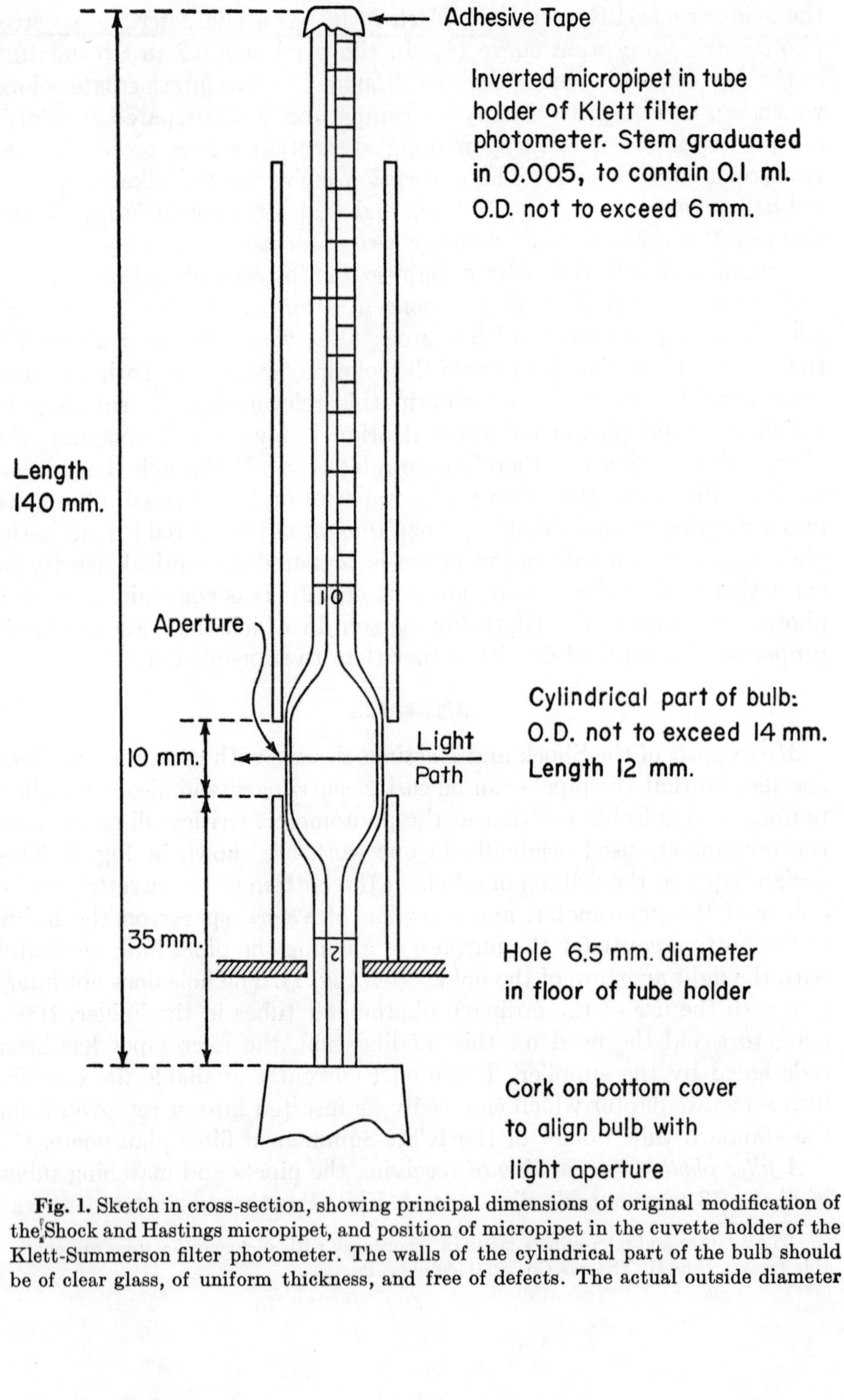

Fig. 1. Sketch in cross-section, showing principal dimensions of original modification of the Shock and Hastings micropipet, and position of micropipet in the cuvette holder of the Klett-Summerson filter photometer. The walls of the cylindrical part of the bulb should be of clear glass, of uniform thickness, and free of defects. The actual outside diameter

used in all of our work.[2] Although the micropipet was modified specifically for use in this photometer, it might be used in any filter photometer or spectrophotometer, provided that it could be positioned with the light path restricted to the cylindrical part of the bulb.

Test tubes for use as photometer tubes, matched as nearly as possible to the internal diameter of the micropipets (see specifications in Fig. 1). These can be selected from a quantity of round-bottom Pyrex test tubes of outside diameter 12.5 mm. and 100 mm. length.

A small water bath set at 38° and provided with a rack to hold micropipets and small photometer tubes.

A centrifuge with four brass shields (cups) of standard outside dimensions about 120 mm. by 19 mm. An angle centrifuge cannot be used because the stem of the micropipet is likely to break. A satisfactory small centrifuge is the Clay-Adams Standard Safeguard centrifuge, Model No. CT-1110, having a maximum speed of 2600 rpm.

Heavy rubber bands, approximately 75 mm. long and 6 mm. wide.

Syringes. A 1-ml. tuberculin syringe and 26-gage hypodermic needle for measuring the heparin solution; several 2-ml. syringes for collecting blood samples, with metal caps (Becton-Dickinson No. 425A); several 20-ml. syringes for storing solutions.

Collecting tips for the 2-ml. syringes, made from a piece of single bore #00 rubber stopper about 8 mm. in length, with a hollow cup ground in one end.

Adapters for use in filling the micropipet from the 2-ml. or 20-ml. syringes, made from pressure tubing of ⅛″ bore and ⅛″ wall. The pieces are 10 to 12 mm. in length and must be cut with a sharp knife so that the ends are flat.

Rubber adapters to center the stem of the micropipet in the centrifuge

[2] The instrument available for our use happened to be an early model that differs from current models in its optical system and in the galvanometer. For ease in reading, a box-type spot galvanometer had been substituted for the needle galvanometer that is a standard part of the Klett-Summerson instrument. However, the pipets have been successfully used in many other unmodified photometers of this manufacture. Any model can be used as long as the light aperture of the adapter, when in position, is within the light aperture of the instrument.

(O.D.) of the bulb averaged about 13 mm. A further improvement in design, made by Arthur H. Thomas Co., is incorporated in the current model of the micropipet. The neck has been shortened so that it is unnecessary to modify the Klett instrument by drilling a hole in the floor of the tube holder, as shown above. A removable metal sleeve has also been made available to slip into the tube holder. The purpose of this is to ensure accurate dimensions of the aperture and proper centering of the pipet.

shield. For use in the shields specified previously, these are made from pressure tubing of ¼″ bore and 3/16″ wall, and are 15 mm. in length.

CALIBRATION

The volume contained in the stem of each micropipet to the nominal 0.1 ml. mark should be checked in order to insure accuracy of sample measurement. This calibration can be carried out to the nearest 0.0005 ml. by weighing the measured volume of mercury, by titrating with dilute alkali the measured volume of standard 1N acid and several rinsings of the stem, or by use of a calibrating microburet.

The micropipets and selected matching test tubes must also be calibrated with respect to their photometer reading, at both low and high readings. The micropipet is placed in the holder bulb down, and pipets and test tubes are always rotated so that the identifying mark faces the front of the instrument. With the green filter in place (Klett No. 54) readings are made (a) with water and (b) with an alkaline phenol red solution of 3.75 mg./l. or one of similar optical density. It is convenient in estimating the water corrections to make the original balance point with a scale setting of +10 divisions on the Klett instrument, since readings are not possible on the negative side of the zero setting. *Failure to reproduce scale readings within one or two divisions on the Klett, or large correction values, may indicate that the aperture is not centered properly with respect to the cylindrical part of the bulb.*

REAGENTS

1. For Collection of Blood

Mercury, clean and free of acid or alkali.

Heparin sodium, 1% in 0.9% NaCl solution (Abbott No. 3672).

2. For Hemoglobin Determination

0.1% Na_2CO_3 solution (1 Gm. per liter).

0.012M $CuSO_4 \cdot 4NH_3 \cdot H_2O$. Dissolve 2.998 Gm. of $CuSO_4 \cdot 5H_2O$ and dilute to 1 liter with approximately 2M NH_4OH.

3. For Use in Micropipets

Phenol red, 0.1% stock solution. Grind 1 Gm. of phenol red with 28.2 ml. of 0.1N NaOH until dissolved and dilute to 1 liter with distilled water. Filter if necessary. Allow to stand several days before using. Store in refrigerator.

Phenol red, 0.0075% working solution. Dilute 75 ml. of 0.1% phenol red to 1 liter with boiled distilled water. Store in refrigerator.

NaCl, 18% stock solution. Dissolve 180 Gm. of NaCl and dilute to 1 liter with distilled water. Store in refrigerator.

Saline-phenol red solution. Dilute 10.5 ml. of 0.0075% phenol red and 5.0 ml. of 18% NaCl to a total of 100 ml. with boiled distilled water. This solution should be freshly prepared at least once a week and, until used, is stored in a closed container or in a 100 ml. buret with a soda lime tube in the top.

4. For CO_2 Determination

(as described in Peters and Van Slyke (5))

Caprylic alcohol.

1N Lactic acid. CO_2-free stock solution, stored in refrigerator.

0.1N Lactic acid. Prepare fresh, free of CO_2 and air.

18N Sodium hydroxide (saturated). CO_2-free stock solution.

1N or 5N Sodium hydroxide. Prepare CO_2-free by dilution of 18N sodium hydroxide with boiled distilled water. The 1N solution must be fresh and air-free. The 5N solution is more stable because of lower solubility for gases (5, p. 284), but causes more rapid stopcock deterioration.

BUFFER STANDARDS AND CALIBRATION CURVE FOR pH MEASUREMENT

Stock solutions of M/3 Na_2HPO_4 (47.33 Gm./L.) and M/3 KH_2PO_4 (45.36 Gm. per liter). These solutions are prepared by dissolving the anhydrous reagent grade salt[3] in freshly boiled redistilled water, and are stored in the refrigerator in glass-stoppered Pyrex bottles. This concentration has been reduced from that used by Van Slyke *et al.* (2)[4] to lessen the amount of crystalline precipitation in the cold. Since the alkaline Na_2HPO_4 tends to pick up CO_2 if exposed to room air, the bottles are unstoppered only at the time of preparing desired solutions. The stock solutions appear to be stable for at least two years.

M/3 Mixed phosphate solutions. These are prepared in the proportions indicated in Table 1, so that the indicated *p*H will be obtained when each solution is diluted 1 to 5 to a final phosphate concentration of M/15. At 20° the *p*H will be 0.03 higher than the figures shown in Table 1 for 37°.

---

[3] The Merck Company provides anhydrous salts of high purity specially processed for buffer solutions.

[4] The concentrations in Gm./L. given by Van Slyke *et al.* on page 746 of this reference (2) actually refer to molar concentrations, not 0.5 molar, as stated.

Table 1. STANDARD M/15 PHOSPHATE BUFFERS
Based on data of Hastings and Sendroy (6)

pH^{a} *at 38°C.*	$pK_2'^{a}$ *at 38°C.*	R^{b}	$Na_2HPO_4^{c}$(mM/L.)	$KH_2PO_4^{c}$(mM/L.)	μ^{d} (ionic strength)
6.79	6.79	1.000	33.3	33.3	0.133
6.80	6.79	1.025	33.7	32.9	0.135
7.00	6.78	1.660	41.7	25.0	0.150
7.20	6.77	2.68	48.6	16.1	0.164
7.40	6.76	4.35	54.3	12.4	0.175
7.60	6.75	7.05	58.3	8.3	0.183
7.80	6.74	11.42	61.3	5.4	0.189
8.00	6.73	18.50	63.3	3.4	0.193

[a] Electrometric measurements with the H_2 electrode, referred to a *p*H of 1.08 for 0.1N HCl at 38°. The same values can be used at 37°.

[b] *R* is the molar ratio of Na_2HPO_4 to KH_2PO_4 used.

[c] These figures for final concentration of the buffer components, or any suitable multiple or fraction thereof, can be used as the number of ml. of each M/15 salt solution required for the preparation of the M/15 phosphate buffer of stated *p*H.

[d] The value of pK_2' is affected by variations in the ionic strength, μ, defined as

$$\tfrac{1}{2} \Sigma c_n V_n^2,$$

where c_n is the concentration of each ion, in Eq./L., and V_n is the valence of that ion.

The column headed *R* in Table 1 gives the molar ratio of Na_2HPO_4 to KH_2PO_4. If a mixed phosphate solution to make a *p*H 7.40 standard is desired, 10.00 ml. of M/3 KH_2PO_4 solution should be mixed with 10.00 *R* or 43.5 ml. of M/3 Na_2HPO_4. If a final volume of 66.7 ml. is sufficient for each mixed phosphate solution, the figures for the ultimate concentrations of Na_2HPO_4 and KH_2PO_4 (in mM/L., Table 1, columns 4 and 5) can be used for the number of milliliters for each solution. These solutions are also stable if stored in Pyrex bottles in the refrigerator. The *p*H and pK_2' values corresponding to a given Na_2HPO_4/KH_2PO_4 ratio in Table 1 are taken from the experimental results of Hastings and Sendroy (6) and are based on H_2 electrode measurements at 38°. They are identical with the ones used by Van Slyke *et al.* (2). There is no significant difference in pK_2' due to use of a temperature of 37° rather than 38°.

Standard M/15 phosphate buffers. Measure 20.00 ml. of mixed phosphate buffer, 10.00 ml. of the working solution of phenol red (75 mg./L.) into a 100 ml. volumetric flask and dilute to 100.0 ml. with freshly boiled redistilled water. This gives a standard M/15 phosphate of the designated *p*H at 37° containing 7.5 mg./L. of phenol red. Although such standard solutions are not so stable as the more concentrated phosphate mixtures, we have observed no significant change in photometer reading and *p*H over periods as long as two months, if the solutions are kept in Pyrex bottles in the refrigerator when not in use.

Calibration curve. At least two calibrated pipets or test tubes are filled for each standard buffer solution. If the pipets are used, the tips are dried and covered with adhesive tape as described in "Procedure." It is convenient to use one of the matched test tubes as a permanent water blank for the zero setting on the photometer in lieu of a calibrated pipet. Each buffer solution must be heated to 38° before reading in the photometer with a green filter, maximum transmission 540 mμ. In the length of time necessary to place a pipet or test tube in the photometer and obtain a reading, the fall in temperature is generally no more than 1°. The zero setting is checked with the water blank after each reading; readings may be repeated, if desired, after rewarming. The appropriate pipet or tube correction is subtracted from each reading, and a graph is constructed of the mean photometer reading against *p*H.

It has been our practice to recheck the complete calibration curve only at infrequent intervals. However, the level of the curve is checked with each *p*H determination by reading at least one buffer, usually the one at *p*H 7.40, and a stable, colored reference solution, the $CuSO_4 \cdot 4NH_3 \cdot H_2O$ used in the hemoglobin determination. The level of the curve set by this buffer reading usually does not vary more than two or three scale divisions from day to day.

Because the pK′ of phenol red in the saline-plasma mixture differs slightly from the pK′ in phosphate buffer, it becomes necessary to apply a correction to the *p*H reading of the unknown solution to make it correspond to the buffer calibration curve. The pK′ of phenol red in various salt solutions has been accurately determined by Sendroy and Hastings (7); values for the M/15 phosphate buffers and 0.9% NaCl solution (with

Table 2. pK′ of Phenol Red—Salt Corrections
Based on data of Sendroy and Hastings (7)

pH at 38°C.	*pK′ PO_4 buffer*	*pK′ 0.9% NaCl*	*Difference*[a]	*pH Range at 37°C.*	*Correction*[b]
6.80	7.658	7.618	+0.040	under 6.94	−0.04
7.00	7.659	7.628	+0.031	6.94–7.18	−0.03
7.20	7.660	7.637	+0.023	7.19–7.42	−0.02
7.40	7.660	7.645	+0.015	7.43–7.67	−0.01
7.60	7.662	7.651	+0.011	7.68–7.91	0.00
7.80	7.660	7.657	+0.003	over 7.91	+0.01
8.00	7.653	7.662	−0.009		

[a] Difference between pK′ of phenol red in M/15 phosphate buffer and pK′ in a solution containing 124 mM/L., NaCl and 30 mM/L. $NaHCO_3$, at the stated *p*H.

[b] Correction to be applied to the *p*H read with 0.9% NaCl solution as a diluent, in order to allow for the difference in pK′ of phenol red in this solution as compared with the M/15 phosphate buffer standards.

H_2CO_3-$NaHCO_3$ buffer) are shown in Table 2, as taken from their work. The correction is given for various ranges of observed *p*H. Ordinarily this correction has been ignored as negligible in the past, but for the most accurate work it should be applied.

PROCEDURE

A syringe of 2 ml. capacity, graduated in 0.1 ml., is used for the blood collection. A constant amount, 0.05 ml., of heparin saline solution is measured in a tuberculin syringe and then injected through a 26-gage needle into the barrel of the 2 ml. syringe. After ejection of the air, about 0.3 ml. of mercury is drawn into the syringe and the rubber collecting tip is attached to it.

Two greased syringes of 20 ml. capacity are used for filling the micropipets with diluent. A satisfactory grease for the syringes is Arthur H. Thomas stopcock grease; silicone grease is too alkaline for this purpose. About 2 or 3 ml. of mercury are drawn into each syringe. Saline, 0.9%, to be used in the control pipets, is drawn into one syringe and the saline-phenol red solution into the other. A rubber adapter which will serve as a connecting piece between syringe and pipet is attached to each syringe. Before filling the pipets, the saline-phenol red solution is adjusted visually to *p*H 7.4 ± 0.2 by adding a fractional drop of dilute alkali or acid.

Collection of Blood Sample

To produce peripheral vasodilatation and fully "arterialize" cutaneous blood, the patient's hand (or the heel in infants) is first placed in warm water at 45° for 3–5 minutes. A sterilized spring lancet or blade is used to make the finger cut. Blood is collected in the rubber funnel tip as it falls drop by drop from the finger and is drawn into the syringe. The flow of blood should be free, but gentle pressure may be applied if necessary. The initial air bubble, if any, is ejected and the syringe is shaken gently to mix the blood with the heparin as the collection proceeds. About 1 ml. of blood should be collected in 1–3 minutes. If the first cut does not supply enough blood for the sample, a second cut may be made and the blood pooled with that of the first cut. The total amount of blood must be noted to the nearest 0.05 ml. so that the heparin dilution can be calculated. The rubber collecting tip on the syringe is replaced by a metal cap. The syringe is placed cap down in a beaker of ice. When the procedure is properly carried out, the exposure of blood to air during collection is without significant effect on the *p*H and CO_2 content.

Instead of the fingertip, the ear lobe can be used as a source of cutaneous blood, after warming by dry heat as described by Lilienthal and Riley (3).

Determination of Hemoglobin Concentration[5]

The collecting syringe is shaken gently for thorough mixing. The metal cap is removed and the blood in the syringe tip is discarded. A rubber syringe adapter is attached to the syringe tip. A drop of blood is forced from the syringe and is drawn by suction into a 0.02 ml. (20 cu.mm.) pipet calibrated to contain that amount. This sample is delivered into a photometer tube containing 5.0 ml. of 0.1% Na_2CO_3 solution. The pipet is rinsed several times with the Na_2CO_3 solution and the tube is stoppered and inverted repeatedly. A tube containing 0.012M $CuSO_4 \cdot 4NH_3 \cdot H_2O$ is used as a standard. The solutions are read in a photometer against a distilled water blank. A 540 mμ (green) filter is used.

$$\text{Hb, in mM/L.} = \frac{\text{Reading Hb}}{\text{Reading } CuSO_4 \cdot 4NH_3 \cdot H_2O} \times \frac{\text{volume blood} + \text{volume heparin}}{\text{volume blood}} \times 9.34$$

$$\text{Hb, in Gm./100 ml.} = \frac{\text{Reading Hb}}{\text{Reading } CuSO_4 \cdot 4NH_3 \cdot H_2O} \times \frac{\text{volume blood} + \text{vol. heparin}}{\text{volume blood}} \times 15.6$$

The factors 9.34 and 15.6 in these equations are derived from the data of Drabkin (8), who proposed the use of $CuSO_4 \cdot 4NH_3 \cdot H_2O$ as a standard solution for photometric estimation of hemoglobin and other pigments. In the Klett-Summerson photometer with a 540 mμ filter, Drakbin found a ratio of 0.963 for the reading of a standard hemoglobin solution (8.98

[5] A detailed description is given for the hemoglobin determination because this is a slightly better index of blood nonbicarbonate buffers than is the packed cell volume, and because the reference standard can be used to check the photometer reading of the phenol red solutions. In our hands the copper sulfate photometric standard was stable and reproducible, and gave good results. However, more recent work by Drabkin and others on behalf of the National Research Council has indicated that slight variations may occur in the water content of the crystalline $CuSO_4 \cdot 5H_2O$ that make it undesirable as a primary photometric standard. Published recommendations have appeared in this journal, Vol. 1, page 151, to determine hemoglobin as cyanmethemoglobin, with the use of a stable, primary cyanmethemoglobin standard that is now available through Division of Medical Sciences, National Academy of Sciences–National Research Council. The use of this new standard is to be preferred.

mM./L. or 15.00 Gm./100 ml., diluted 1–251) and the reading of 0.012M copper sulfate standard. The reading of the standard, which varies somewhat from instrument to instrument, and serially in the same instrument, therefore corresponds to that of a solution containing 8.98/0.963 = 9.34 mM./L. of hemoglobin, or 15.00/0.963 = 15.6 Gm./100 ml. of hemoglobin, after dilution 1–251.

Filling of Micropipets

Before filling each micropipet with an aliquot of the blood sample collected, the collecting syringe is shaken gently and a small portion of blood is discarded by touching a clean cloth to the blood surface. The calibrated end of the micropipet is placed end to end against (not inside) the rubber adapter, and blood is forced carefully from the syringe until the pipet is filled slightly beyond the 0.1 ml. mark. Manipulation is facilitated by holding the barrel of the syringe and the pipet in the left hand while the right hand slowly pushes the syringe plunger (Fig. 2). When the pipet has been filled, it is grasped by the right hand with the forefinger covering the open stem above the bulb; contact with the syringe is then broken. The blood is adjusted to the 0.1 ml. mark by drawing off the excess with a clean cloth or by gently tapping the pipet end with a finger. The pipet is

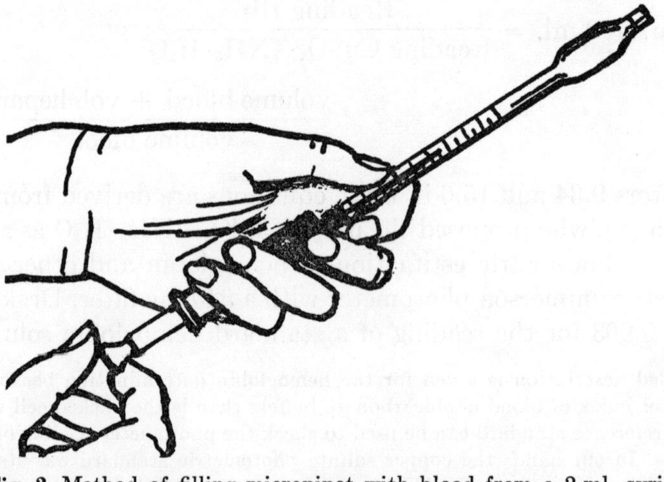

Fig. 2. Method of filling micropipet with blood from a 2-ml. syringe. The stem of the pipet is held between the thumb and forefinger of the left hand. The barrel of the syringe is held between the palm and fourth and fifth fingers of the same hand. The flat bottom of the pipet stem must be firmly apposed to the flat end of the rubber adapter on the tip of the syringe. Filling is controlled by gentle pressure on the plunger of the syringe with the right hand. The same procedure is used in filling the micropipet to the 2.0 ml. mark with diluent from a 20-ml. syringe.

then tilted slightly, bulb down, until there is a small air space between the blood and the calibrated end of the pipet. The outside of the calibrated end is wiped clean.

Saline-phenol red solution in the greased 20 ml. syringe is used as diluent for three pipets, and 0.9% NaCl for the fourth, which serves as a color blank for the *p*H determination. The dilution is accomplished by the filling technic just described; but to avoid trapping air in the pipet bulb, the syringe and pipet should be gradually raised to a vertical position while filling and then lowered to a horizontal position when the solution is slight above the 2.0 ml. mark. Care must be taken to hold the pipet firmly against the rubber adapter, maintaining the pressure fit. After adjusting the volume, a small air space is again left in the end of the pipet. The outside is dried carefully, and the tip of the calibrated end is sealed with a small piece of adhesive tape.

Centrifuging and Determination of Packed Red Cell Volume (Vc)

One of the heavy rubber bands is placed lengthwise about each pipet and flat over the adhesive tape seal to protect the pipet in centrifuging. The calibrated end of the pipet is placed in the cup adapter made from rubber pressure tubing. The pipets in this way are held firmly in the centrifuge cups. Centrifugation is carried out at 2600 rpm for 15–20 minutes. The rubber bands should be removed carefully after centrifugation since they sometimes stick to the adhesive tape seal.

The volume of packed red cells (*Vc*), noted to the nearest 0.5 per cent in the calibrated stem of the pipet, must be corrected for the heparin dilution.

$$\text{Vc} \times \frac{\text{volume blood} + \text{volume heparin}}{\text{volume blood}} = \text{corrected Vc}$$

pH Determination

To check against the standard curve, two pipets or test tubes are filled with *p*H 7.40 phosphate buffer containing phenol red. All the pipets and tubes except the saline blank are heated in a water bath to 38°. Readings are taken on each pipet after placing it bulb down in the holder of the photometer, checking stem orientation each time. A green filter with maximum transmission at 540 mμ is used. All readings should be taken promptly or the red cells in the stem of the inverted pipet may flow into the bulb.

The reading of each micropipet must be corrected by applying the appropriate pipet calibration. The final corrected reading, R, is calculated as $R = R_2 - R_1$, where R_2 is the corrected reading for the blood-phenol red sample and R_1 is the corrected reading for the blood-saline blank. The *p*H is estimated by the interpolation of R on the standard curve of the *p*H of the phosphate buffers at 37° versus the photometer scale reading. This value, plus the appropriate pK′ correction (see Table 2), gives the final *p*H value.

Determination of Whole Blood CO_2 Content $(CO_2)_b$

The CO_2 content of the blood diluted with saline-phenol red is determined in a Van Slyke manometric blood gas apparatus by the basic method of Van Slyke and Neill, as adapted to the characteristics of the sample (1, 5).

One drop of caprylic alcohol is drawn into the capillary and 3 ml. of 0.1N lactic acid are measured in the cup of the apparatus. After removing the adhesive tape seal from the pipet, a small piece of rubber tubing is placed on the tip of the calibrated end to provide a watertight seal between the pipet and the lactic acid. The contents of the pipet are delivered directly into the extraction chamber, delivery being halted with a small air bubble in the stopcock capillary. The air bubble is dislodged with a wire dipped in caprylic alcohol, and 2.5 ml. of the lactic acid are drawn into the machine. The stopcock is sealed with mercury and the mercury level in the chamber is lowered to the 50 ml. mark. After extraction the CO_2 is reabsorbed with 1 ml. of 1N NaOH. Pressure readings are taken at the 0.5 ml. volume.

A blank CO_2 determination is made in the same manner on a 2.0 ml. sample of the saline-phenol red solution used to dilute the blood.

The difference in pressure due to the blood, ΔP, is calculated by subtracting the blank correction from the difference in the pressure readings for the blood diluted with saline-phenol red, $P_1 - P_2$ (see "Sample calculations").

The CO_2 content of the blood in mM/L., $(CO_2)_b$, is obtained by multiplying the pressure difference, ΔP, by the appropriate factors for temperature, pipet calibration, and heparin dilution.

$$(CO_2)_b = P \times \frac{\text{Temperature Factor}}{\text{Pipet Factor}} \times \frac{\text{volume blood} + \text{volume heparin}}{\text{volume blood}}$$

Temperature factors as calculated by Peters and Van Slyke (5) are reproduced in Table 3, page 304.

Centrifugation of Excess Blood for Determination of Plasma Constituents

Additional determinations, such as plasma Na, K, Cl, and CO_2 can be made if a larger sample of blood (1.5 to 2.0 ml.) is collected at the time of the finger or ear lobe puncture. When it is planned to collect a blood sample larger than 1.2 ml., it is advisable to grease the plunger of the collecting syringe before adding the heparin saline solution.

After the aliquots required for the *p*H, CO_2, and hemoglobin determinations have been taken from the syringe, the contents are mixed; the syringe is held vertically, tip down, while the mercury is carefully ejected. The blood is transferred to the bottom of a 1-ml. micro centrifuge tube through a 2-inch 21-gage needle. The centrifuge tube should be filled from the bottom to avoid trapping an air bubble. A small rubber stopper pierced by a short 24-gage hypodermic needle is quickly inserted in such a way that any trapped air and a small amount of excess blood are forced up through the needle. The needle is then removed and the tube is ready for anaerobic centrifugation. The brief exposure of the blood to room air while the tube is being filled does not result in a significant change in *p*H or CO_2 content, as is shown later. After centrifugation the stopper is removed and the plasma is carefully withdrawn through a 21-gage needle into a greased 2-ml. syringe. The empty needle is removed, the syringe held tip up, and the air bubble (from the needle) is ejected. The plasma can be stored anaerobically if the syringe tip is protected with a metal cap.

Sampling is accomplished by forcing a drop of plasma up into a collecting piece placed on the syringe tip and drawing up a 0.05 or 0.1 ml. aliquot into a suitable type of calibrated pipet such as the Linderstrom-Lang-Hølter semiautomatic constriction pipet. The pipet designed by Kirk is also suitable and in the sizes from 0.05 to 0.2 ml. can be utilized as an accurate delivery pipet despite the fact that it is designed "to contain."[6] In this pipet the volume to deliver is about 2 per cent less than the contained volume. Filling and delivery in these pipets are accomplished with the aid of mouth suction and pressure through a rubber tube and mouthpiece, or with the aid of a pipet controller (9).

If desired, the plasma CO_2 content can be measured, with 0.1 ml. aliquots delivered under water in the cup of the Van Slyke apparatus as described previously. The relative accuracy of this determination is greater than that of the whole blood CO_2 because the blank correction is

---

[6] The Linderstrom-Lang-Hølter and Kirk micropipets used by us were obtained from Arthur H. Thomas Co., Philadelphia, Pa.

more stable and the concentration of total CO_2 is about 20 per cent higher in plasma.

Unless plasma CO_2 is to be included, all plasma samples can be drawn directly from the centrifuge tube. If a potassium determination is desired, the blood must be transferred to the micro centrifuge tube before icing the collecting syringe to prevent the exchange of potassium across cell membranes.

Plasma sodium and potassium concentrations can be measured with the internal standard flame photometer (10). For the determination of chloride we have used Sendroy's titrimetric iodate method, with modifications as described by Van Slyke and Hiller (11) on 0.05 ml. aliquots. Protein concentration could be estimated in one drop by means of the gradient tube (12) or falling-drop method (13). A variety of substances in plasma can be determined by suitable micro methods, up to the limit of plasma available, which would be about 0.5 ml. for a 1.5 ml. sample of blood.

Because the plasma is diluted with a heparin solution containing sodium and chloride, appropriate corrections must be applied to the measured concentrations of these ions, and to the concentrations of other substances estimated in heparinized diluted plasma. The corrections are calculated from the amount of heparin solution used in relation to the amount of plasma, and, in the case of sodium and chloride, from the concentration of these ions in the heparin solution.

SAMPLE CALCULATIONS

1. Dilution Factor

Suppose the total volume of blood and heparin diluent (measured in collecting syringe) to be 1.50 ml. Volume of heparin solution measured from tuberculin syringe—0.05 ml. Volume of blood = 1.50 − 0.05 = 1.45 ml. Consequently, the dilution factor for use in calculating hematocrit value and whole blood concentrations is 1.50/1.45 or 1.034.

2. Hemoglobin Concentration

Suppose that the corrected mean reading for the standard $CuSO_4 \cdot 4NH_3 \cdot H_2O$ solution in the Klett-Summerson photometer is 200, and the mean reading for the hemoglobin diluted 1/251 is 185. The hemoglobin pipets used have a calibrated volume of 20.2 cu.mm.

$$\text{Hb conc} = (9.34)\ (186/200)\ (20.0/20.2)\ (1.034) = 8.9 \text{ mM/L.}$$

3. Hematocrit Value

Suppose that the mean value in four micropipets is 0.440.

$$\text{Corrected Vc} = (0.440)\ (1.034) = 0.455$$

It is not useful to measure or calculate the hematocrit value more accurately than to the nearest 0.005.

4. Photometric pH

Suppose the mean reading of the plasma-indicator-saline mixture in three micropipets (with the individual pipet calibration applied to each reading) to be 156. The corrected blank reading is 10. The mean corrected reading for the *p*H 7.40 phosphate buffer is 152, and for the *p*H 7.20 buffer, 111.

Sample reading, corrected for blank = 156 − 10 = 146. The *p*H can then be read from a suitable graph on which photometer readings are plotted against *p*H, or estimated by the following equation in the *p*H range in which the relation is virtually linear:

$$p\text{H} = 7.40 - [(152\text{-}146)/(152\text{-}111)][0.20] = 7.40 - (6/41)(0.20) = 7.37$$

Finally, the correction from Table 2 must be applied (the difference of pK′ of phenol red in 0.9% NaCl solution as compared with M/15 phosphate buffer):

$$\text{Corrected } p\text{H} = 7.37 - 0.02 = 7.35$$

5. Whole Blood CO_2 Concentration

Assume the following data. Volume of micropipet = 0.099; calibration of chamber volume = 0.495 ml. Blank pressure difference for 2.0 ml. of saline-phenol red = 14.0 mm. Calculated blank for 1.9 ml. of saline-phenol red = (14.0)(1.9/2.0) or 13.3 mm. At 24° the two pressure readings obtained for the diluted blood sample are P_1 = 182.6 mm. and P_2 = 114.0 mm.

$$\text{Corrected } \Delta P = (182.6 - 114.0) - 13.3 = 68.6 - 13.3 = 55.3$$

The factor in Table 3 at 24°, for a chamber volume of 0.5 ml. and a sample of 0.100 ml. is 0.304.

$$(CO_2)_b = (55.3)(0.304)(0.100 \times 0.100/0.099)(0.495/0.500)(1.034)$$
$$= (16.8)(1.034) = 17.4 \text{ mM/L.}$$

It is convenient to prepare a table of temperature factors that includes

Table 3. FACTORS FOR CALCULATION OF WHOLE BLOOD CO_2 CONTENT

Temperature (°C.)	*Factor*[a] (mM/L./mm.)	*Temperature* (°C.)	*Factor*[a] (mM/L./mm.)
15	0.320	25	0.302
16	0.318	26	0.300
17	0.316	27	0.299
18	0.314	28	0.297
19	0.312	29	0.296
20	0.311	30	0.294
21	0.309	31	0.292
22	0.307	32	0.290
23	0.305	33	0.289
24	0.304	34	0.287

[a] Factor by which the gasometric pressure difference on the Van Slyke-Neill apparatus, in mm. of Hg, is to be multiplied to obtain the whole blood CO_2 content in mM/L. These factors are calculated for a sample size of 0.1 ml., a solution volume of 4.5 ml., a chamber volume of 0.5 ml., and an "i" factor of 1.037. See Peters and Van Slyke (5). These factors are more convenient to use than the ones given by Shock and Hastings (1), because they give directly the CO_2 concentration in the blood sample instead of the blood-saline mixture.

the correction for the chamber volume. The sample and pipet corrections must be calculated in each individual determination; the dilution factor is usually applied only to the mean of the replicate CO_2 determinations.

6. Obtaining the Derived Acid-Base Factors

The calculated CO_2 pressure and total CO_2 or bicarbonate concentration of plasma can be obtained from the nomograms of Van Slyke and Sendroy (14) and Hastings and Shock (15). The whole blood buffer base concentration can be obtained from the nomogram of Singer and Hastings (16), which also gives values for CO_2 pressure and plasma total CO_2 or bicarbonate. In the application of all of these nomograms to whole blood CO_2 concentrations it is necessary to use the hemoglobin concentration or hematocrit value as one auxiliary parameter, and a known or assumed O_2 saturation as the other. Unless the patient is cyanotic or the sample shows obvious signs of unsaturation, it is assumed that cutaneous or arterial blood is fully oxygenated. If the oxygen saturation is less than 90 per cent, slight errors in CO_2 pressure and buffer base concentration will be introduced unless account is taken of this factor. In the example cited here, with Hb 8.9 mM/L. or Vc 0.455 and an assumed 100 per cent saturation, the whole blood CO_2, 17.4 mM/L., is found in Scale 1 of the nomogram of Singer and Hastings, and the *p*H, 7.35, on Scale 4. A straight line is drawn through these two points and the derived variables are read off.

Plasma $(CO_2)_p$ = 21.0 mM/L. (right-hand edge, Scale 1)

Plasma $(HCO_3^-)_p$ = 19.8 mM/L. (Scale 2)

Whole blood $(BB^+)_b$ = 43 mEq./L. (Scale 3)

P_{CO_2} = 37 mm. (Scale 5)

This represents for an adult a mild metabolic acidosis with a CO_2 pressure at the lower edge of the normal range. However, in an infant, these acid-base conditions could all be within a normal range.

RESULTS

Accuracy of Modified Microtechnic

The respective errors of the various methods involved in the microtechnic have been estimated by an analysis of the deviations in a large number of sets of replicate determinations. The results in Fig. 3 show the distribution of the deviations from the mean. The standard error for the mean of duplicate hemoglobin determinations is ±0.029 mM/L. or less than half of one per cent of the average concentration, a relative error equal to that of the calibration of the 20 cu.mm. pipets. The standard error of the mean of quadruplicate packed cell volumes was ±0.0023. The standard error of the *p*H in triplicate was ±0.0051, and that of the whole blood CO_2 content in duplicate ±0.16 mM/L. Confidence limits have been calculated on the basis of the difference between means (obtained with the usual number of replicates) that has only a 5 per cent probability of being due to chance variation; the ratio of this difference to the standard error of the difference, or $\sqrt{2} \times$ standard error, is 1.96 (17). This least significant difference is less than 0.1 mM/L. or 0.15 Gm./100 ml. for hemoglobin, 0.006 for cell volume, 0.014 for *p*H and 0.44 mM/L. for whole blood CO_2 content. The accuracy of this whole blood CO_2 determination can be compared with that of the determination of CO_2 content in 0.2 ml. aliquots of plasma, measured in a stopcock pipet. The standard error of the duplicate plasma determination was ±0.11 mM/L., and the least significant difference 0.3 mM/L.

Effect of Collection or Transfer of Blood with Momentary Exposure to Air

In Table 4 results are presented of a representative experiment in which heparinized blood was transferred dropwise from a 20-ml. syringe to four separate 2-ml. syringes in such a way as to simulate the collection of cutaneous blood. Two of the small syringes (A and C) were previously prepared with 0.05 ml. of heparin saline solution, and two (B and D) con-

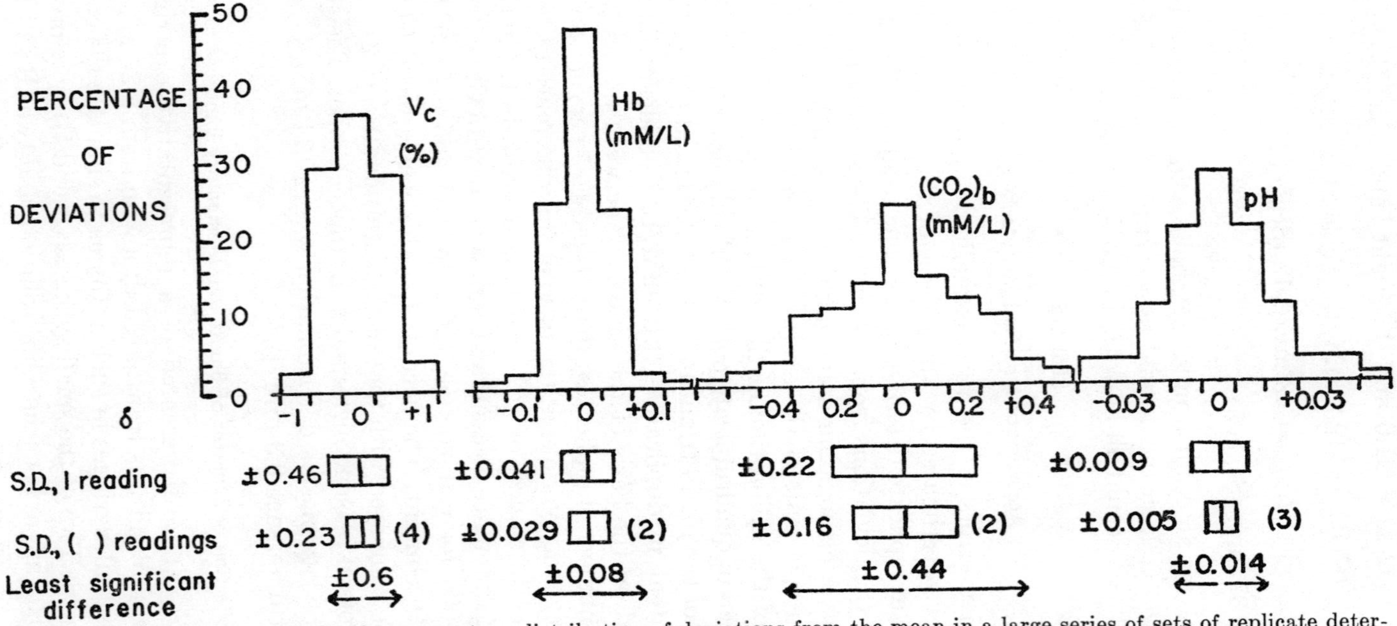

Fig. 3. Frequency diagram showing percentage distribution of deviations from the mean in a large series of sets of replicate determinations utilizing the microtechnic. Below this distribution for each variable are given the standard deviation for a single reading, the standard error of the mean of the usual number of replicates in a single determination, and the least significant difference between two determinations (at the 95 per cent confidence level).

Table 4. TEST OF COLLECTION: DROPWISE TRANSFER OF BLOOD

Specimen	*Hb* (mM/L.)	*Vc*	*pH at 37°*	$(CO_2)_b$ (mM/L)	*Heparin to blood* (ml./ml.)	*Transfer time* (min.)
Control[a]	8.05	0.400	7.300	24.1	0.3/20	—
A	8.00	0.400	7.295	23.8	0.05/0.95	1
B	—	0.410	7.295	23.8	No heparin	1
C	8.30	0.410	7.285	24.0	0.05/0.95	4
D	8.10	0.405	7.290	23.8	No heparin	4

[a] Venous blood, drawn and stored in a 20-ml. syringe containing 0.3 ml. heparin solution. By glass electrode the *p*H of this blood was 7.47 at 26°, or 7.315 at 37°, with temperature factor of Rosenthal, *J. Biol. Chem.*, **173,** 25 (1948).

tained no heparin; all syringes contained some mercury for mixing the blood in the sampling process. Two of the transfers were accomplished "rapidly" (about 1 ml. of blood in 1 minute) and two "slowly" (1 ml. in 4 minutes), to simulate easy and difficult fingertip collection. As is evident from Table 4, very slight decreases were observed in *p*H and CO_2 content in the transferred blood as compared with the control blood. In syringe C the *p*H decrease of 0.015 was barely significant; all other differences in *p*H and CO_2 content were smaller than the least significant differences determined above. The factor of dilution of blood with heparin saline introduces an additional uncertainty in the measurement of cell volume and hemoglobin and CO_2 concentrations. This may explain the rather high hemoglobin concentration in Sample C (wetting of the syringe surfaces might reduce the effective amount of heparin saline dilution of the blood, in some instances). This experiment also shows that the heparin solution has had no significant effect on the *p*H of the blood to which it was added. Other experiments have confirmed this lack of effect, even when relatively much larger amounts of heparin solution were used.

Table 5. "VIRTUAL" ANAEROBIC TECHNIC: TRANSFER OF BLOOD FROM SYRINGE TO CENTRIFUGE TUBE

Method of transfer	*pH at 37°*	$(CO_2)_b$ *(in blood)* (mM/L.)	$(CO_2)_p$ *(in plasma)* (mM/L.)
Anaerobic control—syringe to syringe	7.34	24.30	28.60
"Virtual" anaerobic—Single transfer[a]	7.34	24.25	28.45
"Virtual" anaerobic—5 transfers[a]	7.32	24.00	28.10
Difference per transfer[a]			
Single transfer	0.00	−0.05	−0.15
Multiple transfers	−0.004	−0.06	−0.10

[a] Venous blood, exposed briefly to air during transfer from syringe to small centrifuge tube and back again, after stoppering tube so as to exclude air. Mixing of blood carried out with mercury. Blood heparinized in first syringe.

In another experiment we observed the effect of transferring about 8 ml. of blood from a syringe into an open centrifuge tube (a Pyrex round-bottom tube, 1.25 by 10 cm.). The blood was exposed to air during the filling process until a rubber stopper and needle were inserted as described previously, so as to eliminate any air bubble, and exposed again when the sample was taken up into a second syringe for storage. A portion of the blood in the syringe was then transferred aerobically to a 5-ml. centrifuge tube, stoppered so as to exclude air, centrifuged, and the plasma drawn off and stored in a third syringe for analysis of plasma CO_2 content. The *p*H and the whole blood CO_2 content were determined on the blood in the second syringe, and control analyses performed on the original blood not subject to aerobic transfer. The results are shown in Table 5. In addition to the single tube transfer (as described above) the experiment was repeated with 5 successive transfers to separate tubes before the blood was drawn up in the storage syringe. The differences observed as a result of this multiple transfer were divided by 5, to give figures which should be a more accurate approximation of the differences due to a single transfer. Per single transfer the *p*H was found to decrease 0.004 (an amount too small to be detected in the single transfer), the whole blood CO_2 content decreased about 0.06 mM/L., and the plasma CO_2 content, 0.10 mM/L. These changes are well within the confidence limits found for the microtechnic and we can conclude that this method of aerobic transfer of blood for centrifugation introduced no appreciable error for clinical and most other purposes.

Comparison of Arterial and Cutaneous Blood Samples

Results are presented in Table 6 for the analysis of seven pairs of blood samples, one arterial and one cutaneous in each pair. The arterial sample was drawn in a 10-ml. syringe to which 0.3 ml. of heparin solution had previously been added. The syringe was attached to a manifold connected with a needle placed in the femoral artery. Because of risk of clotting in the long connecting tube of fine bore it was generally not possible to prolong collection of the arterial sample to correspond exactly with the time required for collection of the cutaneous sample. The average time for the latter was 2.0 minutes, and for the former about 0.5 minute. Slight mean differences were observed in packed cell volume and *p*H, and virtually none in CO_2 content. The only significant mean difference was that for hemoglobin, which was 0.19 mM/L. higher in cutaneous than in arterial blood. Although significant, this difference is small enough to ignore for most acid-base analyses, in which cutaneous blood can be considered almost identical with arterial blood.

Table 6. Simultaneous Arterial and Cutaneous Blood Samples
Comparison of Acid-Base Properties

	Arterial	*Cutaneous*	*Difference*
Hemoglobin (mM/L.)	8.50	8.60	−0.10
	7.80	8.05	−0.25
	8.45	8.60	−0.15
	8.20	8.20	0.00
	6.65	7.00	−0.35
	6.65	7.05	−0.40
	7.85	7.85	0.00
Mean			−0.19
S.E.			±0.064
*p*H	7.41	7.41	0.00
	7.53	7.55	−0.02
	7.35	7.35	0.00
	7.45	7.46	−0.01
	7.39	7.37	+0.02
	7.52	7.52	0.00
	7.33	7.35	−0.02
Mean			−0.004
S.E.			±0.0053
Red cell volume (mM/L.)	0.425	0.435	−0.010
	0.400	0.415	−0.015
	0.420	0.420	0.000
	0.395	0.395	0.000
	—	—	—
	0.345	0.365	−0.020
	0.400	0.395	+0.005
Mean			−0.007
S.E.			±0.0058
Whole blood CO_2 (mM/L)	23.3	23.6	−0.3
	32.2	32.4	−0.2
	21.3	21.3	0.0
	25.7	25.6	+0.1
	21.0	21.6	−0.6
	26.4	26.0	+0.4
	21.6	21.1	+0.5
Mean			−0.01
S.E.			±0.147

DISCUSSION

The suitability of this microtechnic for clinical studies of acid-base balance will be discussed from three aspects: the use of cutaneous blood; errors of collection and handling; and analytical accuracy.

Advantages of Cutaneous Blood

Our results confirm those of Lundsgaard and Møller (18), Saito (19) and Lilienthal and Riley (20) that cutaneous blood (drawn from hyperemic skin) is nearly identical with arterial blood in its acid-base properties. A comparable similarity has also been demonstrated for oxygen saturation (3, 18, 19). The only significant difference that we found was a slightly higher hemoglobin concentration, 0.2 mM/L. greater in cutaneous than in arterial blood. Part of the difference may have been due to dilution error but, regardless of the cause, the difference has a negligible effect on the use of this parameter in the calculation of CO_2 pressure and whole-blood buffer base concentration. Such a similarity of chemical properties is a fortunate circumstance for clinical studies, because the sampling of cutaneous blood is a much simpler process than an arterial puncture. The advantage of ease of sampling is thus combined with the further advantage of having arterial or cutaneous blood, rather than venous blood, for analysis of the state of acid-base balance of the patient. The respiratory factor in this state is most conveniently defined by the alveolar, or its equivalent, the arterial, CO_2 pressure, which can be readily calculated from the pH and CO_2 concentration of arterial blood or plasma. The usual arterio-venous differences with regard to O_2 saturation, CO_2 pressure, pH, and CO_2 content are greatly influenced by unpredictable variations in local venous flow. Consequently venous blood has the disadvantages of a wider range for "normal" values, a CO_2 pressure higher than in alveolar air, and a variable O_2 saturation, which introduces an additional factor in the calculation of P_{CO_2} and buffer base (14, 16). All these drawbacks are avoided by the simple expedient of using cutaneous blood for acid-base studies.

Collection, Handling, and Storage

The method described in this paper for the collection, handling, and storage of cutaneous blood samples is based on previous work (3, 21) and has here been shown to produce essentially no change in pH and CO_2 pressure, and only an insignificant decrease in bicarbonate and buffer base concentration amounting to less than 0.2 mEq./L. The anticipated effects of exposing blood to room air are a fall in P_{CO_2} and bicarbonate, a rise in pH, and no change in buffer base. However, a variety of effects may be produced by other sources of error, such as temperature change, the presence of an anticoagulant, glycolysis, hemolysis, and change in permeability of the red cell membrane. The combined error of a given method of handling blood therefore depends on a number of factors in addition to exposure of the blood to air; in this method the results suggest a combination of slight accumulation of fixed acid, such as lactate, in the blood, and loss of displaced bicarbonate. The fact of importance in clinical chemistry is that the combined handling error is negligible if (1) heparin is used as anticoagulant, (2) the blood is chilled and stored in a closed syringe, and (3) exposure to air during collection or transfer is restricted to the conditions described herein.

Since the transient exposure to air does not introduce serious error, a technic of this sort might be called a "virtual anaerobic" technic. Undoubtedly the best method of avoiding this type of error is the "strict anaerobic" technic of Austin *et al.* (22), in which blood is handled in tonometers over mercury. However, these precautions are scarcely feasible or necessary in clinical studies of acid-base balance. On the other hand, such a "virtual anaerobic" technic appears to offer definite advantages over the common practice, in hospital laboratories, of relying on the sometimes uncertain protection (23–25) afforded by handling blood under oil, or of adhering to the outmoded "plasma CO_2 combining power" method (26), which was abandoned in Van Slyke's laboratory more than 30 years ago (27). Centrifuging blood under oil in the ordinary centrifuge tube is almost certain to produce appreciable loss of CO_2 (23), whereas use of a syringe (21) or a completely filled tube entails no appreciable loss (23; Table 6). Even with 1-ml. samples it is a convenience to avoid having to sample blood or plasma under oil; and we have demonstrated a definite decrease in accuracy of measuring 0.1 ml. aliquots when this is done from a sample under oil.

A certain amount of training is required for the analyst to attain proficiency in the collection of cutaneous blood samples and in the filling of the micropipets. The experience gained in acquiring such proficiency and in teaching others leads us to believe that the method is entirely suitable for any hospital laboratory where one or more individuals can be trained in its use, under the supervision of a clinical chemist.

Accuracy

The accuracy of the individual determinations is satisfactory for all clinical and many experimental purposes, as shown by the results in Fig. 3, and various papers describing each method (1, 2, 7, 28). The standard errors of measurement shown in Fig. 3 are estimates of reproducibility rather than of absolute error, which may be somewhat larger. For example, the hematocrit method is subject to errors due to trapping of solution between cells and to anisotonicity of the 0.9% NaCl diluent with respect

Table 7. Comparison of Colorimetric and Potentiometric pH in Human Plasma at 38°
Data from the Literature

Source	*No. comparisons*	*Difference, $pH_{col} - pH_{pot}$*		*Remarks*
		Mean	*S.D.*	
Hastings and Sendroy[a] 1924 (6)	5	+0.007	±0.011	3 comparisons at 20°. In vitro equilibration.
Myers and Muntwyler 1928 (38)	41	+0.020	±0.037	Venous plasma, as drawn from patients. Microcolorimeter for *p*H.
Fosbinder and Schoonover 1930 (39)	28	+0.002	±0.011	Plasma diluted 1–20 with KCl-phenol red and equilibrated in vitro.
Austin, Stadie, and Robinson 1925 (36)	2	+0.035	±0.015	One comparison with *p*H calculated from Henderson-Hasselbalch equation.
Van Slyke, Weisiger, and Van Slyke 1949 (2)	26	−0.002	±0.022	Equilibrated in vitro, *p*H range 6.89 to 7.65. Photocolorimetric *p*H.
Weighted Mean	102	+0.008	..	

[a] Hastings and Sendroy found a difference of −0.015 ± 0.013 in 13 comparisons in horse plasma, and −0.010 ± 0.009 in 4 comparisons in dog plasma.

to the actual red cell contents in a given blood. This uncertainty is not important in the calculation of acid-base factors, but of the two parameters, the hemoglobin concentration is a more accurate determination than the hematocrit value. The precision of the manometric blood-gas apparatus is well established for this as well as macro determinations (1, 28, 29). Unsuspected errors have been shown to be far greater in other methods commonly used in clinical laboratories (30), and best results cannot be obtained without careful attention to detail and accurate calibration of photometer tubes and pipets.[7] The methods described in this paper have been successfully employed in a number of clinical studies (32–34).

The only part of the microtechnic to which objections have been raised in the past is the colorimetric *p*H determination. In comparison with the electrometric method (H_2 or glass electrode), the colorimetric method has been charged with being unreliable when applied to plasma or serum

[7] Stock volumetric pipets as purchased may deviate considerably from the stated volume and this is particularly true of the 20-cu.mm. hemoglobin pipets (31). In our experience the individually tested hemoglobin pipets supplied by Arthur H. Thomas Co. have been quite satisfactory; in one batch of 24 pipets calibration showed a maximum deviation from the 20-cu.mm. volume of only 0.3 cu.mm.

(35–37), and this point deserves comment. Large discrepancies found have been ascribed to variability in the effects of dilution, protein concentration, and other errors on the final result. When available reports of comparisons between electrometric and colorimetric *p*H are examined, it becomes evident that details of procedure have varied widely. Some comparisons have been made with dog instead of human blood, with serum instead of plasma, with the colorimetric *p*H read at room temperature instead of 38°. The only comparisons of relevance here are those made following the basic Hastings and Sendroy technic, on which the Shock and Hastings and current modifications are based. A summary of relevant studies of this type on human plasma is given in Table 7. Results are in terms of the difference between the colorimetric and potentiometric *p*H, both determined at 38°. Most of the papers do not present figures for the mean and standard deviation, which we have calculated from the data for the individual differences. It is evident that there is generally good agreement in the several series, and the weighted mean difference is less than +0.01 *p*H unit. If the correction in Table 2 is applied, assuming an average comparison *p*H of 7.40, the mean difference is seen to fall between 0.00 and −0.01. The reproducibility of the difference, as adjudged by the generally small standard deviation, is good. In a series of 15 comparisons of glass electrode with H_2 electrode *p*H, Van Slyke *et al.* found a mean difference of −0.002 and a standard deviation of ±0.016 (2), a reproducibility only slightly better than for the photometric *p*H. On the basis of these result it would appear that the difference between the photocolorimetric and potentiometric *p*H determinations at 38° lies between −0.04 and +0.04 in over 90 per cent of cases.

The discrepancies referred to previously have not been reported on human plasma, but generally on dog serum, and in connection with variability of the "C" correction, the difference between the colorimetric *p*H at 20° and photometric *p*H at 38°. Species differences and differences between serum and plasma with respect to the "C" correction have been observed by Cullen and many others (35, 36, 40–42). The "C" correction is +0.30 for human serum and +0.23 for human plasma, and Robinson *et al.* demonstrated that the correction varied with the serum protein concentration (43). Some of the results on dog and human serum have been characterized by large standard deviations, ranging from ±0.07 to ±0.11 (35–37). On the other hand, Hastings and Sendroy (6) found little variation from the plasma of one species to another when the colorimetric-potentiometric difference was measured at 38°. The same is true of this difference in human serum as compared with plasma, at 38°

(38, 41). From all this and other evidence (44) it seems clear that the final result in a colorimetric *p*H determination is influenced by a number of possible errors, which are generally larger when serum is used or when the reading is made at room temperature. For human plasma read at 37–38°, these errors either become very small or are self-compensating (44), as is demonstrated by the evidence in Table 7.

In their practical operation for the determination of *p*H in blood, both the H_2 electrode and glass electrode have serious disadvantages that must be weighed along with their advantages, in comparing them with the photocolorimetric method. For clinical work economy of sample size is often an important consideration, and in this the photometric method is superior to the usual glass electrode. The apparatus required for the photometric determination is cheaper and probably more reliable than the glass electrode and *p*H meter, but the technic of the determination is somewhat more complex. The standard error of measurement in the photometric *p*H determination appears to be *smaller* than that for any commercially available *p*H meter utilizing the glass electrode. After experience with both methods our preference in clinical work is definitely for the photometric.

Some of the features of the "virtual anaerobic" technic described here are applicable to the handling and centrifuging of larger amounts of blood, 2–20 ml., for the determination of *p*H and CO_2 concentration by other methods.

SUMMARY

1. A modification has been described for the Shock and Hastings technic of determining simultaneously, in 0.1 ml. aliquots of blood, the *p*H, CO_2 content, and packed cell volume. Advantages of the modification are collection and handling of the blood in a way that avoids the use of oil, and a modified design of the micropipets so that *p*H readings can be obtained in a filter photometer.

2. The standard error of measurement of a single reading was ± 0.009 for the *p*H, and ± 0.22 mM/L. for the whole blood CO_2 concentration. The reproducibility of the photocolorimetric *p*H measurement was slightly better than that obtainable with the most accurate commercially available glass electrode.

3. Results have been presented to show that blood can be handled in the presence of brief, limited, exposure to air with no detectable change in *p*H and only negligible change in CO_2 content (decrease of less than 0.2 mM/L.). Errors attributable to collection and handling of cutaneous blood by this "virtual anaerobic" technic are not of significant magnitude.

4. Results have also been presented in confirmation of the fact that arterial and cutaneous blood are virtually identical in acid-base properties. A sample of as little as 0.5 ml. of cutaneous blood, analyzed by the microtechnic, provides the necessary and sufficient data for a description of the state of acid-base balance. This includes calculation of the physiologically important variables, arterial CO_2 pressure, and whole-blood buffer base concentration, thus furnishing a measure of the respiratory factor and the metabolic factor in any acid-base disturbance. With a sample size of 1.5 ml. it is also possible to determine other individual constituents of plasma, such as sodium, chloride, and total protein.

5. The technic is useful in the study of clinical disturbances of acid-base balance, especially in infants and children.

REFERENCES

1. Shock, N. W., and Hastings, A. B., *J. Biol. Chem.* **104**, 565 (1934).
2. Van Slyke, D. D., Weisiger, J. R., and Van Slyke, K. K., *J. Biol. Chem.* **179**, 734 (1949).
3. Lilienthal, J. L., Jr., and Riley, R. L., *J. Clin. Invest.* **23**, 904 (1944).
4. Clark, W. M., *The Determination of Hydrogen Ion Concentration* (ed. 3). Baltimore, Md., Williams and Wilkins, 1929.
5. Peters, J. P., and Van Slyke, D. D., *Quantitative Clinical Chemistry* (ed. 1). Baltimore, Md., Williams and Wilkins, 1932, Vol. II, Ch. VII and XXVII, pp. 804–809.
6. Hastings, A. B., and Sendroy, J., Jr., *J. Biol. Chem.* **61**, 695 (1924).
7. Sendroy, J., Jr., and Hastings, A. B., *J. Biol. Chem.* **82**, 197 (1929).
8. Drabkin, D. L., "Spectroscopy: Photometry and Spectrophotometry." In Glasser, O. (Ed.), *Medical Physics* (ed. 1), Chicago, Yr. Bk. Pub., 1950, vol. II, pp. 1072–3.
9. Lazarow, A., *J. Lab. Clin. Med.*, **33**, 1603 (1948).
10. Wallace, W. M., Holliday, M., Cushman, M., and Elkinton, J. R., *J. Lab. Clin. Med.* **37**, 621 (1951).
11. Van Slyke, D. D., and Hiller, A., *J. Biol. Chem.* **167**, 107 (1947).
12. Lowry, O. H., and Hunter, T. H., *J. Biol. Chem.* **159**, 465 (1945).
13. Barbour, H. G., and Hamilton, W. F., *J. Biol. Chem.* **69**, 625 (1926).
14. Van Slyke, D. D., and Sendroy, J., Jr., *J. Biol. Chem.* **79**, 781 (1928).
15. Hastings, A. B., and Shock, N. W., *J. Biol. Chem.* **104**, 575 (1934).
16. Singer, R. B., and Hastings, A. B., *Medicine* **27**, 223 (1947).
17. Snedecor, G. W., *Statistical Methods* (ed. 4). Ames, Iowa, Iowa State College Press (1953).
18. Lundsgaard, C., and Møller, E., *J. Exp. Med.* **36**, 559 (1922).
19. Saito, K., *J. Biochem. (Japan)* **25**, 89 (1937).
20. Lilienthal, J. L., and Riley, R. L., *J. Lab. Clin. Med.* **31**, 99 (1946).
21. Davenport, H. C., *Science* **105**, 103 (1947).
22. Austin, J. H., Cullen, G. E., Hastings, A. B., McLean, F. C., Peters, J. P., and Van Slyke, D. D., *J. Biol. Chem.* **54**, 121 (1922).
23. Peters, J. P., and Van Slyke, D. D., *Loc. cit.* (Ref. 5), pp. 55–57.
24. Hendrix, B. M., and Bernasdoni, B., *Texas Reports Biol. and Med.* **2**, 241 (1944).
25. Looney, J. M., and Childs, H. M., *J. Biol. Chem.* **104**, 53 (1934).
26. Van Slyke, D. D., and Cullen, G. E., *J. Biol. Chem.* **30**, 289 (1917).
27. Peters, J. P., and Van Slyke, D. D., *Loc. cit* (Ref. 5), p. 251.
28. Van Slyke, D. D., and Sendroy, J., Jr., *J. Biol. Chem.* **73**, 127 (1927).

29. Van Slyke, D. D., Hiller, A., Weisiger, J. R., and Cruz, W. O., *J. Biol. Chem.* **166**, 121 (1946).
30. Belk, W. P., and Sunderman, F. W., *Am. J. Clin. Path.* **17**, 853 (1947).
31. Andersch, M. A., and Sacks, M. S., *Tech. Bull. of the Registry of Medical Technologists* **6**, 105 (1945).
32. Singer, R. B., *Am. J. Med. Sci.* **221**, 199 (1951).
33. Singer, R. B., *Medicine* **33**, 1 (1954).
34. Harvie, F. R., and Singer, R. B., *Am. J. Dis. Child.* **89**, 149 (1955).
35. Bennett, M. A., *J. Biol. Chem.* **69**, 697 (1926).
36. Austin, J. H., Stadie, W. C., and Robinson, H. W., *J. Biol. Chem.* **66**, 505 (1925).
37. Johnston, C. G., *J. Biol. Chem.* **79**, 297 (1928).
38. Myers, V. C., and Muntwyler, E., *J. Biol. Chem.* **78**, 243 (1928).
39. Fosbinder, R. J., and Schoonover, J., *Biochem. J.* **24**, 1805 (1930).
40. Cullen, G. E., *J. Biol. Chem.* **52**, 501 (1922).
41. Myers, V. C., Muntwyler, E., Binns, D., and Danielson, W. H., *J. Biol. Chem.* **102**, 19 (1933).
42. Robinson, H. W., Price, J. W., and Cullen, G. E., *J. Biol. Chem.* **100**, LXXXIII (1933).
43. Robinson, H. W., Price, J. W., and Cullen, G. E., *J. Biol. Chem.* **114**, 321 (1936).
44. Hastings, A. B., Personal communication, 1944.

Estimation of Lipid Fractions of Blood Plasma

System Using the Allen Volumetric Method

Andre C. Kibrick and S. J. Skupp

Abnormalities in the values of the lipid fractions of blood plasma, except for cholesterol, are not generally employed as a guide in following various clinical conditions, since the laboratory procedures available for their estimation have been quite cumbersome. This deficiency in convenient methods for determining the various lipids of blood is particularly unfortunate at this time when one considers the important role that the various lipids may play in such conditions as atherosclerosis and heart disease (1). In 1934 Allen devised a volumetric method for estimating blood fat of cattle which involved final measurement of the column of fat in a graduated capillary tube (2). Although such volumetric methods were applied to clinical chemistry at about that time (3), they have since been discarded for the most part.

We have recently reinvestigated the reliability of the Allen method on human plasma. By calibrating the tubes for recovery of known amounts of fat instead of using the content of the capillaries, we have obtained satisfactory values for the total of free cholesterol, esterified cholesterol, and neutral fat—that is, for all the lipid fractions except phospholipids which are not determined by this procedure. In the present paper we

---

From the Clinical Laboratories of the New York Veterans Administration Hospital in affiliation with New York University College of Medicine.

This investigation was supported in part by a research grant from the National Institute of Arthritis and Metabolic Diseases, the National Institutes of Health, U. S. Public Health Service.

Reviewed in the Veterans Administration and published with the approval of the Chief Medical Director. The statements and conclusions published by the authors are the result of their own study and do not necessarily reflect the opinion or policy of the Veterans Administration.

Received for publication April 25, 1955.

present data on the reliability of the Allen method and describe its application to a simple system for determining the major lipid fractions of blood plasma.

ADAPTATION OF ALLEN METHOD

The method for the volumetric determination of blood fat was performed essentially as described by Allen (2) on 3-ml. samples of plasma. The 2-neck tubes[1] were the same, and carried graduated capillaries in which the column of fat could be measured with calipers on the millimeter graduations. The samples were measured into the tubes by applying gentle suction to the capillary necks. A 5-ml. amount of reagent[2] was then added in the same way and mixed thoroughly with the plasma by rotation. The unstoppered tubes were heated in a water bath at 85° for 20 minutes with occasional shaking. They were then centrifuged for 5 minutes at 800 rpm., and warm water (75°) was added with a hypodermic needle attached to an elevated reservoir until the tuber were filled to the bottom of the graduated neck. After centrifuging again for 2 minutes, warm water was added until the filling neck overflowed and automatically brought the fat column to the proper level for reading. The tubes were again centrifuged for 5 minutes and placed in a 60° water bath for a few minutes before measuring the fat column with calipers.

The tubes were initially calibrated with mercury according to standard procedure, and the values obtained agreed precisely with the factors obtained by titration of the amount of standard acid contained in the capillaries with standard alkali. However, when the Allen method was performed on known amounts of olive oil, more than 100 per cent recovery of the oil was obtained by using the calibration factors. This was true when the oil was measured into the tubes by taking an aliquot of an ether solution and the ether then evaporated off, or when the oil was carefully weighed on a microbalance and added without solvent. In about 50 experiments the values of olive oil recovered usually ranged between 122 and 129 per cent. An average value of 25 per cent was therefore used to correct the mercury calibration factors.

The validity of the calibration values derived from the recovery of olive oil was checked in several ways. There was no indication of contamination

---

[1] Allen tubes for 3 ml. and for 0.25 ml. of plasma were obtained from E. Machlett and Son, New York. The micro tubes for 0.25 ml. are still being tested and will be reported in a later publication.

[2] The reagent consists of 110 Gm. sodium carbonate and 200 Gm. sodium salicylate dissolved in water and made up to a volume of 1 liter. To this are then added successively 30 ml. of 50% sodium hydroxide and 100 ml. of *n*-butyl alcohol.

of the fat layer with constituents of the Allen reagent. Neither butyl alcohol nor salicylate was found as a contaminant, when the recovered fat was tested with ammonium molybdate or ferric nitrate. The absence of significant amounts of either of these constituents of the reagent was confirmed by the fact that the iodine numbers of olive oil and other fats and oils were exactly the same on samples of the fat layer obtained after performing the Allen method (4) as when the original oil and fat were used as samples. The iodine number of butyl alcohol and sodium salicylate is 0 and 99, respectively, which differ quite markedly from that of olive oil and some of the other fats and oils. Since the values of the iodine number are the same before and after separation by this procedure, the method appears to separate oil and fat in the same degree of purity as the original lipid samples.

Since the apparent volume of the fat layer is larger than that of the original weight of the oil taken, we are forced to the conclusion that the volumes of oil measured in capillaries of this size are affected by spreading factors that may be unique for oils and fats (5). This conclusion is consistent with the results obtained by Chung, Saarinin, and Shaw (6) with the Allen method.

We have confirmed the original findings of Allen that the fat layer contains all the lipids of plasma with the exception of the phospholipids. In many determinations of the fat layer for phosphorus, not more than 5–7 per cent of the phosphorus of the phospholipids of the plasma was ever found. In addition, no fat was separated when the Allen method was performed on lecithin. The cholesterol of plasma was always quantitatively recovered in the fat layer, and, as mentioned above, neutral fat and oils are also quantitatively recovered. In the case of the fatty acids esterified with cholesterol we had more trouble. It was considered quite possible that the mild alkaline hydrolysis which is part of the Allen procedure would liberate the fatty acids, and we have found that free fatty acids are not contained in the fat layer. This point was finally resolved when we found the same amount of both total and esterified cholesterol in the fat layer of plasma as was present in the plasma itself.

The Allen method is conducted essentially as described by Allen with either 3 ml. or 2 ml. of plasma, and the calibration is made as described above, based on recovery of olive oil. The only other change in the method is that the hydrolysis and entire procedure are conducted in open tubes, which eliminates the necessity of using toothpicks to stopper the tubes.

Besides the Allen method, our system of analysis comprises the determination of cholesterol and cholesterol esters in plasma (7) and the determination of lipid phosphorus (8). From the values so obtained the following calculations are made.

CALCULATIONS

1. Lipid P × 25 = phospholipids
2. Esterified cholesterol $\times \frac{277}{386}$ (9) = cholesterol fatty acids
3. Allen fat − cholesterol − cholesterol fatty acids = neutral fat
4. Allen fat + phospholipids = total lipids
5. $\frac{831}{869}$ × neutral fat + cholesterol fatty acids + 0.64 phospholipids = total fatty acids

RESULTS

Total Fatty Acids

In Table 1 we compare the values of total fatty acids found by these calculations in a representative series of plasma samples with values of the total fatty acids obtained by the colorimetric method with dichromate (10) and by the iron perchlorate method for esterified fatty acids (11).

The values of the various lipid fractions found by this system of analysis agree in general with values found in the literature. In several samples we oxidized the total unsaponified lipid residue of plasma by the method of Bloor (12) with dichromate and calculated the values of the various fractions by using their respective factors in milliliters of dichromate. The values agreed quite well with those obtained by our system of analysis. This is especially encouraging in the case of the neutral fat since this fraction has been most neglected in the literature and since it is the least reliable due to the fact that it is always measured by difference.

Neutral Fats

We show in Table 2 the values of neutral fat found in duplicate by our method in 14 apparently healthy normal individuals. It is interesting that all of the values except for Number 8 fall close to zero. Number 8 was a man of about 45 years old, who proved to be an alcoholic and may have had some liver dysfunction. Some of the values may be seen to be slightly negative and must be considered zero. Considering the good agreement between the results of duplicate determinations, the slightly negative values in the table are an indication of the sensitivity of the method with respect to the calculated value for neutral fat.

are quite low

Among the few high values is

for correction see page 421

Table 1. Total Fatty Acids in Plasma

Comparison Between Values Determined by the Present System and Those Determined by the Colorimetric Dichromate and Iron Perchlorate Methods

Sample	*Total fatty acids*	
	Allen (mg./100 ml.)	*Dichromate* (mg./100 ml.)
1	373	402
2	322	328
3	309	300
4	323	350
5	309	336
6	373	396
7	422	425
8	317	313
9	309	291
10	421	441
11	313	343
12	304	343
13	392	392
14	264	274
15	297	296
16	309	320
17	268	282
18	172	189
19	281	264
20	297	296
21	307	315
22	177	197
23	386	378
24	265	269

Table 2. Values of Neutral Fat in the Plasma of 14 Normal Individuals

Subject #	*Neutral fat* (mg./100 ml.)
1	3, 4
2	18, 35
3	47, 65
4	24, 38
5	−17, 2
6	13, 25
7	13, 11
8	142, 123
9	133, 88
10	88, 88
11	−12, −9
12	11, 36
13	13, 15
14	−14, 0

Values are given for duplicate determinations.

DISCUSSION

The advantage of the described system of analysis is its simplicity. Values of neutral fat are calculated with a reasonable degree of validity, and the other fractions are estimated by standard methods. The simplicity and lack of technical difficulty of our method are not so true of other methods. Although total fatty acids may be determined colorimetrically in plasma quite readily by oxidation with dichromate (9), the estimation of other lipid fractions by dichromate oxidation is still difficult technically and involves uncertainties due to calculation from the dichromate factors of the various fractions. The determination of total fatty acids of plasma is also possible by the method of Bauer and Hirsch as a measure of the esterified fatty acids (10). Although this method is reliable when all factors are carefully controlled, very small differences in the time in which reagents are added at each step seriously affect the results. In addition, the method yields only the total fatty acids and can not be used to estimate the other lipid fractions.

SUMMARY

The Allen volumetric method for plasma fat has been modified by calibration to include the percentage of olive-oil recovery. The values obtained from calibration with mercury are corrected for the 125 per cent recovery of the oil. The validity of the entire procedure has been discussed.

A simple system of estimating the lipid fractions of plasma has been described. Total lipids are the total of Allen fat + (25 × lipid P). Neutral fat is Allen fat-cholesterol-cholesterol fatty acids. Total fatty acids are $\frac{831}{869} \times$ neutral fat + cholesterol fatty acids + (0.64 × phospholipids).

The values of total fatty acids have been compared with those obtained by oxidation with dichromate and by determining the esterified fatty acids with iron perchlorate.

The values of neutral fat found in 13 apparently normal individuals are shown to range from 0 to 88 and to give an average value of 28 mg./100 ml.

REFERENCES

1. Gofman, J. W., Glazier, F., Tanplin, A., Strisower, B., and DeLalla, O., *Physiol. Rev.* **34**, 589 (1954).
2. Allen, N. N., *Proc. Soc. Exp. Biol. Med.* **31**, 991 (1934).
3. Collins, D. H., *Quart. J. Med.* **2**, 267 (1933).
4. Kibrick, A. C., and Skupp, S. J., *Clinical Chemistry* **1**, 324 (1955).
5. Markeley, K. S., *Fatty Acids, Their Chemistry and Physical Properties* (*ed. 1*), New York, Interscience, 1947.

6. Chung, A. C., Saarinin, P., and Shaw, J. C., *J. Dairy Sci.* **33,** 918 (1950).
7. Kibrick, A. C., Roberts, T., and Skupp, S., *Arch. Biochem. & Biophys.* **32,** 9 (1951).
8. Youngberg, G. E., and Youngberg, M. V., *J. Lab. Clin. Med.* **16,** 158 (1930).
9. Hawk, P. B., Oser, B. L., and Summerson, W. H., *Practical Physiological Chemistry (ed. 13)*, New York, Blakiston, 1954, p. 589.
10. Kibrick, A. C., and Skupp, S. J., *Arch. Biochem. and Biophys.* **44,** 134 (1953).
11. Bauer, F. C., and Hirsch, E. F., *Arch. Biochem.* **20,** 242 (1949).
12. Bloor, W. R., *J. Biol. Chem.* **82,** 273 (1939).

Iodine and Thiocyanogen Numbers of the Fatty Acids of Blood Plasma

Andre C. Kibrick and S. J. Skupp

LITTLE IS KNOWN about the degree of unsaturation of the fatty acids of human blood (1). A spectrophotometric method has recently been applied to plasma by Wiese and Hansen (2) which consists of conjugation of the double bonds by heating in alkaline solution at 180° and measuring the conjugated forms in the ultraviolet spectrum region. The authors themselves admit that this procedure is subject to much uncertainty since standards are not available for fatty acids with more unsaturated bonds than arachidonic acid. The application of this time-consuming method in clinical chemistry would, therefore, not be warranted at this time.

In order to study the degree of unsaturation of the fatty acids of blood we have chosen, therefore, to use the values of iodine and thiocyanogen numbers, which have proven useful in the analysis of oils and fats (3). In 1931 Yasuda (4) proposed the use of the Rosenmund and Kuhnhenn reagent (5) to determine the iodine number of the fatty acids analyzed according to Bloor (6). We have also found that the iodine number of the fatty acids of blood plasma may be determined in this way, but have improved the oxidative method of Bloor for colorimetric estimation of the fatty acids (7). However, we have found that the thiocyanogen number (8) can not be determined in fatty acid extracts prepared by the method of Bloor. In the present paper, we describe a method to determine both iodine number and thiocyanogen number of some of the fatty

From the Clinical Laboratories of the New York Veterans Administration Hospital in affiliation with New York University College of Medicine.

This investigation was supported in part by a research grant from the National Institute of Arthritis and Metabolic Diseases, The National Institutes of Health, U. S. Public Health Service.

Reviewed in the Veterans Administration and published with the approval of the Chief Medical Director. The statements and conclusions published by the authors are the result of their own study and do not necessarily reflect the opinion or policy of the Veterans Administration.

Received for publication April 12, 1955.

acids of blood plasma by employing the fat isolated mechanically by the volumetric method of Allen (9).

METHOD

Reagents

1. Allen reagent (9).
2. Rosenmund-Kuhnhenn reagent (7) for iodine number.
3. Thiocyanogen reagent (8).
4. 0.1N sodium thiosulfate.
5. Potassium iodide, 1 %. Prepare as needed.

Fat is isolated in Allen tubes from 3 ml. of plasma by the method of Allen as described by the present workers. The fat column is measured in millimeters and calculated as fat content from calibration constants obtained in the usual manner with mercury. The experimental values are also corrected for the percentage recovery of known amounts of olive oil (10). The tubes are then returned to the 60° water bath. Fat is removed with 23-gage 3–4-inch hypodermic needles attached to a syringe, and about 5 mg. are weighed in microcombustion boats on a micro or semimicro balance. The boats containing the fat are then placed in 50 ml glass-stoppered Erlenmeyer flasks. For iodine numbers, 2 ml. of the Rosenmund-Kuhnhenn reagent and 3 ml. of chloroform are added. After mixing, the flasks are allowed to stand for 15 minutes in the dark. The excess reagent is then titrated with 0.1N thiosulfate, using a micro buret, after the addition of 0.5 ml. of 1 % potassium iodide.[1] For thiocyanogen numbers, 2 ml. of reagent and 3 ml. of carbon tetrachloride are added, and the mixture is allowed to stand for 48 hours in a dark water-cooled cabinet at 18–20°. The excess reagent is then titrated with 0.1N thiosulfate. In each case reagent blanks which do not contain fat are titrated in the same way. Since the cholesterol[2] in the isolated Allen fat absorbs iodine, its concentration in the plasma samples must be determined by a reliable method (11).

Calculation

$$(\text{Blank titer} - \text{Unknown titer}) \times 12.69 = \text{mg. iodine absorbed by fat.}$$

$$\frac{\text{Wt. of fat in titration flask}}{\text{mg. Allen fat/100 ml. plasma}} \times \text{mg. cholesterol/100 ml. plasma} = \text{mg. cholesterol in flask.}$$

[1] Iodine numbers have also been determined in the Allen fat with the Wijs reagent.

[2] Experimental iodine number of cholesterol = 0.69. Experimental thiocyanogen number of cholesterol = 0.12.

$$\frac{\text{mg. iodine absorbed} - (0.69 \text{ mg. chol.}^{2} \text{ in flask})}{\text{mg. fat in flask}} \times 100 = \text{Iodine number}$$

$$\frac{\text{mg. iodine absorbed} - (0.12 \text{ mg. chol.}^{2} \text{ in flask})}{\text{mg. fat in flask}} \times 100 = \text{Thiocyanogen number}$$

The method was checked on olive oil and other fats and oils and was found to give the same results as both macro and micro determinations on samples of the fats or oils before going through the Allen procedure. We also determined simultaneously the iodine number of a large number

Table 1. Comparison Between the Values of Iodine Number Determined by the Present Method and the Yasuda Method

Plasma sample #	*Iodine number*	
	Present method	*Yasuda method*
1	107	107
2	100	110
3	104	102
4	123	111
5	103	97
6	108	102
7	109	101
8	102	106
9	120	115
10	105	113
11	102	106
12	109	101

Table 2. Values of the Iodine and Thiocyanogen Numbers Determined in 14 Normal Individuals

Subject #	*Iodine number*	*Thiocyanogen number*	*Difference*
1	123	107	16
2	132	76	56
3	151	73	78
4	133	92	41
5	111	64	47
6	127	102	25
7	134	86	48
8	93	71	22
9	124	111	13
10	116	64	52
11	127	118	9
12	138	90	48
13	157	122	35
14	128	91	37

[2] Experimental iodine number of cholesterol = 0.69. Experimental thiocyanogen number of cholesterol = 0.12.

of plasma samples by this method and by the method of Yasuda. Table 1 shows some representative results. It is seen that the present method yields values not much different from those obtained by the Yasuda method in spite of the absence of the fatty acids of the phospholipids in the Allen fat.

In Table 2 we show the results of iodine and thiocyanogen numbers obtained by our method on the fat isolated from plasma in 14 supposedly healthy laboratory workers.

DISCUSSION

The iodine number, which represents the average degree of unsaturation of the fatty acids, might be expected to be affected in liver dysfunction since there is considerable evidence that the liver is the major site of desaturation (12). Wachstein has found high values in parenchymatous or obstructive jaundice (13), and Nicholls and Perlzweig have found high values in hyperthyroidism (14), a condition in which fat metabolism may be affected.

It was considered likely that a knowledge of both the iodine and thiocyanogen numbers in the same lipid fraction would yield more information about the desaturation mechanism. The iodine number is a measure of the total number of unsaturated bonds of the fatty acids, whereas the thiocyanogen number apparently measures the number of these bonds in acids containing only one unsaturated linkage and one less than the total number of unsaturated bonds in acids containing two or more (3). Oleic acid may be present in considerable amount in blood and tissues. We have found about 50 per cent of the fatty acids to be unsaturated and about 25 per cent to contain more than one unsaturated bond by other methods (15). Since linoleic and linolenic acids are present in only a small amount in normal rat tissues (16), this indicates an appreciable content of other unsaturated acids. Hence, the simple calculation from the values of the iodine and thiocyanogen numbers that can be made for commercial oils (8) are not possible for biologic material of this type. However, the difference between the values of the two numbers reflects the content of fatty acids containing more than two unsaturated bonds.

It is seen in Table 2 that the iodine numbers in our small series of normals range from 111 to 157. Number 8 may be excluded since it represents an adult male of about 45 who was later found to be an alcoholic and to have other indications of liver damage. The differences between the values of the iodine and thiocyanogen numbers found in our small series of normals are rather disappointing. The presence of both small and large relative amounts of fatty acids containing more than two unsaturated bonds in this lipid fraction indicates that it has little significance in disease. The difference between the two numbers may well be a reflection of the diet.

This investigation is being continued to learn the significance of the values of the iodine number in liver disease and in other clinical conditions in which there is a disturbance of fat metabolism. We are also endeavoring to improve the present procedure to yield the iodine and thiocyanogen numbers of the total fatty acids of plasma and of the fatty acids of each lipid fraction.

SUMMARY

A method has been described for the determination of both iodine and thiocyanogen numbers of the fat isolated from human blood plasma by the Allen volumetric method. The values found in 13 normal individuals varied from 111 to 157 for iodine number and from 64 to 122 for thiocyanogen number. The differences between the two numbers varied between 9 and 78.

REFERENCES

1. Peters, J. P., and Van Slyke, D. D., *Quantitative Clinical Chemistry (ed. 2)*, Baltimore, Md., Williams & Wilkins, 1946, Vol. 1, p. 474.
2. Wiese, H. F., and Hansen, A. E., *J. Biol. Chem.* **202,** 417 (1953).
3. Jamieson, G. S., *Vegetable Fats and Oils (ed. 2)*, New York, Reinhold, 1943.
4. Yasuda, M., *J. Biol. Chem.* **94,** 401 (1931–32).
5. Rosenmund, K. W., and Kuhnhenn, W., *Z. Untersuch* **46,** 154 (1923).
6. Bloor, W. R., *J. Biol. Chem.* **82,** 273 (1939).
7. Kibrick, A. C., and Skupp, S. J., *Arch. Biochem. & Biophys.* **44,** 134 (1953).
8. Jamieson, G. S., *Ind. & Eng. Chem., Anal. Ed.* **8,** 233 (1936).
9. Allen, N. N., *Proc. Soc. Exp. Biol. Med.* **31,** 991 (1934).
10. Kibrick, A. C., and Skupp, S. J., *Clinical Chemistry* **1,** 317 (1955).
11. Kibrick, A. C., Roberts, T., and Skupp, S., *Arch. Biochem. & Biophys.*, **32,** 9 (1951).
12. Cantarow, A., and Trumper, M., *Clinical Biochemistry (ed. 4)*, Philadelphia, Saunders, 1950, p. 136.
13. Wachstein, M., *Z. Klin. Med.* **131,** 625 (1936–37).
14. Nicholls, E. G., and Perlzweig, W. A., *J. Clin. Invest.* **15,** 195 (1928).
15. Skupp, S. J., and Kibrick, A. C., unpublished data.
16. Riechehof, I. G., Holman, R. T., Burr, G. O., *Arch. Biochem.* **20,** 331 (1949).

The Correspondence with Beer's Law for the Optical Density of Stained Protein Patterns on Filter Paper as a Function of Surface Protein Concentration

V. H. Rees and D. J. R. Laurence

THE SCANNING TECHNIC for evaluating data from electrophoresis on filter paper, which was first described by Grassmann, Hannig, and Knedel (1) and by Eisenreich and Eder (2), has now become established as routine procedure in many laboratories. Although many types of scanning have been described, they have in common the advantage that the colorimetric determinations are made on the paper strip upon which the protein pattern has been developed. The difficulties of quantitative elution of the colors are thereby avoided. Crook, Harris, and Warren (3, 4) have emphasized that the simple Beer's logarithmic law which is obtained in homogeneous solutions cannot be assumed to hold for the paper matrix without detailed experimental justification, and they have proposed an alternative relationship for such data. The problem of quantitation has also received the attention of many other workers, and several, notably Griffiths (5), Latner (6), Grassmann and Hannig (7), Sommerfeldt (8), and Cooper and Mandel (9) have found the application of Beer's law to be justified experimentally over the working range of the method, as long as transmission densitometry is used.

The verification of Beer's law has now become of especial interest since Laurence (10) and Cooper and Mandel (9) have described the use of a light-sensitive circuit with an output linear with the optical density. This circuit permits the automatic recording of paper electrophoretic patterns to give a tracing from which proportions of the separate fractions

---

From the Department of Chemical Pathology, Postgraduate Medical School of London, Ducane Road, London, W. 12, England.

The criticism and advice of Professor E. J. King and Dr. I. D. P. Wootton have been of greatest assistance in this work.

Received for publication April 12, 1955.

can be estimated directly by means of a planimeter, as long as Beer's law can be assumed. The value of automatic recording would be greatly reduced if the results require rectification afterwards by application of a correction curve; also the scale of the recording could no longer be adjusted electronically without restriction, if deviations from the logarithmic law must be considered.

The comparisons made by Rees and Laurence (11) between the results of automatic recording and a fluorimetric method showed indirectly that the scanning method was satisfactory, but there remained the possibility of several errors in the scanning method leading to a correct result by compensation. A detailed investigation has therefore been made of the relationship between protein concentration and optical density of the protein-dye complex. The investigation was limited to transmission densitometry only and has no bearing on the problem of the varying dye uptakes of different protein species.

THEORETICAL CONSIDERATIONS

In this paper certain terms are used as follows:

1. The surface protein concentration is the number of micrograms of protein contained in 1 sq. cm. of the filter paper, or the corresponding incremental definition if the pattern density varies continuously.

2. The optical density is $\log_{10} (I_0/I)$ where I_0 is the incident light intensity and I is the intensity of the light emerging after absorption.

3. According to Beer's law the optical density of any region should be proportional to the surface protein concentration. The application of the law is therefore tested by plotting optical density against surface concentration of protein and the result should be a straight line through the origin.

4. Simple considerations trace most deviations from Beer's law to fluctuations in absorbing power within the light beam. Examples are the use of light of several wave lengths which are absorbed to different extents, the influence of stray light which is not absorbed at all, and the effect of scattering to produce paths of differing lengths through the absorbing region. All these effects cause the optical density observed to be less than that predicted from experiments at low densities, since the observed result is the logarithm of average light intensities, whereas the required result is an average logarithm of light intensities which is always the greater. Therefore if the optical density of the paper is plotted as ordinate against surface protein concentration as abscissa, expected deviations are a bending "downward" of the curves.

MATERIAL AND METHODS

Known amounts of protein were added along filter paper strips either (1) uniformly over known areas limited by silicone barriers (termed the "wedge method," as the developed strip resembles an optical step wedge) (Fig. 1*a*) or (2) as transverse lines (the "stripe" method) (Fig. 1*c*). Wedge methods have been used by Crook *et al.* (4) and by Latner (6) and stripe methods by Griffiths (5), by Sommerfeldt (8), and by Grassmann and Hannig (7). The strips were then stained, washed and oiled, and examined by transmission densitometry. The densitometer tracing for the wedge method is a series of flat-topped segments (Fig. 1*b*). The distance between the top and the base line was calibrated in terms of optical density and the surface area of protein on the filter paper measured by means of a planimeter. As the amount of protein is known and the distribution is uniform, the optical densities of the various segments of the wedge could be plotted against surface protein concentration (μg./cm.^{2}).

The densitometer tracing for the stripe method is a series of density contours reminiscent of the patterns obtained in a conventional separation of plasma proteins (Fig. 1*d*). The areas within these contours above the base line are obtained with a planimeter and compared with the corresponding dilutions of the protein sample.

FILTER PAPER STRIPS. Whatman No. 1 (for chromatography) in strips size 29 × 4 cm.

PROTEIN SAMPLES. Plasma from hospital patients diluted with 0.9% saline to 2–3% w/v and also 2% solutions of bovine serum albumin.

SILICONE. Dow Corning 1107 with acetone (1:1).

Wedge Method

A filter paper strip was placed on a glass plate and 7 transverse pencil lines were drawn 2 cm. apart, commencing 8.5 cm. from one end, to form a set of 6 adjacent compartments 4 × 2 cm. transverse to the length of the paper. The silicone-acetone mixture was applied along the pencil lines from a Petri dish, using the edge of a standard histologic glass slide cut to 4 cm. in length. The filter paper was then heated for 5 minutes in an oven at 105° to fix the silicone and used within 30 minutes. The paper was held horizontally by its ends in a frame. The 6 compartments were each moistened with 0.05 ml. of 0.9% saline and allowed to dry at room temperature. A series of 6 dilutions of the protein sample (at concentrations of 1.0, 0.8, 0.6, 0.4, 0.2, 0.1, taking the original sample concentration as 1.0) were made in 0.9% saline. Exactly 0.04 ml. of these solutions was applied, one to each of the compartments of the filter paper, using a calibrated blood pipet. The sample was applied to the center of a compartment and was sufficient in amount to ensure a thorough and even wetting of the paper. Because of the silicone barriers, the samples were confined strictly within single compartments and the edges of the protein patterns were sharp. The strip was allowed to remain uncovered at room temperature for 5 minutes and then placed in the oven at 105° for 15 minutes, still horizontally supported. The dried paper was then stained as described.

Stripe Method

A filter paper strip was damped with 0.9% saline and lightly blotted to remove excess. The strip was then placed across a wire frame consisting of 5 parallel wires 3 cm. apart stretched across a laboratory wire basket. On each wire was a dry filter paper circle (Whatman No. 1, 11 cm. diameter) sharply folded to form an inverted V. The action of the frame was to drain saline from the transverse lines of the paper strip in contact with the frame. A number of 2-fold dilutions of the protein sample in 0.9% saline were madc and exactly 0.02 ml. of these dilutions were applied by means of a pipet to the paper strip centrally between the wires of the frame as transverse stripes. The effect of the moisture gradient so produced in the strip was to spread the stripes laterally, producing a gradual increase in protein concentration towards the center of the stripe. Care was taken that the stripes were evenly applied and of constant length. The pattern was allowed to become almost dry in the air and then heated at 105° for 15 minutes in the oven. The dried paper was stained as described.

Dyeing

Amidoschwarz 10B (Bayer) and azocarmine B (Gurr) were employed in dyeing.[1] Amidoschwarz was used as a saturated solution (about 1.5% w/v) in 10% acetic acid–90% methanol, and azocarmine as a 0.75% solution in 10% acetic acid–45% methanol–45% water. Staining was for 10 minutes at room temperature. The background color was washed away with 10% acetic acid–90% methanol, and in the case of amidoschwarz the further washing described by Rees and Laurence (9) was used. The strips were washed finally with methanol and dried at 105° for 5 minutes in both cases.

[1] G. T. Gurr, Ltd., London.

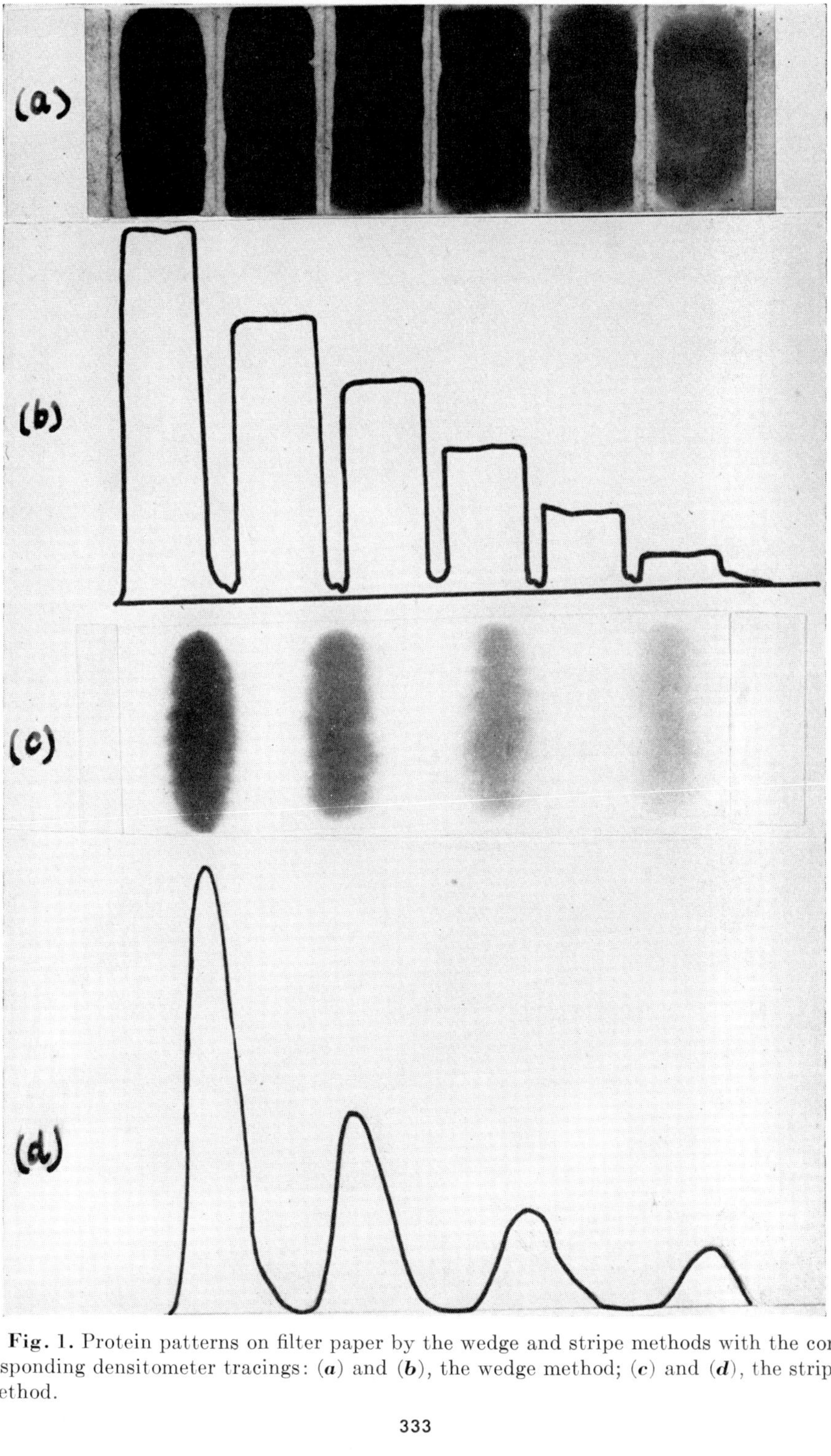

Fig. 1. Protein patterns on filter paper by the wedge and stripe methods with the corresponding densitometer tracings: (***a***) and (***b***), the wedge method; (***c***) and (***d***), the stripe method.

Oiling

The oil applied was a mixture of 1 part of α-bromonaphthalene (B.D.H.) and 2 parts of liquid paraffin (B.P.). This mixture (5 parts) was diluted with xylene (2 parts) and 1% of sorbital mono-oleate (Croda) was added to bind the oil to the paper. The paper strips were drawn through a pool of the oil on a glass plate so that the oil was taken up by the paper from the lower surface only, to avoid trapping air bubbles. The oiled paper was then slightly bowed and stood upright on a longer edge on a flat filter paper sheet to drain. After 20 minutes, most of the xylene had evaporated and the paper was lightly oiled, yet could be subject to slight pressure without exuding oil.

Scanning

The automatically recording densitometer described by Laurence (10), was used to examine the oiled papers. The paper was placed in a holder and covered with a thin glass plate to hold it flat. It was then driven between an illuminated slit and a photocell at a constant rate and the optical density was obtained from the photocell response and plotted by a Murday type recorder[2] on recorder paper moving at the same rate.

Calibration of Densitometer

The densitometer was calibrated using an Ilford[3] calibration strip on 35-mm. film, which is a neutral filter step wedge, with which an individual calibration chart in optical densities is provided by the manufacturers. In order to obtain an accurate calibration for low optical densities, the Ilford wedge was cut into 3 segments. The central segment containing a reference mark to identify it on the calibration chart was used in recording with both the higher and the lower density segments on appropriate scales of amplification. Deflections for the densest segment (M) were noted on a microammeter, which is independent of amplification used in the recording. The corresponding microammeter deflections (m) for any given segment could be obtained by measuring the deflection on the recorder chart in millimeters (d) and using Equation 1

$$m = Md/D \tag{1}$$

where D is the deflection of the densest segment in millimeters. In this way a calibraton curve of the reading of the microammeter related to optical density was obtained. This curve could be used to obtain the

---

[2] Evershed & Vignoles, Ltd., London.
[3] Address: London, W.C.1.

optical density scale for any given recording in subsequent work. The microammeter deflection corresponding to the densest part of a recording was noted and from this the deflections for all parts could be calculated using Equation 1. These microampere deflections could then be converted to optical densities using the calibration curve.

Specifications of the Densitometer

The following characteristics of the recording densitometer must be mentioned in the present context. The light source is a 6W, 6V festoon lamp with a linear filament about 1 cm. long, and the light from this filament converges on the slit 2 cm. × 0.5 mm. through a double plano-convex molded condenser lens system. The lens system is 6.5 cm. in diameter and 2.5 cm. in thickness, the lamp is 10 cm. from the nearest face of the lens, while the slit is 7.5 cm. from its nearest face. The light falls on the slit as a convergent beam and is focused on the filter paper strip to give a sharp image about 1.8 cm. × 0.25 mm. as the window in the holder carrying the filter paper allows only the central 1.8 cm. of the 4 cm. wide filter paper strip to be scanned. The light passes through the paper strip and through a light filter, to be received by the photocathode of an R.C.A. 931-A multiplier photocell (cathode dimensions, 1.0 × 0.3 cm.) parallel to the slit and about 2 cm. from it. A mirror placed between the lens system and the slit deflects the beam through a right angle in order to conserve space.

Light Filters

The light filters used in this work were as follows. For amidoschwarz 10B, Ilford gelatine filters Mercury Yellow #808 (one thickness) and Red Absorbing #802 (two thicknesses) were combined with a neutral filter of density 0.5. For azocarmine B, the Ilford gelatine filter Bright Spectrum Yellow-Green #625 was combined with a neutral filter of density 0.8.

Removal of Oil

The oil was removed from the papers after scanning, using a 1:1 mixture of acetone and ether.

Planimetry

The Ott planimeter[4] was used throughout. In the wedge method, the area of the sharply defined protein-containing regions was measured.

[4] Bender and Hobein, Munich, Germany.

In the stripe method, the area of the densitometer tracing above the base line was measured.

Elution

Experiments relating surface concentration or amount of protein with optical density of the dyed protein complex have a direct relation with the requirements of the scanning technic. These experiments nevertheless can be further analyzed by adding an elution procedure. In this way it is possible to obtain the dye in free solution where there is no doubt that Beer's law is obeyed, provided a suitable light filter is used. By comparing the density of the eluted dye with the amount of protein from which it is eluted, the relationship of dye uptake with amount of protein can be tested. A colorimetric comparison of the density of eluted dye with the density of dye determined *in situ* on the filter paper relates optical density with surface concentration of the dye. After removal of the oil, the colored segments from strips prepared by the wedge method were cut out and extracted into 7 ml. of a suitable solvent, and the dye concentration estimated in a Gallenkamp photoelectric colorimeter. For amidoschwarz 10B the solvent was phenol saturated with water and containing 1% of anhydrous sodium acetate, an Ilford filter Spectrum Orange #607 being used for the estimates. For azocarmine B, the solvent

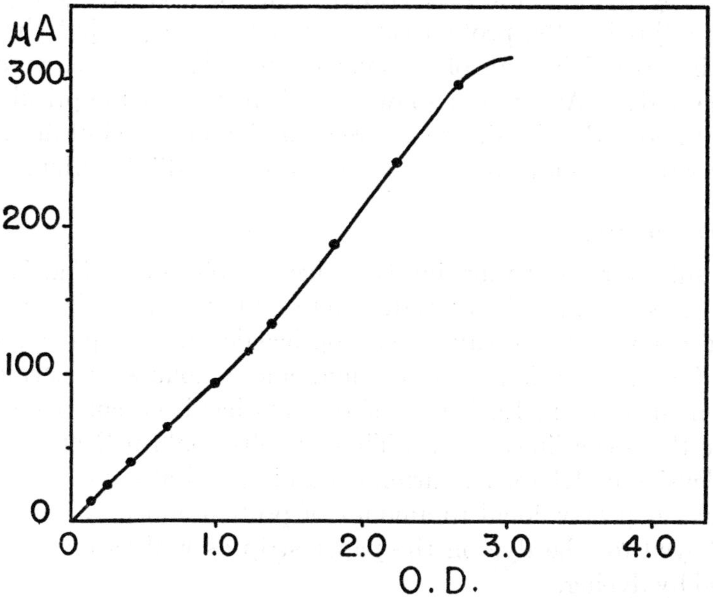

Fig. 2. Calibration curve for the automatically recording densitometer.

was 0.10N sodium hydroxide, and an Ilford filter Bright Spectrum Blue Green #623 was used.

RESULTS

A calibration curve for the recording densitometer is given in Fig. 2. This shows that between densities of 0 and 1.5, the deflection of the densitometer is linear with optical density within 1 per cent, but that above density 1.5 a curvature upwards appears. As most of the data to be given in this section will refer to the linear region of response the data have been plotted on a scale linear for microamps and the optical density scale which is on the same ordinate is therefore somewhat expanded above a density of 1.5.

Wedge Methods

Amidoschwarz Staining

Figs 3 and 4 show results from the wedge method plotted in the standard manner. Figure 3 shows results with 3 separate wedges prepared from a serum sample with an equal concentration of albumin and globulins and amidoschwarz 10B staining. The data are in accordance with Beer's law. In Fig. 4 the results from a series of 9 wedges stained with amidoschwarz are plotted and in this case the variation between strips has been removed, leaving only the variation within the strips. This has been done by plotting the best straight line for each wedge separately and then adjusting the protein concentration scales so that these lines are superimposed. The scale of protein concentration was then an average for all the wedges. Again Beer's law is confirmed up to an optical density of 1.4, but above this density there are a number of large but inconsistent departures from the law in the expected "downward" direction.

Azocarmine B Staining

The results for an azocarmine B wedge are plotted in Fig. 5. In this case all the segments of the wedge were eluted and therefore 3 corresponding sets of results are available—optical densities on paper, colorimeter readings in solution after elution, and amounts or surface concentrations of protein. Each pair of the sets has been compared and in each case there is a linear result. These results confirm Beer's law to an optical density of 1.1 for azocarmine staining and also confirm that the dye uptake is proportional to amount of protein added and that Beer's law is obeyed for the dye on the paper strip as well as for the protein estimated by dyeing.

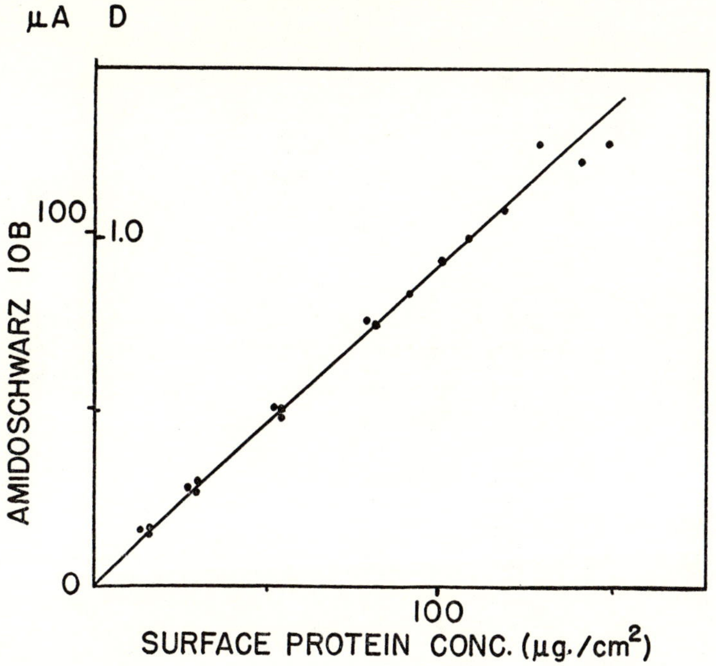

Fig. 3. Optical density related to surface protein concentration. Results with 3 wedges. (Amidoschwarz staining)

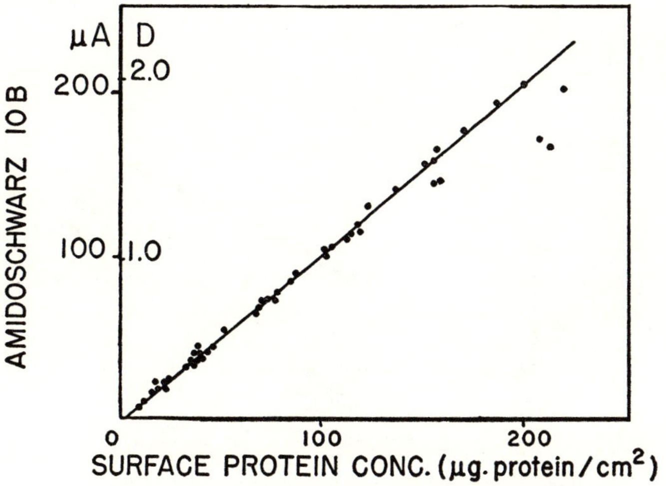

Fig. 4. Optical density related to surface protein concentration. Results with 9 wedges. The interwedge variation has been removed. (Amidoschwarz staining)

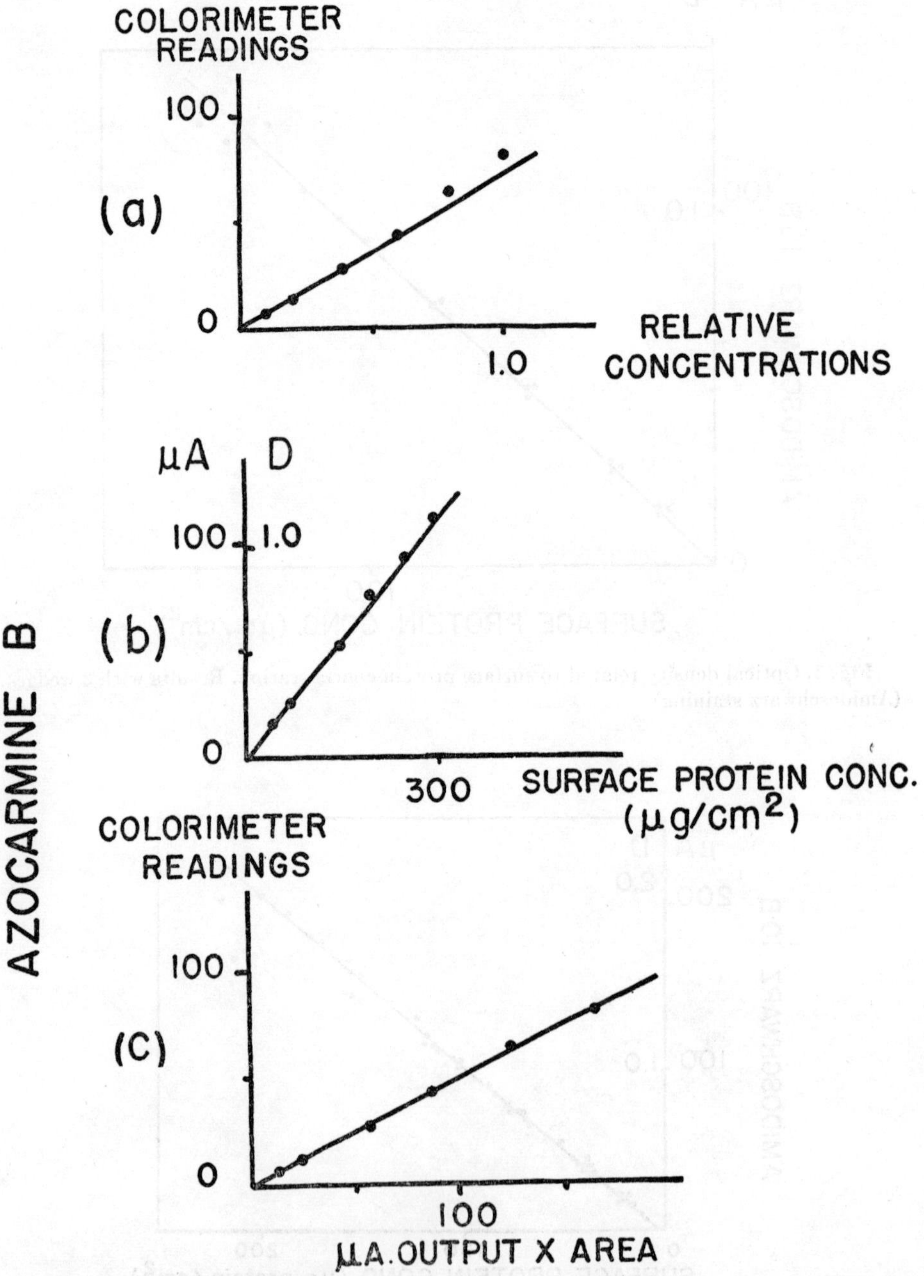

Fig. 5. Elution experiments with azocarmine B: (***a***), linearity of dye uptake with amount of protein added to the paper; (***b***), optical density related to surface protein concentration; (***c***), amount of dye eluted related to dye estimated *in situ* on the paper by densitometry.

Bovine Serum Albumin

Beer's law was also confirmed for bovine serum albumin tested for densities up to 1.0 using amidoschwarz staining, and an elution experiment was also made for amidoschwarz staining with a linear result, similar to that in Fig. 5.

Effect of Oiling and of the Light Filter

Fig. 6 shows the results with an amidoschwarz 10B wedge of omitting the oiling procedure by scanning the dry paper and of omitting the light filter. In the former case the neutral 0.5 density filter was removed and in the latter case a neutral 1.2 density filter was added in order to restore the light intensity to the usual value. If the dry paper is scanned a general increase of about 2- or 3-fold in optical density occurs due to multiple reflections in the dry paper [*cf.* Laurence (10); Price and Ashman (12)]. Also the increase is greater for low than for high densities and a curvature downward results in an overestimation of low densities. This effect has been noticed by Grassmann and Hannig (7). If the light filter is omitted, the optical density is decreased about 2-fold due to the

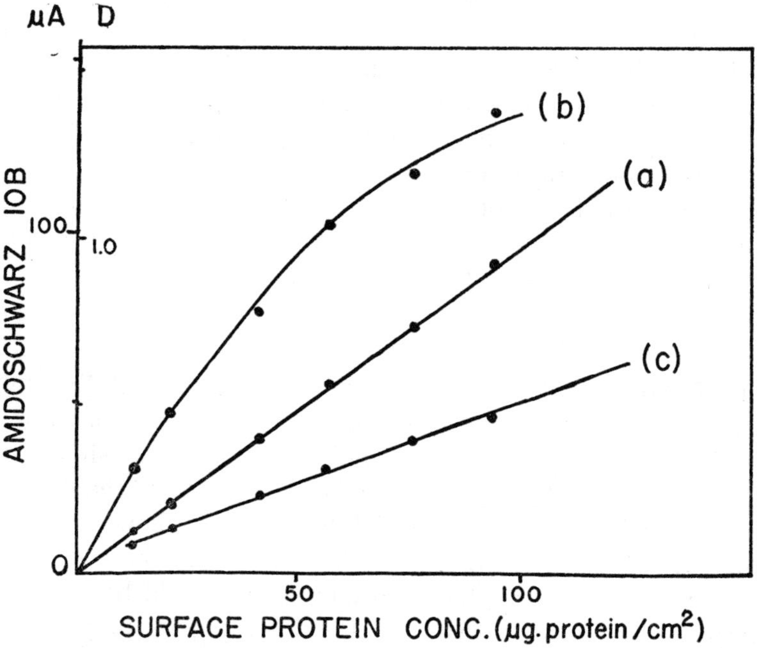

Fig. 6. Results without oiling and without a light filter: (***a***), oiled paper with light filter; (***b***), dry paper with light filter; (***c***), oiled paper with no filter. (Amidoschwarz 10B staining)

inclusion of less absorbed spectral regions of the incident light. The expected curvature downward is not apparent in this curve, which however shows a positive intercept on the density axis as found by Wenzel and Hanson (13). This latter deviation from Beer's law was not consistently obtained without a light filter and is difficult to explain.

In order to check that the light filter used was sufficient to counteract the pronounced sensitivity of the photocell to blue light, a new filter was constructed, containing three thicknesses of the Ilford Mercury Yellow 808 gelatine sheet, two thicknesses of the Red Absorbing 802, and a neutral 0.2 density filter. No differences could be detected between the results with the normal and with the new filter.

It is clear from these results that the optical density obtained for any wedge depends on the light filter and oiling procedure used, as well as on the surface protein concentration. Therefore, in order to specify the range over which linearity is found it is necessary to give details both of optical density and of protein concentration.

Results with Direct-Reading Scanner

A comparison has also been made of the results from an amidoschwarz wedge scanned by the recording scanner and by a commercial direct reading scanner with a logarithmic scale fitted with a barrier layer cell[5] but with no light filter. A linear result was obtained with either scanner, but with the commercial instrument the densities obtained were about 40 per cent less than with the recording instrument. With the commercial instrument a comparison was made between the wedges oiled as described above and "fully" oiled by removing all air in the paper immersed in the oil, using a rotary oil pump. Full oiling of the paper resulted in a further decrease of 30 per cent in the optical density.

Stripe Method

Figure 7 shows results with the stripe technic. A set of 4 protein solutions was prepared by serial 2-fold dilutions of a plasma sample. The results of scanning the four corresponding protein stripes should be areas in the ratio 8:4:2:1. By equating the largest area to 8, the deviations of the smaller areas from the expected 4, 2, and 1 are shown in the form of a histogram. There is no systematic deviation from the expected values and the scatter of the results is no more than would be expected with this technic. The peak density on the filter papers prepared by this

[5] Evans Electroselenum Ltd., Harlow, Essex, England.

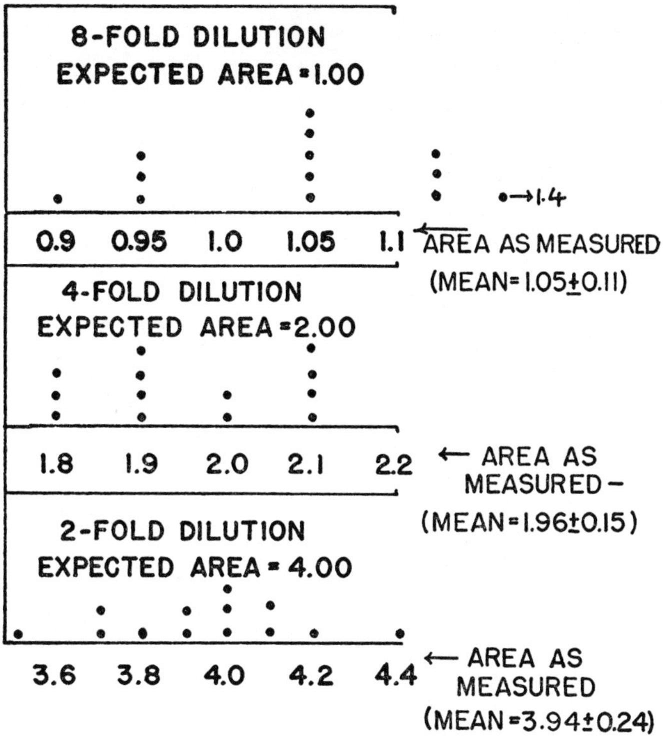

Fig. 7. Results with the stripe method. Deviations from expected "scale of two." The results shown are 13 observations for each dilution. The areas are standardized so that the area of the undiluted sample equals 8 units. (Amidoschwarz 10B staining)

method varied between 0.9 and 1.3. Although the stripe method is preferred as a test of the dynamic response of the recording system, it is a less critical test of Beer's law than the wedge method, as only a small part of the total stained area is near the peak density.

DISCUSSION AND CONCLUSIONS

The results obtained here consistently failed to show deviations from Beer's law for optical densities less than 1.4, and the use of scanning as a convenient method for differential protein estimations would appear to be justified. The methods described may enable other workers to make similar tests of the method with a minimum of preliminary development, and some may succeed in obtaining significant failure of Beer's law in their apparatus. The use of apparatus of this type would enable the variation of the deviations with arrangement of the optical system, etc., to be worked out, but the following experimental conditions are already known to lead to significant deviations:

1. Use of dry paper instead of lightly oiled paper.
2. An inadequate light filter for the photocell.
3. An illuminated slit too long to be completely covered by the protein pattern.
4. Variations in protein density over the slit, either because the slit is too wide or because the protein pattern has been applied unevenly.
5. Use of low quality filter paper containing "pin holes."
6. A dye uptake which is not proportional to protein content of the paper [Martin and Franglen (14)].

The failure of Crook, Harris, and Warren (4) to substantiate Beer's law does not indicate the most general situation for the application of the scanning method.

SUMMARY

The application of Beer's logarithmic law to the scanning of dyed protein patterns has been investigated by methods described in detail. No deviations could be found for optical densities less than 1.4 for amidoschwarz 10B or less than 1.1 for azocarmine B staining. The scanning method can be used for evaluation of protein fractions if care is taken.

REFERENCES

1. Grassmann, W., Hannig, K., and Knedel, M., *Deut. med. Wochschr.* **76,** 333 (1951).
2. Eisenreich, F., and Eder, M., *Klin. Wochschr.* **29,** 60 (1951).
3. Crook, E. M., Harris, M., and Warren, F. L., *Biochem. J.* **51,** 26 (1952).
4. Crook, E. M., Harris, M., Hassan, F., and Warren, F. L., *Biochem. J.* **56,** 434 (1954).
5. Griffiths, L. L., *J. Clin. Pathol.* **5,** 294 (1952).
6. Latner, A. L., *J. Lab. Clin. Med.* **43,** 137 (1954).
7. Grassmann, W., and Hannig, K., *Klin. Wochschr.* **32,** 838 (1954).
8. Sommerfeldt, S. C., *Scand. J. Clin. & Lab. Invest.* **5,** 299 (1953).
9. Cooper, G. R., and Mandel, E. E., *J. Lab. Clin. Med.* **44,** 636 (1954).
10. Laurence, D. J. R., *J. Sci. Instr. and Phys. in Ind.* **31,** 137 (1954).
11. Rees, V. H., and Laurence, D. J. R., *J. Clin. Path.* **7,** 336 (1954).
12. Price, T. D., and Ashman, P. B., *Nature* **175,** 45 (1955).
13. Wenzel, M., and Hanson, H., *Hoppe-Seyle Z. Physiol. Chem.* **292,** 137 (1953).
14. Martin, N. H., and Franglen, G. T., *J. Clin. Path.* **7,** 336 (1954).

p-Toluenesulfonic Acid, Cholesterol Determination, and Explosions

Betty Jo Jones and Ferrin B. Moreland

WE HAVE BEEN USING the method of Pearson, Stern, and McGavack (1) for the determination of cholesterol for some time. It has proved to be a convenient and accurate procedure and the reaction had always gone smoothly. One day recently, however, the tubes were set up for the determination as usual, using a freshly prepared solution of *p*-toluenesulfonic acid. Solutions made from the same bottle of solid acid[1] had previously been used with smooth results. However, on this occasion, a minute or two after the serum, acetic acid, *p*-toluenesulfonic acid solution, and acetic anhydride were measured into the tubes and not mixed, a series of explosions occurred and most of the contents was blown out of the tubes. The serum blank and its zero reference tube, not containing acetic anhydride, did not blow up. A fresh solution of *p*-toluenesulfonic acid was prepared from the same solid used above, with a repeat performance of the explosions. A new solution made from a different batch of solid[2] gave smooth results. Unfortunately the offending *p*-toluenesulfonic acid was discarded before it could be analyzed to determine the change which caused the trouble. On cursory examination the bottle of solid reagent had appeared somewhat moist, particularly on the inside of the screwcap.

This note is not intended to discourage use of the Pearson, Stern, and McGavack method, which is still our method of choice for determining total cholesterol, but merely to advise caution in keeping away from above the tubes after the reagents are added, when a new solution of *p*-toluenesulfonic acid is first used. It might be well to set the rack of tubes under a shelf or to cover them with a board immediately after the components are piped in, when an unproved solution is used.

REFERENCE

1. Pearson, S., Stern, S., and McGavack, T. H., *Anal. Chem.* **25**, 813 (1953).

Present addresses: B. J. J., 203 Hermann Professional Bldg.; F. B. M., Biochemistry Department, Baylor University College of Medicine; Houston, Texas.

Received for publication June 29, 1955.

[1] Eastman 984 (this sample had been in our laboratory for about 1 month).

[2] Matheson Pract. 2736 (this sample had been in another laboratory for over 2 years).

the Clinical Chemist

INTERNATIONAL CONGRESS ON CLINICAL CHEMISTRY

The Executive Committee of the American Association of Clinical Chemists has approved arrangements for an International Congress on Clinical Chemistry to be held in New York City during the week of September 9, 1956. The Congress will bring together eminent scientists from all over the world, in a program designed to exhibit the contributions of outstanding clinical chemists both here and abroad.

Albert E. Sobel, Chemist to the Jewish Hospital of Brooklyn and Adjunct Professor of Biochemistry at the Polytechnic Institute of Brooklyn, as well as past president of the Association, has been appointed coordinating chairman of the Congress. Committees will be announced as they are selected.

A tentative program will soon be published and will consist of symposia and contributed papers. Members of the Association and our overseas colleagues are urged to make plans to attend this Congress and participate in the scientific and social programs to be arranged.

ERNST BISCHOFF AWARD

The 1955 Ernst Bischoff Award has been presented to Michael X. Sullivan, Professor of Biochemistry at the Georgetown University in Washington, D. C. The presentation was made at the annual dinner of the Association on September 15, 1955, in Minneapolis, Minn.

SEVENTH ANNUAL MEETINGS

The Seventh Annual Meetings of the American Association of Clinical Chemists were held in Minneapolis from September 14–16, 1955. The scientific program was in participation with the Division of Biological Chemistry of the AMERICAN CHEMICAL SOCIETY, as it has been in every previous annual meeting of the Association. A report on the highlights of the meetings will appear in the next issue of CLINICAL CHEMISTRY.

REPORTS FROM THE SECTIONS

Southern California

C. Dubbs

The fourth symposium of the season was held on April 5, 1955, at the Los Angeles County Hospital. A. G. Redeker, M.D., and W. G. Bergren, Ph.D., of the University of Southern California Medical School, discussed clinical and analytical aspects of porphyrins, especially coproporphyrin, porphyrobilinogen, and the uroporphyrins. Isolation and fractionation methods were described, including paper ionophoresis and chromatography on paper and columns of alumina and Florisil.

The final meeting, held on June 7, 1955, at the Carolina Pines Restaurant, featured election of new officers. Rex Sterling, Ph.D., chemist, Los Angeles County Hospital, succeeded Dr. H. O. Carne as chairman. Kenneth D. Johnson, Ph.D., A. L. Chaney Chemical Laboratory, was elected program chairman as well as chairman-elect to succeed Dr. Sterling. Roscoe R. Schaffert, biochemist, Veterans Administration Center, Los Angeles, was elected secretary-treasurer to succeed Maxine Wertman.

As a result of the California attorney general's opinion [*Clin. Chem.* **1,** 134, (1955)] that special licensure for clinical chemists is not permitted by the California Clinical Laboratory Act, this local section has begun efforts toward obtaining corrective legislation.

Texas

The Texas Section of the American Association of Clinical Chemists is sponsoring a symposium and session of contributed papers at the American Chemical Society Southwest Regional Meeting to be held in Houston, Texas, December 1 to 3, 1955. The symposium is tentatively titled "Instrumental Methods in Clinical Chemistry". Preliminary announcement of the meeting was made in *Chemical and Engineering News*, August 15, page 3417. This ACS weekly will carry the final program. A dinner meeting is also planned as one of the events.

All clinical chemists planning to attend the meetings are requested to notify the Chairman, Dr. Ferrin B. Moreland, Department of Biochemistry, Baylor University College of Medicine, Houston, Texas.

PRINCIPLES OF LEGISLATION

The following is reprinted with permission of the American Chemical Society from the *Chemical and Engineering News* [**33,** 3105 (1955)]. It appeared as part of the Board of Directors Minutes of the American Chemical Society and embraces eight basic principles for legislation. The Committee on Clinical Chemistry of the American Chemical Society meeting in Cincinnati during April 1–2, 1955, prepared the statement. The Committee consists of Max M. Friedman, Joseph H. Gast, Rollo N. Harger, John G. Reinhold (chairman), Joseph I. Routh, Bradford N. Stanerson, Arnold G. Ware, and Hans Zinsser.

Principles of Legislation for Regulation of the Practice of Clinical Chemistry

In 1953, the ACS Committee on Clinical Chemistry presented to the Board of Directors for approval a statement of principles of legislation for regulation of the practice of clinical chemistry; no action was taken. The report was published with a request for comment.

The committee has given careful consideration to the communications received. A revised statement was presented to the Board of Directors in June 1955. Its action is given in Minute 13. In accordance with the instructions therein, the following is published:

This report has *not* been endorsed by the Board of Directors nor have the eight numbered principles for legislation been approved. It is published for the purpose of eliciting comment. Letters should be sent to John G. Reinhold, Pepper Laboratory of Clinical Medicine, University of

Pennsylvania, Philadelphia 4, Pa., with copies to the Executive Secretary of the ACS, 1155 Sixteenth St., N. W., Washington 6, D. C.

Principles of Legislation for Regulation of the Practice of Clinical Chemistry—Drafted by the Committee on Clinical Chemistry of the *American Chemical Society*.

I. The primary objective of legislation to regulate the practice of clinical chemistry is the protection of the public health.

II. Clinical chemistry is the practical application of chemical science for the purpose of providing factual data to authorized persons for use in evaluating the state of health or cause of death.

III. A license to practice clinical chemistry must be based on good character and high standards of professional competence. The competence of a clinical chemist should be judged by his ability in chemistry. He should not be compelled to qualify in other disciplines in order to practice clinical chemistry. A duly licensed clinical chemist may perform venipuncture or skin puncture for test purposes upon specific authorization from any person with authority granted under any provisions of law relating to the healing arts.

IV. Legislation to regulate the practice of clinical chemistry should require as minimal qualifications: (1) During the first five years after the act becomes effective, (a) graduation with a chemistry major from a four-year course of a college or university approved for training in chemistry by the examining board, (b) a minimum of five years of practical experience in a laboratory approved for training in clinical chemistry by the examining board. (2) Five years after the act becomes effective and thereafter, licenses should be issued only to those having (a) an earned doctorate, from a college or university approved by the examining board, in chemical science, or in biological science, medicine or public health, provided training in chemistry sufficient to establish competence is assured, and (b) one year of practical experience in a laboratory approved for training in clinical chemistry by the examining board. (3) Persons meeting the requirements of education and good character shall in addition demonstrate their competence as clinical chemists by passing an examination. (4) Persons who have directed a laboratory of clinical chemistry within two years before the date the act takes effect shall be considered eligible to practice clinical chemistry without examination.

V. Provision should be made for the supervision by licensed clinical chemists of chemical work done in laboratories where work is related to health (clinical laboratories) or for periodic evaluation of the work of such laboratories by an authorized agency such as the State Board of Health.

VI. Authorization to practice clinical chemistry shall include the right to direct a laboratory restricted to clinical chemistry. Authority to direct a clinical laboratory embracing other branches of laboratory science should be granted only to those qualified in each. However, practice should be restricted to those fields in which a scientific director has qualified.

VII. A majority of the members of a board for examining candidates and for administration of an act for the regulation of clinical chemistry should be clinical chemists. Legislation which covers several specialties related to health should recognize these in board appointments. Because of the importance of clinical chemistry among the laboratory sciences related to health, the board administering a general act should include clinical chemists.

VIII. The requirements outlined shall not apply to employees of federal, state, or municipal governments or to scientists whose work consists primarily of research.

AAAS CLINICAL CHEMISTRY SYMPOSIUM

Albert E. Sobel, Program Chairman for the Association on scientific participation in a Symposium to be held under the auspices of the subsection, the American Association of Clinical Chemists, participating in the Atlanta Meeting of the American Association for the Advancement of Science, announced the following program for the meetings.

The Symposium, entitled "Recent Concepts in Clinical Chemistry," will be held in the Dixie Ballroom of the Henry Grady Hotel, Atlanta, Ga., on Monday, December 26, 1955.

Symposium Program

Opening Remarks by the Chairman, Albert E. Sobel, of the Jewish Hospital of Brooklyn, N. Y.

Role of the Clinical Chemist in the Hospital— Joseph H. Gast, Baylor University College of Medicine, Houston, Texas

New Concepts in Acid-Base Balance —Samuel Natelson, Memorial Hospital, Rockford, Ill.

Studies on Lipid Metabolism—D. B. Zilversmit, University of Tennessee, Memphis, Tenn.

Blood Proteins—Henry G. Kunkel, Rockefeller Institute, New York, N. Y.

Meeting Program

Symposium: "Recent Concepts in Clinical Chemistry" *December 26, 1955, 2 p.m., Henry Grady Hotel, Dixie Ballroom.*

AACC Dinner: *December 26, 6 p.m., Henry Grady Hotel, Dixie Ballroom.*

Contributed Papers: *December 27, 9 a.m., Henry Grady Hotel, Room B.*

Contributed Papers: *December 27, 2 p.m., Henry Grady Hotel, Room B.*

LECTURING ABROAD

Harry Sobotka, Mount Sinai Hospital, New York City, is visiting the Near East during September and October. He will give a number of lectures and hold conferences on subjects of physical biochemistry at the University of Athens and the National Technical University in Athens, Greece, at the University of Ankara and Istanbul, Turkey, and at the University of Jerusalem and at the Weizmann Institute in Rehovot, Israel.

NEW CATALOGUE SUPPLEMENT

The Arthur H. Thomas Company, Philadelphia, Pa., announces publication of a 264-page supplement to their 1472-page general catalogue. The Supplement follows the tradition of the catalogue and provides factual, detailed, and up-to-date listings of items added to their stock since publication of the catalogue in 1950. Also included is a price list covering all current items in both catalogue and supplement.

ERRATUM

In the article, "A Note on Quantitative Urobilinogen Determinations", by Bernard Balikov, Vol. 1, 264 (August 1955), the abscissa label of Fig. 1, page 265, should read "2% glacial acetic acid assumed to yield 100% recovery."

ABSTRACTS

Editor: ELLENMAE VIERGIVER. *Contributors:* JOSEPH A. ANNINO, GLADYS J. DOWNEY, CLYDE A. DUBBS, ALEX KAPLAN, MARGARET M. KASER, MIRIAM REINER, HERAERT THOMPSON

Uptake of radioactive iodine in the thyroid of patients with impaired liver function. R. Mueller, C. C. Brausch, E. A. Hirsch, R. S. Benua, and B. M. Dobyns. (*Western Reserve University School of Medicine, Cleveland, Ohio*)

The I^{131} thyroidal uptake was 50 per cent or higher in 20 of 50 patients with liver disease without evidence of thyroid disease. Among the patients with liver disease, elevated I^{131} thyroidal uptakes were associated most frequently with spider angiomata, jaundice, and microscopic evidence of severe cellular liver damage. No correlation could be established between elevated I^{131} thyroidal uptakes and either the presence of ascites or the results of any single test for liver function.

In spite of the elevated I^{131} uptakes by the thyroid in some patients with liver disease, there was no evidence of increased production of thyroid hormone, either by clinical findings or by the basal metabolic rate, the serum protein-bound iodine level, or by the height of thyroid cells. Although abnormal kidney function may be present in patients with cirrhosis, the normal urinary excretion of radioiodine found in sample patients in this series indicates that renal disturbance at the time of the tests was not the case of the elevated I^{131} thyroidal uptakes.—*J. Clin. Endocrinol. & Metab.* **14,** 1287 (1954).

M. R.

The influence of single doses of propylthiouracil on the kinetics of iodine accumulation by the thyroid glands of normal and hyperthyroid subjects. S. H. Ingbar (*Walter Reed Army Medical Center, Washington, D. C.*)

An evaluation was made of the influence of propylthiouracil in single doses of 25, 50 and 100 mg. on the intrathyroidal mechanisms of hormone formation in 10 euthyroid and 8 hyperthyroid patients. No reduction of the ability of the gland to concentrate inorganic iodide was observed. A diminution in the thyroidal rate of transfer of iodide from the plasma into the glandular hormone pool occurred in all patients as the result of an inhibition of the rate of protein binding of thyroidal iodide. The magnitude of the inhibitory effect was found to be proportional to the control level of the protein-binding rate and to the dose of antithyroid agent administered.—*J. Clin. Endocrinol. and Metabolism* **15,** 331 (1955).

(M. R.)

Chemical Evaluation of the Functions of the Liver

(Revised)

John G. Reinhold

STRUCTURE OF THE LIVER

The liver of a healthy adult weights 1650 Gm. on the average and it is by far the largest gland in the body. It consists of lobes which vary in size and differ to some extent in the sources of their afferent blood supplies. The liver is encased in a membrane of connective tissue. This extends into the liver at the transverse fissure of the undersurface (porta) in the form of a tree with innumerable branches. This framework of connective tissue supports the parenchymal cells, blood vessels, and bile ducts. The portal vein, hepatic artery, hepatic vein, and bile ducts enter the liver through the porta also, and undergo equally extensive branching. In its finer structure the liver consists of lobules 1–2 mm. in diameter. The lobules consist of numerous tubular secretory units; each formed by parenchymal cells surrounding a bile canaliculus.

The recent investigations of Elias (1949, 1953) have clarified structural relationships of the hepatic lobule to the vascular and biliary systems. Elias finds that the normal adult liver consists of many plates of epithelial liver cells one cell in thickness. The thickness of the plates may increase to 2 or more cells during regeneration of the liver. In lower animals also thicker plates are observed. The plates meet at varying angles to form a labyrinth of communicating cavities of irregular shape. Elias and Sokol (1953) state that the arrangement of the plates depends upon blood pressure and flow within the lobules.

From the William Pepper Laboratory of Clinical Medicine, Hospital of the University of Pennsylvania, Philadelphia, Pa.

The preparation of this review was aided in part by the Office of the Surgeon General, Department of the Army.

The author is very much indebted to Mrs. Ruth Wright and Mrs. C. A. J. Goldberg for assistance in preparing this review.

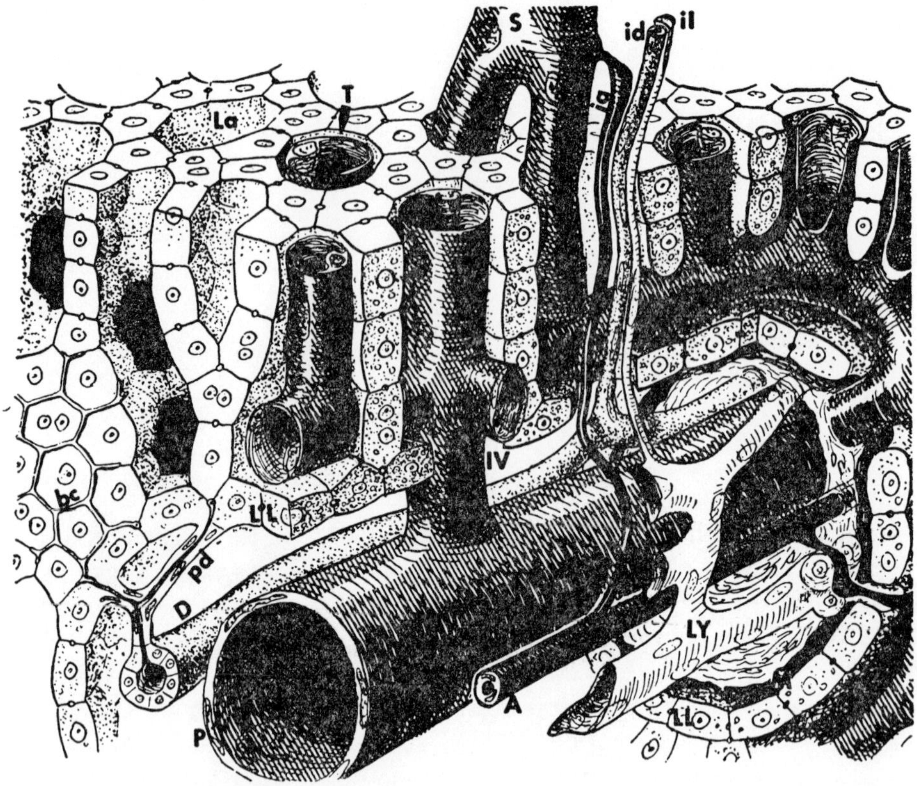

Fig. 1. Sterogram of the normal liver (drawn by Hans Elias). *A*, hepatic artery branch; *bc*, bile capillary; *D*, interlobular bile duct; *ia*, intralobular arteriole; *id*, intralobular ductule (cholangiole); *il*, intralobular lymph vessel; *IV*, inlet venule; *K*, Kupffer cell; *La*, labyrinth; *LL*, limiting plate; *LY*, portal lymph vessel; *P*, portal vein branch; *pd*, periportal ductule; *S*, sinusoid; *T*, tissue space of Disse. (From Popper, H., *Am. J. Med.* 76, 99, 1954. Reprinted with permission of the author and the publisher.)

The bile capillaries, according to Popper (1954), lie in grooves between the epithelial cells and may represent a special adaptation of the cell membranes of the latter. These join to form a "chicken-wire meshwork within the liver cell plates," and in turn continue into small bile capillaries (cholangioles). The cholangioles are lined with epithelial cells differing structurally and cytochemically from the liver cells (Fig. 1). Cholangioles arise from the liver cells embryologically and may proliferate excessively as a result of disease or injury of the liver, and especially during regeneration of the liver. This proliferation and secreting activity associated with it may be reflected in characteristic chemical changes in the blood.

Blood from the portal vein fills the sinusoids in the labyrinthine cavities between the plates of liver cells. This blood is enriched by arterial blood from the hepatic artery entering the sinusoids by way of intralobular arterioles. The latter are equipped with sphincters capable of regulating over wide limits the flow of arterial blood into the sinusoids.

Blood flows through the sinusoids in a direction opposite to that of the flow of bile (Fig. 2). It appears that blood entering the portal vein from the superior mesenteric and the splenic veins maintains discrete lines of flow with relatively little mixing. India ink injected into the former is deposited only in the right lobe of the liver; that injected into the splenic vein is confined to the left lobe [Sérégé, H. J., (1901) cited by Wakim, (1954)]. As a result, the right lobe of the liver receives blood well supplied with nutrients predominantly from the small intestine; whereas the left lobe of the liver receives its blood mainly from the spleen and large intestine. One would expect therefore that the left lobe would be more vulnerable to noxious substances formed in the large intestine by action of micro-organisms.

Attached to the lining of the sinusoids are Kupffer's cells, large star-shaped or pyramidal cells, which are a part of the reticuloendothelial system. As such, they are phagocytic and contribute to the destruction of erythrocytes, hemoglobin breakdown, and bile pigment production. Some estimates place the number of reticuloendothelial cells in the liver at one third of the total number of cells. They may contribute to antibody production, and some workers believe them to be an important source of γ globulins. Cholesterol given to rats by the oral route is concentrated by the reticuloendothelial cells of the liver to a much greater extent than by the parenchymal cells (St. George and Friedman, 1955).

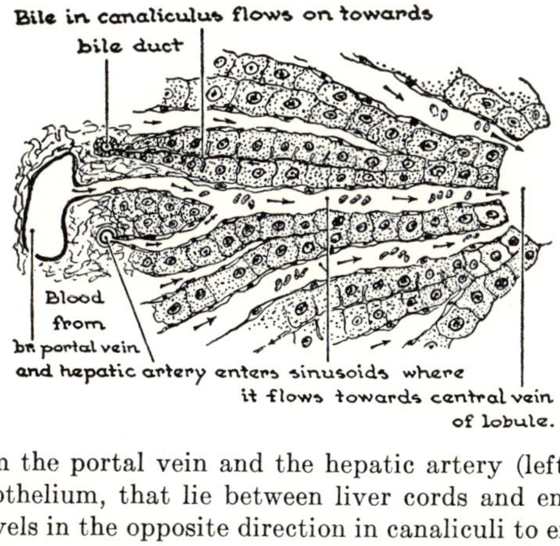

Fig. 2. Blood from the portal vein and the hepatic artery (left) flows into sinusoids, lined by reticuloendothelium, that lie between liver cords and empties into the central vein (right). Bile travels in the opposite direction in canaliculi to empty into bile ducts in portal areas. (From Ham, A. W., *Histology* (ed. 2), Philadelphia, Lippincott, 1953.)

The total volume of blood flowing through the liver was found by Bradley *et al.* (1945) to average 1500 ml. per minute, the range being 1085 to 1845 ml. per minute. Of this, about 12–44 per cent is arterial. However, the arterial blood contributes up to 60 per cent of the oxygen supply.

DISEASES OF THE LIVER AND BILIARY TRACT

Disturbances of metabolism occurring in liver disease may be sufficiently severe to jeopardize survival. They may be the result of (1) failure of the parenchymal cells to carry out vital functions because of infections or noxious agents; (2) decreased mass of functioning parenchymal cells resulting from disease; (3) decreased availability of blood to the liver cells because of (a) distortion of the liver architecture by scar tissue, (b) prolonged disturbance of the mechanisms regulating flow of blood in the liver with consequent shunting of blood around the liver or through it, (c) extrahepatic interference with blood supply, (4) impaired nutrition, (5) reaction of other organs to liver damage, e.g. brain, kidney, pancreas, adrenal, gonads, spleen, (6) injudicious therapy.

In a recent article of outstanding interest, Popper (1954) has revised and amplified many concepts of the morphologic changes occurring in liver disease. Among the changes he describes are:

1. Liver cell degeneration characterized by
   (a) loss of basophilic cytoplasmic nucleic acids, progressing at times to coagulation of the cytoplasm, or
   (b) marked swelling and rarified cytoplasm, found in hypoxia and carbon tetrachloride poisoning.
2. Atrophy, a thinning of the liver cell plates, associated with debilitating disease, senility, starvation, compression caused by biliary obstruction, or deposition of amyloid or of excessive amounts of glycogen.
3. Necrosis, an advanced degree of degeneration, characterized by loss of nuclear staining and ultimate disappearance of the cell. It may be
   (a) localized, with death of one or more cells and appearance of scavenger cells such as segmented leukocytes and lymphocytes.
   (b) central, involving all cells of the central zone of the lobule. This type occurs in severe hypoxia due to congestion or shock. It has been observed also in thyrotoxicosis and heart failure (Myers *et al.*, 1950).
   (c) periportal, involving the periphery of the lobule.
4. Regeneration, in which cells grow rapidly into areas destroyed by necrosis. Regeneration also may be stimulated in parts of the liver remote from the lesion. Proliferation of bile ducts is now regarded as evidence of liver cell regeneration.

5. Fatty metamorphosis, usually starting in the center of a lobule occurring as a result of
   (a) toxic injury
   (b) hypoxia
   (c) hormonal imbalance
   (d) nutritional deficiency
6. Stagnation of bile flow (cholestasis), associated with dilated bile capillaries, many with plugs of bile, and pigmentation of the cytoplasm of liver cells. Prolonged obstruction leads to bile duct proliferation, fibrosis, and degeneration of liver cells. The stagnation may be associated with inflammation of the tissues surrounding the duct. In addition to mechanical blockage, bacterial infection or intoxication by chemicals as different as arsenicals, methyl testosterone (Almaden and Ross, 1954), or chlorpromazine (Loftus *et al.*, 1955) may produce this response.
7. Cirrhosis, according to Popper (1954) "a chronic hepatitis with abnormalities of both parenchyma and mesenchyma, including scarring." An altered reconstruction of lobular parenchyma, due to injury of various etiology, results from two processes common to all types of cirrhosis. One is the formation of nodules in which normal arrangement of blood vessels and blood flow is altered. As a result, liver plates are rearranged. The nodules compress hepatic vein tributaries and cause elevation of blood pressure in the portal system. The second is the development of abnormal shunts between portal vein branches and hepatic vein tributaries. [For a more detailed discussion of the pathogenesis of cirrhosis see Popper's (1954) review.]
8. Inflammation, a common response to systemic disease, viral hepatitis, cirrhosis, and disease of the biliary or gastrointestinal tracts. Massive accumulations of inflammatory cells and marked proliferation of Kupffer's cells may be responsible for some of the chemical changes in blood occurring in liver disease.

Infectious disease of the liver, such as viral hepatitis, is characterized by degeneration and necrosis and regeneration of parenchymal cells as shown by variations in size and staining characteristics. Necrosis and complete disappearance of cells and destruction of the normal architecture of the lobule by scar tissue may follow. Scavenger cells, histiocytes, lymphocytes and plasma cells infiltrate the damaged regions. Edema may occur and, together with the disorganization of structure, contribute to decrease the blood supply. Regeneration of the parenchymal cells can occur rapidly and produce an astonishingly large mass of cells within as little time as 24 to 48 hours. Regeneration is favored by a well-maintained blood supply, and lacking this, fails to occur (Grindlay and Bollman, 1952).

Viral hepatitis ordinarily runs its course within 1–3 months with apparently complete recovery. It may however, become chronic in about 1 per cent, persisting for many years, at times in an asymptomatic form. Formerly, viral hepatitis was often mistaken for a disease of the bile ducts and the term "catarrhal jaundice" in the older literature is a result of this confusion.

The term cholangiolitic hepatitis has been applied by Watson and Hoffbauer (1946) to a syndrome in which inflammation of the smaller bile passages predominates. It differs strikingly in its effect on the chemical composition of the blood from those diseases that involve primarily the parenchymal cells. Chemical changes are similar to those found in biliary obstruction and all the resources of medical knowledge may be required to make a differentiation. Abscesses and cysts of the liver caused by infections or parasites may lead to significant changes in liver function (Brem, 1955).

Deposition of fat in the liver may occur as part of a general adiposity resulting from overnutrition, as a result of dietary deficiencies, or as an effect of the action of toxic substances. Dible (1951) has recently evaluated the significance of liver fat and has demonstrated experimentally that liver fat tends to be increased in proportion to body fat. Fatty liver resulting from overnutrition has little importance insofar as the function of the liver is concerned. However, deposition of fat caused by toxic substances is evidence of a serious disturbance of hepatocellular function. Among the nutritional deficiencies associated with fatty liver are those induced by lack of betaine, choline, methionine, threonine, B_{12}, or folic acid. Low protein intakes contribute to the production of fatty livers.

Extensive deposition of fat often precedes fibrosis. Popper (1954) describes the gradual appearance of connective-tissue septa in large, fatty livers, occurring around the lobules and also extending into the lobules.

Although liver disease of nutritional origin is uncommon in the United States (if the chronic alcoholic is excepted), it is a major problem in many parts of the world, notably the tropical regions of Africa and Asia and in the Caribbean area. It may be accompanied by infiltration of fat, necrotic changes, and cellular infiltration, and in certain instances by accumulation of exudate in the liver. In certain parts of Africa, primary carcinoma of the liver may be a major manifestation of nutritional deficiency; in others, cirrhosis has been reported in four of five necropsies.

Liver damage may occur as a result of severe strains on metabolism associated with many diseases. In infectious mononucleosis it may be sufficiently severe to constitute a grave hazard to the patient. Marked jaundice and severe alterations in liver function are seen in such patients. Malaria, lobar pneumonia, typhoid fever, various anemias, syphilis, and cholera serve as other examples. Diabetes and thyrotoxicosis also may lead to marked liver damage. Surgical operation and anesthesia cause impairment of liver function in some patients (Fairlie and others, 1951). Liver failure may occur in pregnancy.

A failing heart and the resulting accumulation of blood in the liver and other viscera (chronic passive congestion) may lead to marked impairment of the efficiency with which the liver functions.

Proliferation of the connective tissue of the liver may result from liver disease of infectious, nutritional, toxic, hypoxic, or neoplastic etiology, or it may occur spontaneously because of diminished blood supply resulting from circulatory and other factors. The overgrowth of connective tissue in turn leads to disorganization of the liver structure and this again to further interference with the blood supply. The end result is a shrunken liver consisting largely of connective tissue, and with a markedly decreased mass of parenchymal, reticuloendothelial, and vascular tissue. The designations *portal cirrhosis*, *atrophic cirrhosis*, and *Laennec's cirrhosis* have been used at various times to denote such scarred livers. Although not all scarred livers fit the pathologist's definition of Laennec's cirrhosis, this descriptive term appears to be preferred at present. Laennec's cirrhosis accounts for a large proportion of the liver disease encountered in American hospitals.

Cirrhosis of a completely different etiology, differing also in its morphologic and chemical characteristics, appears after biliary obstruction has persisted for long periods. Known as biliary cirrhosis, it is relatively uncommon. This condition may occur spontaneously also, its etiology being unclear.

Obstruction of the bile ducts often causes jaundice, which may be attributed erroneously to liver disease. It is essential to distinguish jaundice due to biliary obstruction from that caused by liver disease or excessive destruction of blood, because obstruction requires surgical treatment, whereas surgery may not be well tolerated by the patient with liver disease or be needed by the patient who is hemolyzing his erythrocytes. Gall stones entering the common bile duct are the usual cause of biliary obstruction. Other causes include neoplastic disease of the ducts, especially of the ampulla of Vater, or carcinoma of the head of the pancreas. Stricture of the ducts may follow infection, surgical exploration, or other trauma. Disease of the gall bladder frequently is complicated by liver damage. The pancreas often shows evidence of being involved. Failure to establish the presence of biliary obstruction and to correct it may lead eventually to biliary cirrhosis.

Carcinoma or other types of neoplastic disease of the liver may or may not be accompanied by jaundice. Often such lesions present few signs to the physician. Obstruction of the bile ducts within the liver by neoplasm presumably brings about the rise in alkaline phosphatase activity in serum, which provides one of the few diagnostic aids available.

Damage to the liver may be caused by a large number of chemicals and drugs. Carbon tetrachloride has been extensively used for production of experimental liver damage and probably has been involved more often than realized as an insidious cause of clinical liver disease. Atophan, various sulfonamides, para-aminobenzoate, testosterone, arsenicals, and others have been implicated. The effect on liver function, as measured by laboratory studies, may resemble that observed in biliary obstruction rather than parenchymal liver disease.

Liver disease may affect the metabolism and functions of other organs. Effects upon the brain are especially noteworthy. Continuing liver disease of maximal severity may eventually lead to loss of consciousness or convulsions, and the electroencephalogram may show the characteristic pattern seen in the syndrome known as hepatic coma. Hepatic coma is frequently but not necessarily fatal. Recovery may occur spontaneously but also has been attributed to a variety of therapeutic agents. Among treatments reported as successful are injection of nicotinic acid, thiamine phosphate, vitamin B_6, multiple B vitamins, sodium glutamate, and glucose. Exchange transfusion and oxygen therapy also have been used.

Impairment of kidney function commonly accompanies liver disease, and may become a grave problem. The coexistence of hepatic and renal failure is often referred to as the "hepato-renal syndrome." Whether this is a clinical entity has been questioned by many. Lichtman (1954) points out that renal complications in liver disease vary in their pathogenesis. Patek, Segal, and Bevans (1951) find that intercapillary glomerulonephritis occurs much more frequently in cirrhotic patients than in the ordinary population. Farquhar (1949) has described the deterioration of kidney function occurring in viral hepatitis.

CHEMICAL PHYSIOLOGY OF LIVER DISEASE

The list of chemical disturbances observed in liver disease is a long one and will become lengthened as metabolism in liver disease is studied more intensively. Knisely (1951) has listed 18 major asserted chemical functions of the liver with 75 subheadings. Many of these cannot be discussed here for lack of space.

Carbohydrate Metabolism

Studies of hepatectomized animals by Mann (1927) and his collaborators showed conclusively the vital importance of the liver for maintenance of the blood glucose concentration. Although hypoglycemia severe enough to cause symptoms is not a common complication in acute parenchymal liver disease, it does occur in cirrhosis of the Laennec type with sufficient frequency to require that measurement of fasting blood glucose concentrations be included in the study of such patients. Blood sugar concentrations as low as 25 mg./100 ml. are not unusual. A diagnosis of islet cell adenoma of the pancreas occasionally is erroneously made in cirrhotic patients because of recurrent hypoglycemia (Conn *et al.*, 1938). Mellinkoff and Tumulty (1953) describe the occurrence of hypoglycemia in patients with liver disease, including some of those with relatively moderate liver involvement.

Waife *et al.* (1951) showed that insulin resistance occurs in cirrhosis, the fall in blood sugar after a standard insulin injection being delayed as compared with that of healthy individuals. However, hypoglycemia following the insulin persisted for a much longer time than in healthy controls. Thus a markedly impaired ability to mobilize glucose in response to hypoglycemia may be deduced. Injection of epinephrine causes a smaller rise in blood sugar of patients with liver disease than it does in healthy subjects (Geill, 1943; Kinsell and associates, 1949). Hillman (1949) reports this test to have doubtful value in the study of liver function.

Glucose administered to patients with liver disease often causes a greater and more persistent rise in blood glucose than it does in healthy individuals. (Conn *et al.*, 1938; Campbell and Tagnon, 1946). Smith, Ettinger, and Seligson (1953) have studied the metabolism of fructose and of glucose in patients with liver disease. They found evidence of impaired ability to utilize both, but not of sufficient consistency to enable application as diagnostic or functional tests.

Decreased utilization of galactose in liver disease has provided the basis for one of the earlier tests of liver function (Bauer, 1906). The measurement of galactose excretion in urine originally used has been replaced by measurement of blood galactose concentrations (Althausen, Lockhart and Soley, 1940; Althausen, 1949; Zieve, Hill and Nesbitt, 1950). Colcher,

Patek and Kendall (1946) have described an intravenous galactose tolerance test by which the quantity of galactose removed per minute was found to be markedly decreased in liver disease. The cause of the elevated blood galactose and increased output in urine characteristic of severe liver disease has not been established, but presumably it represents interference with the conversion of galactose to glucose. An idiopathic defect in galactose metabolism involving a galactose kinase has been studied by Greenman (1950). The liver is thought to be the source of the enzyme.

Methods for Study of Disturbances of Carbohydrate Metabolism in Liver Disease

Blood sugar determinations after an overnight fast generally will enable detection of hypoglycemia. A diet very low in carbohydrate accentuates the tendency toward hypoglycemia. (Conn. *et al.*, 1938). Glucose tolerance measured by standard 3- or five-hour technics may be used but, as indicated above, offers little useful diagnostic information. Measurement of phosphate concentrations in serum also fails to differentiate clearly between the several causes of impaired glucose tolerance. The galactose tolerance procedures are discussed above. Further studies by means of these improved technics are needed for appraisal of this procedure. The recent literature gives little reason to believe that fructose tolerance tests would be of value in diagnosis of liver disease.

Serum Cholesterol and Lipids in Liver Disease

The serum lipids often show marked changes in diseases of the liver and biliary tract. Although serum cholesterol concentration and the partition between free and esterified cholesterol is most frequently studied, neutral fat and especially phospholipid may also show marked changes. Relationships between free and esterified cholesterol and between free cholesterol and phospholipid, which in health are maintained within narrow limits, are subject to striking disturbances in severe liver disease. Liver disease in which injury to the parenchymal cells is severe is characterized by lowered lipid concentrations which often fall below the minimal concentrations observed in normal individuals of the same age. The onset of jaundice in viral hepatitis is soon followed by falling serum cholesterol and phospholipid concentrations. The decrease of the esterified cholesterol is striking. Both concentration of esterified cholesterol and the percentage of the total cholesterol esterified are lowered. If liver damage is very severe, esterified cholesterol may become undetectable. Recovery is accompanied by rising concentrations of the esterified cholesterol in serum. Free cholesterol often is increased at the same time so that moderately elevated concentrations may exist during the stage of remission.

Lecithin, but not cephalin, concentrations are also increased in serum at this stage (Peterson, 1953). Alterations in serum lipid concentrations and the interrelationships of the various lipids have been described by Man *et al.* (1945), Hoagland and Shank (1946), Havens (1948), and Billing *et al.* (1955). Studies of the lipoproteins of sera of patients suffering from liver disease show that these also are involved in the general disturbance of lipid metabolism. Pierce and Gofman (1951) observed a marked increase in the lipoproteins of the class S_f 10–20. Pierce *et al.* (1954) described high values in the S_f 0–12, 20–100, and 100–400 classes also. The serum lipoproteins of hepatectomized dogs remained unchanged for 6 hours, and then decreased despite increasing hemoconcentration (Lewis, Page, and Thomas, 1953). Nikkila (1953) demonstrated a decrease in α_1 and an increase in β-lipoprotein by the use of zone electrophoresis in hepatitis and also in biliary obstruction. Cirrhosis of the Laennec type, is characterized by low serum lipid concentrations, especially when atrophy of the liver is extensive. Serum cholesterol concentrations of less than 100 mg./100 ml. are quite common. The proportion of esterified cholesterol also is lowered, although exceptions exist. Low phospholipid concentrations also are the rule. Cayer and Cornatzer (1950) found the rate of phospholipid synthesis in cirrhosis to be decreased and this may account for the low values in serum.

Billing *et al.* (1955) found a correlation between total liver lipids and total serum lipids, and also between total liver lipids and serum total fatty acid, phospholipid, and total and free cholesterol in 22 patients with cirrhosis. No correlation could be established by the study of a group of patients with viral hepatitis or in fatty vacuolization, focal necrosis, or granuloma. Colwell (1954) observed that an excessive deposition of fat occurred in the liver during convalescence from viral hepatitis if the patient gained much weight during the convalescence period. Such patients ate diets rich in carbohydrate and fat and relatively poor in protein.

Biliary obstruction regardless of cause is characterized by elevated concentrations of serum lipids. Extremely high concentrations, among the highest known to occur due to any cause, are encountered in patients with biliary obstruction of long duration or with biliary cirrhosis. Ahrens *et al.* (1950) in a review dealing with biliary cirrhosis describe a disproportionate increase in serum phospholipid concentration. They have also clarified the relationship of elevated serum lipid concentrations to xanthelasma and xanthomatosis.

Cholangiolitic hepatitis and toxic hepatitis of the type caused by chemicals and drugs also are associated with elevated serum lipid concentrations.

Some use is made of serum cholesterol analyses for differentiation of primarily parenchymal from primarily biliary lesions in jaundiced patients. However, such analyses offer little information that cannot be obtained more easily and dependably by other methods. Not only do some patients with biliary obstruction fail to show a rise in concentration of serum cholesterol exceeding the broad range of concentrations found in healthy individuals, but abnormally elevated serum cholesterol concentrations occur in many patients with infectious hepatitis or other predominantly parenchymal types of liver disease. Such increased levels are observed especially as regeneration of the liver proceeds.

The finding of low concentrations and ratios of esterified to total cholesterol in a jaundiced patient is strong but not conclusive evidence for parenchymal liver involvement of severe degree. Serial studies of the esterified cholesterol concentration provide means for estimating changes in the state of the liver in parenchymal liver disease of maximal severity. They do not however, reliably indicate the prognosis. Esterified cholesterol measurements are useful in the study of such patients because more sensitive tests, such as bromsulfalein retention, become maximally positive when there is still a substantial amount of functioning parenchymal tissue remaining. On the other hand, for study of patients with less severe liver disease, less elaborate and time-consuming methods than esterified cholesterol determinations are more satisfactory. As an indication for determination of esterified cholesterol, the presence of jaundice or of a marked elevation of serum bilirubin serves reasonably well. Measurement of esterified cholesterol concentration is useful for the preoperative study of patients with biliary tract disease.

Zieve (1953) has demonstrated that the lowered esterified cholesterol concentrations in patients with liver disease and obstruction of the common bile duct are correlated with the degree of jaundice. Although the proportion of cholesterol esterified shown in his data varied widely for any given bilirubin concentration, a fact that suggests some degree of independence, Zieve's study has helped to prove what many workers have long suspected—that esterified cholesterol measurements make a rather limited contribution to the study of patients with liver disease.

The cause of the lowered concentrations of serum lipid observed in many patients with severe liver disease is not known. Contributing factors include (1) the lowered intake of lipid brought about by prescription of diets high in carbohydrate and low in fat for patients with liver disease; (2) decreased synthesis of fat and of other lipids because of reduced mass of parenchymal cells, impaired blood supply and other related mechanical factors leading to impaired efficiency of biochemical transformations; (3) a diminished supply of supplementary factors such as labile methyl, choline, etc., because of diminished intake and decreased synthesis, these together with other factors, leading to (4) deposition of fat in the liver; and (5) impaired absorption of fat from the gastrointestinal tract. Steatorrhea is a frequent finding in patients with liver disease. Gross *et al.* (1950 b) attribute this to deficiency of bile salts, for they were unable to demonstrate a lack of digestive enzyme secretion by the pancreas in patients with viral hepatitis.

The decreased esterification of cholesterol occurring in severe liver disease, when there is extensive destruction or replacement of the parenchyma, also is unexplained. It may be a manifestation of a general decrease in esterase activity since cholinesterase of serum is also depressed. Bollman (1950) has pointed out that the intestinal mucosa is an active site for esterification of cholesterol and that it adds by way of the lymph each day twice the amount of cholesterol ester found in the plasma at any time. However, Friedman and Byers (1955) offer strong evidence that the liver is the organ that chiefly synthesizes and removes cholesterol esters.

The cause of the elevated concentration of lipid in serum, so typical of biliary obstruction, is also obscure. The bile does not appear to be an important route of lipid excretion. Much of the cholesterol and probably all of the phospholipid excreted in the bile is reabsorbed. Balfour (1947) found that the rate of production of phospholipid was increased in biliary obstruction and that the rise in concentration was proportional to the increase in rate of its production. Rosenman, Friedman, and Byers (1952) have postulated that cholesterol concentration in serum rises as a response to an increase in concentration of bile acid (cholate). They believe that changes in concentration of the latter are accompanied by changes in serum cholesterol which serves perhaps to counteract the toxicity of cholate for tissues. Byers, Friedman, and Michaelis (1951) find that the liver itself is the source of the extra cholesterol. Frederickson *et al.* (1954) also observed a nearly 20-fold increase in cholesterol synthesis in rats following ligation of the bile duct. The close relationship maintained between free cholesterol and phospholipid might then be expected to lead to increased concentrations of the latter.

Information concerning bile acids in liver disease is scanty and unsatisfactory. It is to be hoped that recent improvements in the methods for bile acid determination in serum and bile will overcome this deficiency. Studies of fistula bile following release of biliary obstruction in patients showed cholate to be absent from the bile for a number of days (Ravdin *et al.* 1933). The crude methods available in the past for estimating bile acid concentrations in serum indicate that bile acid enters the blood stream to attain concentrations of 10 to 20 mg. per 100 ml. in the presence of biliary obstruction. Elevated values may occur also in liver disease affecting the parenchyma predominantly (Sherlock and Walshe, 1948).

Methods for Study of Disturbances of Lipid Metabolism in Liver Disease

Serum cholesterol and cholesterol ester concentrations may be determined by the methods of Abell *et al.* (1952) or of Sperry and Webb (1950). For phospholipid concentrations the method of Zilversmit and Davis (1950) is convenient. A rapid and simple method for detecting total lipid of serum, the phenol turbidity, has been described by Kunkel, Ahrens, and Eisenmenger (1948). De la Huerga *et al.* (1953) have described a rapid turbidimetric method for total lipid in serum that depends upon liberation of lipid in fine suspension by a reagent consisting of dioxane and dilute sulfuric acid. If a more accurate method is required, that of Sperry and Brand (1955) may be used.

Nitrogen Metabolism

Several studies of the nitrogen metabolism of patients with liver disease have failed to demonstrate any marked imbalance. Kinsell *et al.* (1948) found the nitrogen balance of 2 patients with chronic hepatitis to be positive. Gross *et al.* (1950 a) found a slightly positive nitrogen balance in 7 patients diagnosed as having acute hepatitis and in one with chronic hepatitis. They cite the work of Fawitzsky in 1889 who studied 6 patients with Laennec's cirrhosis and came to a similar conclusion.

The liver is the principal site for transformation of amino acids by synthesis, transamination, etc., into those forms specifically needed. It carries out such transformations less effectively when diseased or otherwise injured.

Amino acid concentrations of plasma (Flock *et al.*, 1953) and of brain and muscle (Flock, Block, *et al.*, 1952) are increased substantially after complete removal of the liver. In liver disease the concentration of amino acid in plasma may be increased in patients with severe involvement of the liver. Hsia and Gellis (1954) found that of 19 children ill with viral hepatitis, about half had moderately elevated concentrations of amino acid in plasma. About two thirds excreted increased amounts in urine. Walshe (1953) found by means of chromatographic methods that some adults showed little change in plasma amino acid in hepatitis, whereas marked changes occurred in others. However, Murphy *et al.* in 1949 failed to demonstrate an increase in plasma amino acids in a group of patients with liver failure. Mellinkoff *et al.* (1954) also found only moderately increased concentrations in viral hepatitis, although the results are somewhat questionable because of the use of serum for analysis instead of plasma. After a meal containing 20 Gm. of protein, amino acid concentrations decreased in serum of patients with hepatitis. In healthy persons the opposite occurred. The cause of the unexpected behavior of the amino acids in hepatitis is obscure, but the suggestion is offered that it may be the effect of insulin present in increased concentration in the tissues because of a diminished rate of destruction of insulin by the damaged liver. Insulin was shown to cause an abrupt fall in amino acids of plasma after hepatectomy (Flock *et al.*, 1953).

Several reports indicate that methionine concentration is increased considerably in plasma in viral hepatitis (Kirsner *et al.*, 1950; Schreier, 1951; Balch *et al.*, 1954; Kinsell *et al.*, 1948). Kinsell *et al.* (1948, 1949) also demonstrated a delayed rate of removal of injected methionine from the blood stream. Walshe (1953) and Walshe and Senior (1955) describe the occurrence of high cystine concentrations in plasma in cirrhosis, with highest values occurring in hepatic coma.

Mitchell, Butt, and Code (1954) found elevated blood histamine concentrations in patients with liver disease. They noted a correlation between pruritus and the extent of the elevation.

The excretion of certain amino acids in urine is increased substantially in parenchymal liver disease (Dunn *et al.*, 1950; Gabuzda *et al.*, 1952; Walshe, 1953). Among those affected in this way are cystine, methionine, taurine, β-aminoisobutyric acid, methyl histidine, and tryptophan. The excretion of some amino acids is lowered. Among these are lysine, histidine, and isoleucine. Dent and Walshe (1951) describe several different patterns of aminoaciduria occurring in liver disease.

Walshe (1953) identified more than 30 amino acids in urine following massive necrosis of the liver. He found the output of amino acids in urine to undergo greater change than did the concentration in plasma. Relatively moderate gains in concentration in plasma led to a marked increase in the output of amino acids in urine. Thus, the change in plasma concentrations of amino acids with high renal clearances often was slight compared with the change in the amounts found in urine. Amino acids with lower renal clearances, including methionine, phenylalanine, and tyrosine, show much more marked changes in plasma concentrations.

Dent and Walshe (1954) state that patients with biliary obstruction, secondary carcinoma of the liver, and liver infiltrations had no abnormality of amino acid metabolism. The extent of abnormality in parenchymatous disease corresponded roughly to the extent of the disease.

Walshe (1951) detected methionine sulfoxide in chromatograms of the plasma of a patient dying of hepatic coma. This compound is a glutamic acid antimetabolite and the suggestion was made that it might be inhibiting the utilization of glutamic acid by the brain. Interference with the metabolism of a substance having such a vital role in brain metabolism would have important consequences. However, it may be an artefact.

Ethanolamine was found in excessive amounts in urine of patients with liver disease by Dent and Walshe (1951, 1953). One patient with a huge hepatoma excreted 0.5 to 1.0 Gm. per day. The presence of large amounts of ethanolamine, a precursor of lecithin, may be related to the failure of phospholipid synthesis referred to above.

In Wilson's disease (hepatolenticular degeneration) amino acid output in urine is substantially increased, whereas little or no change can be detected in concentrations of blood amino acids (Dent and Walshe, 1951).

Some of the tests employed for study of liver function have as their basis the impaired metabolism of amino acid. Among such is the tyrosine tolerance test of Bernhart and Schneider (1943). One of the factors causing delayed excretion of hippuric acid in Quick's test (1933) is said to be the decreased ability to mobilize glycine for conjugations.

The elevated amino acid concentration in blood contributes to the elevation of nonprotein nitrogen characteristic of patients with severe liver involvement. Concentrations of other substances, including creatine, creatinine, uric acid, ammonia, as well as the undetermined nitrogen, also may be elevated. Urea concentrations may be increased, within normal limits, or decreased, the latter being a rare occurrence. The elevation of nonprotein nitrogen is mainly a result of the impairment of kidney function. However, urea nitrogen may not be elevated in proportion to the creatinine and NPN concentrations. In part this is due to impaired efficiency of the reactions involved in its synthesis. A second factor is the lowered protein intake often prescribed for patients with liver disease. Conclusions concerning the kidney function of patients with severe disease of the liver are, therefore, likely to be more reliable if based on creatinine or nonprotein nitrogen determinations than if based on blood urea nitrogen.

Creatine concentrations are markedly increased in the serum of some patients in hepatic coma (Reinhold, unpublished observations). The impaired metabolism of muscle in such patients, with resulting losses of creatine, is thought to be the main cause. Renal failure alone is not responsible. Failure of methylation may contribute.

Blood Ammonia in Liver Disease

The liver is the site of numerous reactions concerned with ammonia metabolism. These include deaminization of amino acids and adenylic acid and synthesis of glutamine. Blood ammonia concentrations in hepatectomized dogs were found to rise rapidly (Gordon, Freeman, and Farmer, 1952), confirming earlier work by Bollman and Mann in 1930. Interest in blood ammonia in liver disease has been revived recently by the finding that patients suffering from cirrhosis, who had received ammonia-containing ion exchange resins, at times became stuporous with signs suggesting those of hepatic coma (Gabuzda, Phillips, and Davidson, 1952). Blood ammonia concentrations were substantially increased (Schwartz *et al.*, 1953). Fuld (1933), Kirk (1936) and others previously have shown that the ammonia content of blood is increased in patients with severe liver disease. Seligson (1953) reported that not all patients in hepatic coma had elevated blood ammonia concentrations.

Riddell and McDermott (1954) found higher blood ammonia concentrations in blood of patients with cirrhosis than in that of normal persons, especially in the period preceding coma. However, a decrease in blood ammonia concentrations of such patients was not necessarily accompanied by an improved clinical condition. Administration of ammonium compounds to cirrhotic patients caused a greater rise in blood ammonia concentrations than in healthy persons (Traeger, *et al.*, 1954). Ammonia concentrations in cerebrospinal fluid exceeding 105 μg./100 ml. were associated with mental disturbances (McDermott, Adams, and Riddell, 1955).

The neurologic effects of elevated ammonia concentrations in the body fluids are of unusual interest. They have been described by Adams and Foley (1953) and by McDermott and Adams (1954).

Bessman and Bessman (1955) found that ammonia is converted in brain and muscle to a bound form. Arterial blood contained somewhat higher concentrations of ammonia than did venous blood returning from the brain. They believe that the uptake of ammonia by the brain causes a diversion of α-ketoglutarate to glutamate. A deficiency in the production of the former is thought to interrupt the citrate cycle and may impair cerebral metabolism. A study by Nelson and Seligson (1953) showed that ammonia enters the circulation mainly from the portal vein, kidneys, and muscles. In shock the liver fails to remove it completely and the blood ammonia level rises.

Studies of the ammonia metabolism of experimental animals (Mann *et al.*, 1954) and of patients suffering from liver disease, especially cirrhosis (Schwartz *et al.*, 1954), have led to a critical re-evaluation of the role of high protein intake in raising blood ammonia concentrations. High protein intake tends to raise blood ammonia concentrations and low protein intake to lower them. It appears from this that the protein intake should be adjusted to the capacity of the patient to dispose of ammonia.

These observations, together with those of Nelson and Seligson (1953), strongly implicate the intestine as the major source of the blood ammonia. Parnas and Klisiecki (1926) came to a similar conclusion nearly 30 years ago. In the normal person most of the ammonia is removed by the liver. However, the considerable proportion of the blood that flows around instead of through the liver of the cirrhotic delivers the ammonia into the general circulation and so raises the ammonia concentration. White *et al.* (1955) believe that there is a defect in hepatic metabolism of ammonia in addition to the enteral factor.

Blood ammonia concentrations may be measured either by the method of Conway (1935) [*see also* Conway and Cooke (1939) and McDermott and Adams (1954)] or by the method of Seligson [described by Reinhold and Gentzkow (1955)]. Although the two methods differ in results, either procedure is capable of providing useful information about blood ammonia concentrations. For both theoretical and practical reasons that of Seligson is the method of preference.

Plasma Proteins in Liver Disease

The liver has a dominant role in plasma protein synthesis. It is the known source of plasma albumin and fibrinogen (Miller, Bly, Watson, and Bale, 1951). Probably proteins other than fibrinogen involved in the clotting of blood also originate in the liver. It is the source of important components included in the alpha and beta globulins (Roberts, 1953; Roberts and Brunish, 1953). The liver also is involved in synthesis of gamma globulin, although there is much evidence indicating that synthesis of gamma globulin is largely extrahepatic.

Albumin concentrations in serum are lowered in patients suffering from cirrhosis, in viral hepatitis during its clinically active stages, in nutritional liver disease, and in neoplastic disease involving the liver. Many authorities consider it to be among the most dependable measurements available for establishing the presence of liver disease (numerous other causes of low albumin concentration usually can be excluded without difficulty) and for following its clinical course. For this purpose it is superior to total serum protein concentration because changes in albumin are commonly masked by an equal and simultaneous rise in globulin so that total protein remains unchanged. The changes occurring in serum proteins of a volunteer in whom viral hepatitis was induced are shown in Fig. 3.

The causes of the decreased albumin concentration include (1) impaired synthesis because of decreased mass of parenchymal tissue; (2) losses by transudation into ascitic and edema fluid; (3) losses by hemorrhage, a frequent complication of cirrhosis; (4) increase in plasma volume (in cirrhosis) and (5) low protein intake.

The lowered concentration of serum albumin is one of the factors re-

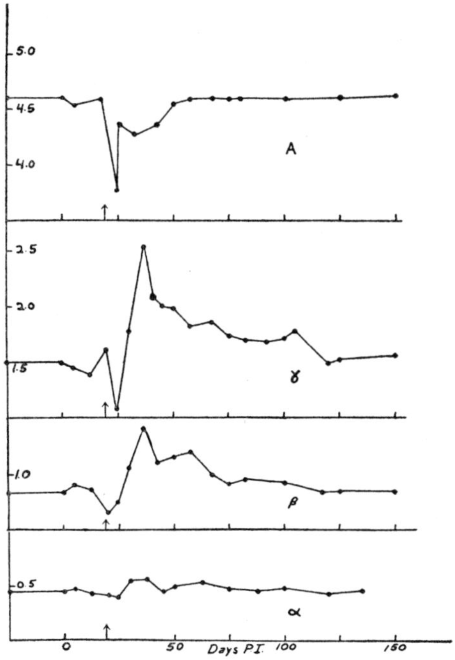

Fig. 3. Changes in serum proteins occurring in a human volunteer during the course of viral hepatitis. At 0 days, this volunteer ingested material containing virus obtained from a patient suffering from infectious hepatitis. The arrow indicates the appearance of clinical symptoms. Note the fall in albumin concentration and the sharp rise in gamma and beta globulin concentrations with gradual return to the original values. Protein measurements were made by the moving boundary method at pH 7.6 in phosphate buffer. (From unpublished studies by Neefe, Chambers, Gilman, and Reinhold.)

sponsible for the occurrence of flocculation in the cephalin-cholesterol flocculation and related tests. A change in constitution of albumin and α-globulin probably contributes. A second major factor is a rise in concentration of γ-globulin. Yet another variable is a rise in stabilizing action associated with biliary obstruction (Ducci, 1950). The physicochemical basis for the flocculation and turbidity tests has been discussed by Saifer (1952).

An increase in γ-globulin accounts for much of the increase in total globulin of serum. Whereas in healthy individuals γ-globulin reaches a maximum of 1.6 Gm./100 ml., in liver disease concentrations double this are common, and concentrations five or more times the maximal normal occur in some patients with hepatitis. Zimmerman, Heller, and Hill (1951) observed a globulin concentration of 9.9 Gm./100 ml. in a patient with subacute hepatic necrosis. Values as high as this have been encountered on several occasions in the writer's laboratory. [*See also* Kunkel, Ahrens, *et al.* (1951).]

The marked rise in γ-globulin occurring in liver disease is similar to that occurring in many other diseases. Robertson (1950) has described extremely high γ-globulin concentrations as a manifestation of sensitization to drugs, and Carter (1949) described equally high γ-globulin concentrations as a result of trichinosis. Teilum (1948) considers the rise to be part of a general response to sensitizing agents. The rise is associated with a marked proliferation of plasmacytes in bone marrow to as much as 25 per cent or more of the total count. Plasmacytes and lymphocytes also accumulate in the liver and other affected areas. These and other observations have led Fagreus (1948), Bjorneboe and associates (1947), and Ehrich (1953) and others to attribute to the plasma cells the formation of γ-globulin. According to their hypothesis the elevation in γ-globulin occurring in response to stressful stimuli, among them liver disease, is a result of the proliferation of this γ-globulin-producing tissue. However, Popper (1951), Franklin (1951), and their coworkers have observed changes in the Kupffer and mesenchymal cells of the liver that correlate with increased γ-globulin concentrations in serum. They believe that these cells are the source of the extra γ-globulin. Yet another explanation has been offered by Miller (1953), who believes that the diminished synthesis of albumin and other plasma proteins leaves a surplus of amino acids which are converted into γ-globulin outside the liver.

The rise in γ-globulin in many patients suffering from liver disease is accompanied by elevation of β-globulin. Extra protein components not normally observed may appear when electrophoretic separation of serum protein is made at *p*H 8.6, (Martin, 1949). That most frequently encounted is the H protein of Viollier (1950) observed in infectious hepatitis. Increased $gamma_1$ concentrations were observed by Franklin and associates (1951) frequently in liver disease and rarely in other conditions. These components have mobilities close to that of fibrinogen. Other abnormal components may appear within the gamma and beta fractions.

Fibrinogen concentrations of plasma fall after removal of the liver (Foster and Whipple, 1922). Stefanini (1949) found low fibrinogen concentrations in patients suffering from liver disease. Schulz (1953) observed occasional high fibrinogen values in viral hepatitis. These fell in the later stages. Low values were the rule in cirrhosis.

Alpha globulins, particularly α_1, show a tendency toward lower concentrations than those existing in health. Much of the mucoprotein of serum is included within the alpha-globulin fraction of the serum protein. Serum mucoprotein has been found by Greenspan *et al.* (1952; 1953; 1954) to be decreased by hepatitis but increased by metastatic invasion of the liver. Mandel *et al.* (1955) find that the results are not always consistent with the diagnosis, and have reservations about the usefulness of the mucoprotein measurement. However in the writer's laboratory, the serum mucopolysaccharide measurement appears to have provided valuable aid to physicians confronted with diagnostic problems in jaundiced patients.

Mucoprotein may be measured by a method such as that described by Rhees, Ellerbrook, and Lippincott (1954). Graff *et al.* (1951) showed that the somewhat laborious method for mucoprotein could be replaced by measurement of protein-bound polysaccharides, a relatively simple procedure when anthrone is used as the reagent. However, see Shetlar (1952).

The concentrations of some of the specific proteins included in the alpha globulin fraction also are decreased. Thus serum pseudo-cholinesterase is markedly decreased in many patients with liver disease. Gray, Probstein, and Heifetz, (1941) showed that serum amylase activities are decreased (exceptions occur if there is an associated pancreatitis or impaired renal function). Others have reported lowered lipase and esterase activities.

Methods for Evaluating Changes in Serum Protein

Practical methods for serum albumin and globulin determinations have been described in a recent article (Reinhold, 1953). Measurements of albumin and globulin concentrations are among the more useful available for the study of liver disease. Zone electrophoresis on paper shows great promise as a method for study of serum proteins of patients with liver disease, Knedel (1951), Brante (1952), Satoskar *et al.* (1954) have described changes in serum protein in diseases of liver and biliary tract measured by zone electrophoresis.

Some patients, especially those with liver damage of moderate degree, do not show significant changes in serum albumin and total globulin concentrations. The quantitative measurement of γ-globulin concentrations may offer some advantage in this connection and the salting-out methods of Wolfson *et al.* (1948) or of Jager and Nickerson (1948) are available for this purpose. De la Huerga and Popper (1949) have described a turbidimetric method for measurement of γ-globulin which is rapid although less accurate than the preceding.

However, the most widely used methods for detecting changes of the type occurring in serum proteins in liver disease are the semi-empirical flocculation and turbidity tests. More than a dozen of these tests have been proposed. Among them the zinc turbidity (Kunkel, 1947), thymol test (Maclagan, 1944) and cephalin-cholesterol flocculation test (Hanger, 1939) are widely used in this country. Saifer's (1952) review may be consulted for information about other flocculation and turbidity tests and for an analysis of their mechanisms. [*See also* Maclagan *et al.* (1952) and Armas-Cruz *et al.* (1952).]

The zinc turbidity test depends upon the poor solubility of zinc compounds of γ-globulin in solutions of low ionic strength. If experimental conditions are carefully maintained, the absorbency of the suspension produced by adding to serum the zinc ion in a solution of barbital buffer will approximately measure the concentration of γ-globulin. The presence of markedly increased concentrations of γ-globulin are demonstrated by a marked increase in turbidity readings. However, smaller changes in γ-globulin concentration are not as dependably demonstrated. This is because the density of the suspension formed is governed in part by the concentration of albumin and, perhaps, of α_1-globulin in addition to the concentration of γ-globulin.

A significant difference between the zinc turbidity readings of healthy Negroes and whites has been demonstrated (Reinhold, Rawnsley, and Yonan, 1955). The average value of the former was 7.30 ± 1.78 units; that of the whites 4.97 ± 1.44 Shank-Hoagland units. This difference is sufficient to affect interpretation of the results of this test when it is applied to Negroes.

Elevated concentrations of γ-globulin are the rule in viral hepatitis, cirrhosis of the Laennec type, and certain other types of liver disease. However, comparable elevations of γ-globulin concentrations occur in many other diseases and this lack of specificity must be considered in interpreting the results. The zinc turbidity is elevated in a few patients, particularly those suffering from chronic liver disease while the thymol and cephalin-cholesterol flocculation tests are negative. Thus it finds some use as a supplement to these ordinarily more sensitive tests. The zinc turbidity often is within normal limits when the thymol and cephalin-cholesterol tests are abnormal, whereas the reverse occurs infrequently.

Thymol Test

The thymol turbidity test was devised by Maclagan (1944). Its basis was the discovery that a saturated solution of thymol in barbital buffer produced marked turbidity when added to the serum of patients suffering from extensive liver disease. On standing, a flocculum appeared in some abnormal sera.

If satisfactory results are to be obtained, the thymol concentration and temperature, and especially the *p*H of the reagent, must be rigorously controlled.

Three methods of preparing thymol barbital reagent have been described. In addition to Maclagan's (1945) original method, de la Huerga and Popper (1949) and Yonan and Reinhold (1954) have described modifications. The directions for preparation of the reagent of Yonan and Reinhold may be found in the original version of the present review (Reinhold, 1953) and will be published shortly as a separate article. Objections to Maclagan's technic are (1) the difficulty of producing reagents of uniform quality and (2) the poor keeping qualities of the reagent. Carne (1953) and Katz *et al.* (1954) recommended the de la Huerga and Popper reagent in preference to that of Maclagan.

The temperature at which the tests are done is a factor of critical importance (Yonan and Reinhold, 1954).

Accurate measurement of thymol turbidities is difficult. Visual comparison as proposed by Maclagan lacks precision and accuracy. Photometric measurement is complicated by two major problems, (1) the optical geometry of the instrument used and (2) the preparation of a standard. Photometers of different design may give significantly different measurements. It appears that most of the work done on the clinical application of the thymol test (in the United States at least) has been done by means of the Evelyn or Coleman photometers. If other instruments are to be used, the relationship of the readings obtained to those of the foregoing should be tested. In the writer's experience, the Beckman DU, and Klett-Summerson instruments may give results that differ markedly from those of the other two. Previously, Hoyer and Jorgensen (1952) have directed attention to the importance of the optical dimensions of the photometer.

Some of the difficulty occurs because the reaction with lipid yields particles differing in size from those formed by reaction with protein (Kunkel and Hoagland, 1947; Reinhold, 1955), and can be avoided if fasting specimens are obtained for examination. Difficulties in the turbidimetric measurements may also be diminished by use of an appropriate standard (Reinhold, 1955).

Confusion caused by the inadvertent introduction of a second unit (Shank and Hoagland, 1946) may be eliminated if results are reported in named units, e.g. "Maclagan" or "Shank-Hoagland." Two of the latter units equal 1 Maclagan unit.

Interpretation

Thymol turbidity readings are affected by ingestion of food containing fat, and measurements made by the use of serum collected from persons in fasting state are more easily interpreted. Reinhold and Yonan, in a study to be published, found thymol turbidities of 68 out of 71 healthy persons who were fasting to read below 4.0 Shank-Hoagland units when a reagent buffered at *p*H 7.55 was used. After a meal, the limit rose to 4.8 units. If the reagent was buffered at *p*H 7.80, readings were roughly 20 per cent lower when sera of healthy persons were tested. Differences between the readings of the reagents buffered at the two different *p*H values may become much greater when pathologic sera are studied.

Mateer *et al.* (1947) introduced the thymol-barbital reagent buffered at *p*H 7.55 with evidence that it was more sensitive than the reagent buffered at *p*H 7.80. Neefe *et al.* (1950) and Latner and Pendleton (1949) have confirmed this finding. Maclagan (1945) appears to have used a reagent at a *p*H of about 7.65 instead of 7.80 as he stated. Since the limits of normal as well as the behavior of the reagent in pathologic sera is directly dependent upon *p*H, it is important that the physician be informed concerning the reagent used. This applies also to the units used for reporting results.

Infants have lower thymol turbidities than adults (Desmond *et al.*, 1949). According to Gellis and Hsia (1953) flocculation tests are not reliable for study of infants aged less than 6 months.

The thymol turbidity test ranks high among liver function tests in its ability to reveal presence of liver disease. It is among the tests frequently positive in viral hepatitis, and is particularly useful during the recovery period for evaluation of progress. Although patients with cirrhosis may show elevated thymol turbidity, often it may fail to become positive in cirrhosis either of the Laennec or biliary type. An evaluation of a group of tests for the purpose of finding which were most effective for detecting the subclinical form of hepatitis in carriers of the virus led to the selection of the thymol test (Fitch *et al.*, 1955; Reinhold, 1955; Kassouny *et al.*, 1955).

The thymol turbidity is generally within the limits of normal in patients suffering from biliary obstruction, if this is of relatively recent origin. Occurrence of elevated thymol turbidity in a patient diagnosed as having biliary obstruction should cause the clinician to re-evaluate carefully the evidence for the diagnosis. On the other hand, lesions of the biliary tract after several months may produce sufficient damage to the liver to cause the thymol turbidity to become positive. Even in these circumstances, however, it is unusual for it to be abnormal. Ducci (1950, 1951) has studied the "stabilizing" action of serum of patients with biliary obstruction on the turbidity tests. The high concentrations of the bile salt-phospholipid-cholesterol complex and perhaps of mucoprotein in serum, characteristic of biliary obstruction, would by dispersing action inhibit the formation of the aggregates causing turbidity and flocculation.

The changes in serum responsible for elevated thymol turbidity readings are complex and difficult to study because the reagent reacts not only with certain proteins but also with certain lipids and lipoproteins. Recant *et al.* (1954) and Cohen and Thompson (1947) reported that β-globulins were the principal reactants in serum. Others have found that γ-globulins are predominant (Maclagan and Bunn, 1947; Ralli *et al.*, 1949; Marrack *et al.*, 1950; Havens and Williams, 1949; Reinhold, 1955). Kibrick *et al.* (1952) actually use γ-globulin added to serum as a standard. A third group believes that both β- and γ-globulins react (Kunkel and Hoagland, 1947; Martin, 1948, 1949; Albertson *et al.*, 1950).

Thymol turbidity may be increased in any disease characterized by marked elevation of γ-globulin. This may occur quite independently of appreciable liver involvement (Carter and Maclagan, 1946). Among the diseases which may be accompanied by elevated γ-globulin are lupus erythematosus, multiple myeloma, lymphogranuloma, sarcoidosis, tuberculosis, diseases due to parasites, and sensitization to drugs. Although liver damage may occur in these and other diseases, either intrinsically or as a complication, it is necessary to confirm its presence by recourse to other liver function tests not directly dependent upon changes in serum protein.

Increased concentrations of lipid in serum may cause significant elevation of thymol turbidity (Shay *et al.*, 1947; Linder *et al.*, 1948; Popper *et al.*, 1948, 1949; Babb and Pedrazzini, 1949; Katz *et al.*, 1954; Reinhold, 1955). The effect of different lipids varies. Neutral fat in the large aggregates present in serum after a fat-containing meal are especially effective in raising the thymol turbidity reading. The effectiveness of the fat diminishes as the serum clears. Other lipids react in different ways (Shay *et al.*, 1947). Dekema (1951) states that phospholipids are among the serum constituents that react with the thymol-barbital reagent to form turbidity. However, experiments carried out in the writer's laboratory suggest that phospholipid at times may have the effect of decreasing turbidity. According to Maclagan (1948) addition of cephalin had a variable effect on thymol turbidity but decreased flocculation.

The significance of elevated thymol turbidity readings of sera rich in fat (lactescent) undoubtedly differs from that of elevated readings in sera of fasting persons. The relationship of such readings to liver disease is not established; however, liver disease, and especially viral hepatitis at certain stages, may be associated with disturbed tolerance for fat (*see* Reinhold, 1955, for references).

Estimation of serum lipid concentrations by means of the phenol turbidity method of Kunkel or of de la Huerga *et al.* (1953) has been used to evaluate the degree of lipidemia and thereby to provide some estimate of the extent of the effect of lipid.

Thymol Flocculation

Flocculation occurs more frequently when the thymol turbidity readings are elevated but it may occur when there is little or no rise in turbidity. Clinical experience also suggests that the occurrence of flocculation depends upon some additional or different factors (Neefe, 1946). In general, the significance of a positive flocculation test is the same as for abnormal turbidity. The flocculation test is less frequently positive than is the turbidity test; however, false positive tests are uncommon and the occurrence of thymol flocculation thus may be accepted with a higher degree of confidence as evidence of liver damage.

The serum of healthy individuals shows no flocculation. Flocculation graded 1 plus or more, therefore, is abnormal.

Cephalin-Cholesterol Flocculation (Hanger, 1938)

Although rough estimates of flocculation usually suffice, several quantitative methods have been described for measuring either the degree of clearing (Kibrick *et al.*, 1952) or the amount of cholesterol in the precipitate (Saifer, 1948; Jennings *et al.*, 1953). However, the principal difficulty continues to be the variation in sensitivity of the reagent as purchased. Although the manufacturers are at present supplying preparations that are greatly improved, the writer encountered one excessively sensitive lot during the past year. Thus the need for standardization of each lot continues. Standardization consists of testing 10 to 15 sera from healthy persons and an equal number from patients suffering from liver disease. A suitable reagent will not form a flocculum in the normal sera but will show flocculation in a high proportion of the sera of patients suffering from liver disease. Once a reagent has been standardized, subsequent lots can be tested by comparison with the acceptable reagent before the latter is used up. It is helpful also to include a sample of a standardized pooled serum with each day's run. Frozen serum may be used for this purpose, care being taken to thaw it rapidly at 45° to avoid fluctuations in turbidity caused by lack of uniform technic.

The photosensitivity of the test as carried out with reagents available 10 years ago was striking (Neefe and Reinhold, 1944; Moses, 1945). Its cause never was established. Torres (unpublished observations, 1952) working in the writer's laboratory was no longer able to demonstrate this sensitizing effect of light on cephalin-cholesterol flocculation of serum with reagents currently on the market. However, Bassir and Hall (1955) report its occurrence in sera of patients with liver disease and also those with no clinical evidence of liver disease. Difco antigen was used by both laboratories, and it appears unlikely that the reagent is responsible for the discrepancy. The technic of Torres differed from that of Neefe and Reinhold by inclusion of Merthiolate as a preservative. It is possible that this alters the photosensitive groups.

Interpretation

It is essential for the physician to know the sensitivity of the reagent used, since in different laboratories the readings of the sera of healthy persons and of patients without liver involvement may vary from negative to 2 plus or even 3 plus. Using the criteria described, reactions of 2 plus or greater offer evidence of disturbed liver function. Hanger believes that a positive test is an indication of active parenchymal disease, and in support of this may be cited the high proportion of patients suffering from acute viral hepatitis who exhibit positive cephalin-cholesterol flocculation. Positive tests occur within a few days of onset of clinical illness, frequently before jaundice or significant elevation of bilirubin appears. Thus it offers valuable support for a diagnosis of viral hepatitis, particularly in hepatitis without jaundice. However, failure of the cephalin-cholesterol test to become abnormal does not exclude the diagnosis. Neefe, Gambescia, Gardner, and Knowlton (1950) found that 20 per cent of a large group of patients ill of viral hepatitis gave negative tests. Abnormal cephalin-cholesterol flocculation readings may or may not persist into the stage of recovery. In this respect it differs from the thymol test, which tends to remain positive for a considerable time.

A high proportion of cirrhotic patients show positive tests. Positive tests are prevalent in a variety of diseases such as malaria, pneumonia, infectious mononucleosis, and others causing damage to the liver. Biliary obstruction of short duration is characterized by negative cephalin cholesterol flocculations, and it may be used along with other observations to aid in determining whether jaundice is due to causes that may require surgical intervention. Inflammatory disease of the bile ducts usually is accompanied by positive tests.

The mechanism producing flocculation of the cephalin-cholesterol reagent appears to differ somewhat from that of the thymol test. Moore, Pierson, Hanger, and Moore (1945) showed that the change in serum responsible was associated primarily with the albumin fraction. Addition of normal serum albumin to serum giving a positive test may alter the response to negative; hence care must be taken to avoid collection of serum for testing during the 12 to 24 hours following administration of albumin parenterally.

A number of attempts have been made to establish a chemical difference between albumin of sera giving positive reactions with cephalin-cholesterol reagent and that of normal sera. Charlwood (1954) found no indication of a significant difference in albumins separated electrophoretically from sera of patients with liver disease. Hanger (1947) finds the inhibiting action of albumin to be variable. Martin (1951) found that albumin from serum of patients with hepatitis had less effect on the thymol turbidity.

A relationship of α_1-globulin to the flocculation of serum proteins by cephalin-cholesterol reagent has been postulated. Grassmann *et al.* (1951) describe a patient with cirrhosis whose α_1-globulin was elevated and attribute the negative cephalin-cholesterol test to this.

Acid-Precipitable Globulin Turbidity Test

A new turbidity test, the acid-precipitable globulin (APG) turbidity test, has been described by Greenspan (1955). Serum is added to an acetate buffer of low ionic strength adjusted to *p*H 4.42. He reports that treatment of sera of patients with obstructive or inflammatory lesions of the biliary tract leads to markedly increased turbidity readings. In hepatitis, the response was similar to that in normal persons but in cirrhosis a tendency toward low readings existed. Alpha$_2$- plus β-globulins are measured by this reagent.

Abnormalities in Blood Clotting in Liver Disease

These are another manifestation of the disturbances in protein metabolism, although associated disturbances in lipid metabolism also may be important. It is now known that the delayed clotting of blood of many patients with liver disease is the result of a combination of defects. Besides the diminished prothrombin that commonly is found in both acute and chronic liver disease, deficiency of accelerator globulin (Ac-globulin, Factor V, labile factor, proaccelerin, etc.), and probably of other factors occurs. Alexander and Goldstein (1950) report not only a lowering of labile factor but also of serum prothrombin conversion factor. Fibrinogen concentration may be low, as already mentioned. Fibrinolysin activity of plasma may be increased.

Selman (1952) has reported on the occurrence of low antithrombin titers in serum hepatitis. A clotting factor, thrombin accelerator, in cirrhosis is defined by Ratnoff (1953).

Hepatectomy causes a decrease in fibrinogen, "thrombogen," and antifibrinolysin (Nolf and Adant, 1951) and in prothrombin, cothromboplastin, labile factor, as well as fibrinogen (Mann, Shonzo, and Mann, 1951). The complexity of the disturbance of clotting function in liver disease is apparent in recent reviews of this topic (Harrington *et al.* 1950; Stefanini, 1953; Alexander, 1955). Alexander (1955) points out that in addition to the defective clotting mechanism, vascular abnormalities and thrombocytopenia contribute to deficiencies in clotting in patients with liver disease. He points out that the multiple abnormalities may have a more than additive effects.

The depletion of prothrombin in biliary obstruction is related to impaired vitamin K absorption. This in turn is due to the failure of bile to reach the intestine in sufficient amounts to maintain absorption of fats and fat-soluble vitamins. Perhaps a similar mechanism contributes to the lowered prothrombin activity in parenchymal liver disease. Vitamin K administered parenterally in large amounts usually has little effect on the lowered plasma prothrombin activity of patients suffering from parenchymal liver disease. On the other hand, it corrects this defect in patients with biliary obstruction, provided liver damage is not excessive.

Methods for Evaluation of Clotting Function

These include studies of plasma prothrombin activity, accelerator factor, fibrinolysin, and, at times, fibrinogen. Numerous technics for prothrombin and fibrinogen measurements are described in the literature.

Estimation of prothrombin activity is an indispensable preliminary to surgical operations on patients with disease of biliary tract, liver, or small intestine, and to needle biopsy of the liver. It is used also to evaluate the response to vitamin K administered to jaundiced patients. A substantial rise in prothrombin activity to values that are within or approaching the normal range suggests that liver function is not greatly impaired: thus the jaundice may be presumed to originate from a lesion of the biliary tract (Lord and Andrus, 1941; Shapiro and Richards, 1945). One of the important shortcomings of this method is the lack of precision of prothrombin measurements, as ordinarily measured, in the 30 to 100 per cent range.

Many patients with parenchymatous liver disease maintain prothrombin activities within normal limits throughout the course of their illness [according to Stefanini (1949), roughly half]. This is true especially if liver involvement is of minimal or moderate severity. For this reason the measurement of prothrombin activity is not as efficient for detection of liver damage as are a number of the other procedures described in this review. However, an occasional patient will have a significantly lowered prothrombin activity due to liver disease when other simple tests, including the serum-bilirubin concentration and flocculation and turbidity group, fail to give an abnormal response.

Impairment of Energy Production and Storage

Liver disease is associated with increased concentrations in blood and urine of the di- and tricarboxyl acids that constitute pathways by which foods are converted into energy. Considerable attention has been given, by Scandinavian workers especially, to the elevation of plasma citrate in patients suffering from liver disease. These studies have been reviewed by Sjöström (1936). Bunker *et al.* (1955) report that patients with liver disease are susceptible to citrate intoxication when transfused with large volumes of citrated blood. Marked elevation of serum citrate occurs as a result of impaired ability to utilize this substance.

Others have found that lactate (Snell and Roth, 1932), pyruvate (Amatuzio and Nesbitt, 1950), alpha-ketoglutarate (Seligson, McCormick, and Sborov, 1952) and succinate (Emmrich, 1948) concentrations also are elevated. These findings suggest the occurrence of a general increase in concentration of such substances. The occurrence of such an increase in turn suggests that the efficiency with which these transformations are being made is impaired in the presence of severe parenchymal liver disease. Thus, the supply of energy available to the cells is decreased. The effects on cellular metabolism would be widespread and important, and would be manifested in decreased rates of synthesis of the various products made by the liver cells as well as impairment of regulatory and other functions. Recant (1954) recently described a defect in ketone metabolism in patients with cirrhosis. This was characterized by average blood ketone concentrations of 0.94 mg./100 ml. in cirrhotics compared with 2.28 mg./100 ml. in normal persons.

Saltzman and Caraway (1953) have described a method for measurement of the efficiency of an oxidation, the conversion of cinnamic to benzoic acids, in vivo. They find a reduced rate in patients with liver disease.

Studies of certain components of the phosphate cycle have been made. Helve (1946) reports no change in major fractions of the blood cell phosphate. However, it is difficult to establish impairment in functioning of the phosphate cycle in vivo by analysis of concentrations because its efficiency is a function of the rate of turnover rather than of concentration. Smith, Ettinger, and Seligson (1953) state that serum inorganic phosphate decreased following injection of glucose and fructose to the same extent in patients with liver disease as in normal persons, while in diabetes mellitus little change in its concentration occurred. The marked rise in serum creatine concentration and increase in creatine excretion previously described suggests that phosphocreatine is being hydrolyzed and presumably not rapidly reformed. As a result, stores of high energy phosphate are being depleted.

Waterlow (1953) has studied the enzyme activity of samples of liver removed by punch biopsy from infants suffering from liver disease of nutritional origin. His material included specimens from patients with kwashiorkor or the closely related nutritional liver disease of Jamaican infants, as well as samples obtained from control subjects. He found a wide variation in susceptibility of various respiratory enzymes to severe malnutrition and associated liver damage. His work, and that of others using animals, emphasizes the importance of low protein intake in causing depletion of certain enzymes.

Measurement of the activities in serum of several enzymes which are liberated from the liver acutely damaged by various agents appears to offer new leads for study of liver disease. Aldolase, the enzyme splitting fructose-1,6-diphosphate into the triosephosphates, has been studied by Bruns and Puls (1954) and by Cook and Dounce (1954). Striking increases in activity were observed in sera of patients suffering from acute hepatitis. On the other hand, little increase over normal activities was found in cirrhosis, latent hepatitis, or biliary obstruction. Phosphohexose-isomerase, an enzyme transforming glucose-6-phosphate to fructose-6-phosphate, behaved in the same manner as aldolase (Bruns and Jacob, 1954; Bruns and Hinsberg, 1954). Wroblewski and LaDue (1954) report that the activity of glutamic-oxaloacetic transaminase rises in serum in patients with severe liver damage. None of these changes are specific indications of liver involvement, for the activity of serum aldolase is greatly increased in activity in muscular dystrophy (Dreyfus *et al.*, 1954; Jacob and Neuhaus, 1954) and glutamic-oxaloacetic transaminase in coronary occlusion (LaDue *et al.*, 1954). Methods for estimating these enzymes may be found in the articles listed. A spectrophotometric method for glutamic-oxaloacetic transaminase is described by Karmen *et al.* (1955).

The relationship between serum and hepatic enzyme activities has been studied experimentally by Koch-Weser *et al.* (1951). They found that in chronic liver damage produced by a diet low in protein and by chemicals in small amounts, serum and hepatic enzymes were lowered in roughly parallel manner. During regeneration of liver when cellular activity was vigorous, augmented activity of serum enzymes was observed. Acutely damaged cells permitted escape of enzymes from liver tissue. A tendency toward high values in serum for 24 to 48 hours was followed by subnormal activities.

Hormone Metabolism

Chronic liver disease is often accompanied by enlargement of the breasts in males and other evidences of altered sex hormone metabolism. A number of studies have been made of the excretion of various hormones in liver disease. Lloyd and Williams (1948) observed that excretion of 17-ketosteroids, androgens, and follicle-stimulating hormone was diminished in cirrhosis of the liver. Dohan *et al.* (1952) found a significant increase in estrogen excretion in cirrhotic male patients. This was especially marked if they showed signs of gynecomastia. Spider nevi were associated with increased estriol excretion. 17-Ketosteroid excretion was significantly decreased. A decrease in gonadotrophin (FSH) was associated with testicular atrophy.

Peterson *et al.* (1954) surveyed steroid excretion patterns in several different diseases of liver and in patients with biliary obstruction. Some patients with hepatitis had normal or even increased 17-ketosteroid excretion, although the prevailing tendency in hepatitis, as in cirrhosis, was toward low values. Corticosteroid excretion was found to be increased in many patients with cirrhosis and the suggestion is made that conversion of these substances to ketosteroids is impaired in liver disease. Bongiovanni *et al.* (1954) report a decreased rate of conjugation of adrenal corticoids in cirrhosis. Brown *et al.* (1954) found the rate of disappearance of infused hydrocortisone to be inversely proportional to liver damage as measured by bromsulfalein retention. Patients with liver disease had normal fasting 17-hydroxycorticosteroid concentrations in plasma but excreted less in urine, evidence perhaps of a homeostatic adjustment. Miller and Axelrod (1954) found that cortisone perfused through rat livers was metabolized more slowly after the liver was made cirrhotic. Even more interesting is the finding that β-hydroxyl derivatives were formed in the cirrhotic but not in the normal liver. Schedl *et al.* (1953) reported differences in type of hormone excreted by patients with cirrhosis.

The liver produces enzymes that oxidize testosterone and related steroids. Injected testosterone is inactivated less rapidly in hepatectomized dogs than in intact dogs (West, 1951). Even mild liver damage decreased the proportion of injected testosterones excreted as 17-ketosteroid by patients (West *et al.*, 1951). Cantarow and associates (1951) found that the conjugation of injected testosterone was decreased in patients with liver disease. Adrenocorticotrophic hormone is inactivated by liver tissue (Eversole and Giere, 1951; Geschwind and Li, 1952).

The association of liver damage with hyperthyroidism was studied by many workers in the 1930's. A review by McIver (1942) summarizes the early findings. Maclagan and Rundle (1952) have confirmed earlier work by Althausen and Weaver (1938) demonstrating decreased galactose tolerance. Changes in rate of galactose absorption from the gastrointestinal tract may be important. Bartels (1938) found that 68 of 78 patients suffering from hyperthyroidism excreted less than 3 Gm. of hippuric acid, the lower limit of excretion found in persons with normal liver function. A recent paper on liver function in hyperthyroidism is that of Lamberg and Gordin (1954).

Disturbances of Water and Electrolyte Balance

Retention, loss, or maldistribution of electrolytes and the resulting disturbances of water metabolism are among the most important and troublesome disorders encountered in patients with liver disease. These are caused in part by impairment of certain functions of the liver related to water and salt metabolism. Impaired synthesis of plasma albumin, depletion of intracellular proteins and electrolytes, disturbed metabolism of the hormones of the pituitary and adrenal as described in a previous section, and interference with the flow of blood through the portal system are some of the numerous derangements that contribute to alterations in salt and water equilibria in liver disease [*see* Strub, Talso, and Kirsner (1955)]. Failure of the liver often is accompanied by impaired function of the kidney, which adds to the gravity of the situation.

Salt and water retention is one of the characteristic complications of Laennec's cirrhosis. Its causes are complex. Mechanical factors such as increased pressure in the portal venous system are important. The resulting alterations in renal hemodynamics impair the efficiency of renal function. The lowered serum albumin concentration, while favorable to glomerular filtration, also favors transudation from the capillaries and thus accumulation of water in the tissues. Hormonal factors are known to be important. Shorr *et al.* (1951) have described a vasodepressor substance, ferritin (or VDM), whose concentration in the body fluids, they claim, is regulated in large measure by the liver. In addition to ferritin, it is possible that the antidiuretic hormone of the posterior pituitary contributes to the oliguria and hyposthenuria that precedes or accompanies salt and water retention. Still other factors may be involved. Increased sodium-retaining activity was found in the urine of patients with cirrhosis (Chart and Shipley, 1953). Luetscher and Johnson (1954) attribute this to the presence of increased quantities of aldosterone.

It is possible that some of the same factors that cause sodium and water retention in nephrosis are operating in cirrhosis. Conditions favoring the loss of cellular protein and potassium, considered by Metcoff *et al.* (1954) to be of primary causative importance in salt and water retention in nephrosis, exist also in cirrhosis. Plasma volume generally is increased in cirrhosis (Bateman *et al.*, 1949; Gilder *et al.*, 1954). Patients suffering from cirrhosis have diminished ability to excrete water administered in the course of a water-loading test. This may be decreased to one third of the control value in the presence of ascites (Ralli *et al.*, 1951). A reversal of the diurnal rhythm of water and sodium excretion has been described by Popper and Rosenbaum (1952).

Rigorous restriction of sodium intake appears to be the most effective method of preventing accumulation of salt and water in excessive amounts by the cirrhotic patient (Eisenmenger *et al.*, 1949; Gabuzda *et al.*, 1954). The patient on such a regimen, in turn, requires regular and frequent chemical study because of the threat of the salt-depletion syndrome. The hazard of the latter is greatest when large amounts of fluid, 2–10 L. or more, are removed by paracentesis. If the patient subsequently dilutes the remaining extracellular fluid by consumption of water, sodium concentrations may fall sufficiently to bring about the abnormalities in blood flow and blood supply to the tissues that characterize the low-salt syndrome (Nelson, Rosenbaum, Strauss, 1951; Holly and McLester, 1951). Serum-sodium concentrations as low as 110 mEq./L. have been observed. Circulatory failure in such circumstances may lead to coma and death.

Artman and Wise (1953) have stressed the importance of potassium depletion in liver failure. Low fluid intake, vomiting, urinary losses, diarrhea, and administration of glucose are listed as contributing causes. They found potassium deficiency to be critical in many patients in hepatic coma. Aikawa *et al.* (1953) found lowered exchangeable potassium in cirrhosis with a deficit in the cells that was refractory to therapy [*see also* Amatuzio *et al.* (1952)].

Elevation of serum potassium also must be guarded against, especially in those patients whose liver disease is accompanied by marked impairment of kidney function.

Stutzman and Amatuzio (1953) called attention to lowered serum magnesium concentrations in portal cirrhosis. Studies of serum magnesium recently made in the writer's laboratory in a patient in hepatic coma have demonstrated a low value of 0.39 mEq./L.

Serum Iron in Liver Disease

Serum-iron concentrations are markedly affected by liver disease. In hepatitis, serum iron rises to 2 or 3 times the highest concentration ordinarily found in health. (Peterson, 1952; Matassarin and Delp, 1952). Low concentrations occur in serum of some cirrhotic patients (Howard, 1950).

Serum iron remains within normal limits in most patients with biliary obstruction. Since elevated values are prevalent in the presence of liver damage, one might expect that measurement of serum iron would aid in differentiation of these two causes of jaundice. Recently, Christian (1954) and Landau (1954) have advocated its use for this purpose. The consensus of those who have attempted such an application is that it has relatively little value.

Serum iron determinations and especially determinations of serum iron-binding capacity, are of special interest in hemochromatosis. In this condition, accumulations of exceptionally large amounts of iron in the body lead to its deposition in liver, skin, and other tissues. The architecture of the liver is distorted as in cirrhosis. Fibrosis of the pancreas with diabetes mellitus is characteristic.

Serum iron concentrations are elevated in hemochromatosis, although not necessarily to concentrations higher than those occurring in health or in hepatitis. However, the measurement of iron-binding capacity in hemochromatosis consistently shows that the serum is almost completely saturated with iron. Gitlow, Beyers, and Colmore (1952) cite saturation values of 74 to 99 per cent as compared with 14 to 69 per cent in cirrhosis and 28 to 58 per cent in normal individuals. In hepatitis and all other conditions, at least a third of the total iron-binding capacity remains unsaturated.

Kleckner *et al.* (1955) have assessed the procedures used for diagnosis of hemochromatosis. In contrast to most observers, they state that serum iron-binding capacity may be saturated also in acute hepatitis, portal cirrhosis, transfusion hemosiderosis, aplastic anemias, etc., as well as in hemochromatosis. Liver biopsy, they state, is the best diagnostic criterion. Hemochromatosis should be distinguished from hemosiderosis, a condition characterized by excessive accumulation of iron in the tissues, largely as hemosiderin, as a result of malnutrition or of excessive iron administered either as blood or therapeutically as iron compounds. It lacks the pathologic changes in liver and pancreas characteristic of hemochromatosis. Klein *et al.* (1955) were unable to establish differences between hemochromatosis and hemosiderosis by analysis of iron in tissues. Kleckner *et al.* (1955) state that a patient with hemochromatosis may have a total iron content of 58 Gm. as compared with a normal of 4 Gm. Extremely high serum iron concentrations may occur in some patients with hemochromatosis (Howard *et al.*, 1954).

Methods for Study of Iron and Iron-Binding Capacity

Among several practical methods for serum iron are those of Barkan and Walker (1940) and of Kitzes *et al.* (1944). Iron-binding capacity can be determined by the method of Cartwright and Wintrobe (1949) and of Ventura (1952).

Spectrophotometric iron-binding capacity measurements are unreliable if serum is icteric, hemolyzed, or lactescent. Peters and Apt (1955) have very recently described a new method based on the adsorption of ionic iron on a resin.

Copper and Diseases of the Liver

Wilson's disease (hepatolenticular degeneration) is associated with abnormalities in metabolism of copper (Glazebrook, 1945; Denny-Brown and Porter, 1951). The copper content of brain, liver, and urine is increased. After treatment with BAL (2,3 dimercaptopropanol) urine-copper concentration decreases. Bearn and Kunkel (1954a) report subnormal serum copper concentrations in 16 of 18 patients with Wilson's disease. The output of copper in urine was decreased also in these patients. Ceruloplasmin, a copper containing protein of serum, described by Holmberg and Laurell (1947), is present in lower concentrations in Wilson's disease than in healthy persons (Scheinberg and Gitlin, 1952; Bearn and Kunkel, 1954a). In Wilson's disease, Bearn and Kunkel (1954b) observed that Cu^{64} administered orally was immediately taken up by serum albumin. However, the transfer to an α_1-globulin that occurred in healthy persons and in patients failed to proceed in patients with Wilson's disease. In Laennec's cirrhosis, serum copper tends to be elevated (Bearn, 1953). The abnormal copper metabolism of Wilson's disease has been reviewed recently by Denny-Brown (1953).

Severe and persistent aminoaciduria is characteristic of Wilson's disease (Uzman and Denny-Brown, 1948; Stein, Bearn, and Moore, 1954).

There is sufficient liver involvement in Wilson's disease to produce abnormalities in the liver-function tests in a high proportion of patients suffering from this condition (Franklin and Bauman, 1953). However clinical and laboratory evidence of liver disease may be lacking in some.

Detoxification Reactions of the Liver

Numerous studies have demonstrated that in liver disease various reactions associated with detoxification are impaired. The best known example is the synthesis of hippuric acid following administration of benzoic acid, extensively studied by Quick (1940). Whereas at least 70 per cent of injected benzoic acid is excreted as hippuric acid within 1 hour by healthy individuals, less than this amount is excreted by patients with liver damage. Quick believes that the factor limiting hippuric-acid synthesis in liver disease is inability to mobilize glycine; however, this has been disputed (Voight, 1951). Voight compared the excretion of hippuric acid by patients with liver disease before and after they had received glycine. In many patients the rise in output was insignificant; moreover, the proportion excreted during the first 2 hours was not increased. A revived interest in hippuric-acid excretion tests in Germany seems to have resulted from the observations of Voight (1951) and Hartmann (1951) that hourly collection of urine after 6 Gm. of sodium benzoate gives a better clue regarding liver function than does the measurement of total excretion. Normally most of the excretion occurs during the first 2 hours. In hepatitis and cirrhosis the excretion is diminished and the greater percentage appears during the third and fourth hours. By applying this technic, Bogenhard (1954) found 90 to 95 per cent positive tests in hepatitis and 74–79 per cent positive in suspected hepatitis. Quick had originally recommended hourly collections, but this practice was abandoned because of emphasis on total output and also because of the extra labor required.

The conjugation of benzoic acid with glycine has been demonstrated in liver homogenates by Borsook and Dubnoff (1947). It occurs also in kidney, spleen, and probably other tissues. Benzoyl-coenzyme A appears to be an intermediate in hippurate synthesis (Schachter and Taggart, 1953).

Deiss and Cohen (1950) have described a similar test in which para-aminobenzoate replaces benzoate, and the conjugation is evaluated by analysis of serum. The para-aminohippurate formed is estimated colorimetrically in a sample of blood collected 1 hour after the test dose.

An increased excretion of hippuric acid in "free anxiety," a condition of exaggerated foreboding or apprehension, was observed by Persky *et al.* (1950). Deiss and Musser (1950) described a similar effect upon para-aminohippurate synthesis. Musser *et al.* (1955) found that administration of glycine had little effect in augmenting synthesis of para-aminohippurate in the presence of free anxiety, in comparison with normal controls. They studied hyperthyroid patients also, and found that a lowered synthesis characteristic of this condition was greatly enhanced by glycine.

Conjugation of various substances with glucuronic acid also is impaired in liver disease (Wagreich *et al.*, 1941; Ottenberg *et al.*, 1943). Snapper and Saltzman (1949) have described a test of liver function that measures glucuronate conjugate excretion after administering sodium cinnamate. Its application to the study of liver disease is evaluated by Sharnoff *et al.* (1951). Saltzman and Caraway (1953) have described a refinement of the cinnamic acid test in which blood cinnamic acid levels are measured.

Hartmann (1951) has evaluated the use of detoxification reactions other than that of benzoate for study of liver disease. Intramuscular injection of guaiacol followed by measurement of sulfate and sulfate-ester excretion showed decreased conjugating ability in hepatitis and cirrhosis, with normal values in cirrhosis. Glucuronate excretion appeared to offer less information. Increased outputs occurred in hepatitis. The xanthoproteic-acid reaction applied to serum gave increased values in hepatic precoma and coma. Salicylate or thiocyanate excretion tests were not useful for study of liver disease. Deamination of tyramine, a pressor amine, occurs in the liver (Hare, 1928) and it is thought that other substances of this type are similarly inactivated.

Methods for the Study of Detoxification Function

Measurement of hippuric acid excretion is most frequently used for this purpose. However, availability of more simple procedures for study of liver disease appears to have decreased the use of the hippuric-acid test. The technic of Quick (1940) may be used. Intravenous administration of hippuric acid is preferred. The conditions under which the test is done are important. The patient should ingest sufficient water to insure adequate urine flow (Machella, Helm, and Chornock, 1942). He must be physically and mentally relaxed.

Hippuric acid is readily excreted by the kidney but marked impairment of kidney function lowers the output. Body weight and sex should be taken into account in interpretation of results (Hepler and Gurley, 1942).

Zieve *et al.* (1950) include measurement of hippuric-acid synthesis in a combined test that also measures galactose utilization and bromsulfalein retention. Zieve and Hanson (1953) found that administration of benzoic acid on 3 consecutive days caused a marked increase in hippurate-forming ability of patients with liver disease. A higher proportion of the benzoate was conjugated on each successive day.

A chromatographic method for quantitative determination of hippuric acid described by Gaffney *et al.* (1954) requires only 10–100 μL. of urine. Kimbel (1955) has developed a micro method for para-aminohippurate in blood.

The para-aminohippurate test of Deiss and Cohen (1950) has the great advantage of avoiding the necessity for urine collections, a major source of difficulty in the hippuric-acid test. Trial of this procedure is desirable. The same may be said of the new cinnamic acid test of Saltzman and Caraway (1953).

Serum Alkaline Phosphatase

Measurement of alkaline phosphatase activity of serum often assists in the differentiation of parenchymal liver disease from that due to obstruction and other lesions of the biliary tract. Biliary obstruction is characterized by an increase in phosphatase activity to two or more times the maximum found in healthy individuals (Roberts, 1933), and by the persistence of such high activities. Some increase occurs also in patients suffering from viral hepatitis; however, the rise is moderate and transitory. Toxic hepatitis caused by chemicals or drugs is usually accompanied by elevated phosphatase activities. Several reports indicate that chlorpromazine (thorazine) therapy may cause phosphatase activity and bilirubin concentration of serum to rise to the same extent as in biliary obstruction (Zatuchni and Miller, 1954; Loftus *et al.*, 1955). In cirrhosis of the Laennec type, no marked rise in alkaline phosphatase activity occurs ordinarily, but at times, high activities may be encountered.

The rise in phosphatase associated with obstruction of the bile ducts occurs regardless of the nature of the obstruction, whether due to calculus, stricture, or neoplasm. Elevation of serum alkaline phosphatase may provide one of the few clues to the presence of neoplastic growth in the liver (Rothman *et al.*, 1936; Flood *et al.*, 1937; Ricketts *et al.*, 1950; Shay and Siplet, 1954). Inflammatory disease of the bile ducts (cholangiolitic hepatitis) causes striking increases in serum alkaline phosphatase (Watson and Hoffbauer, 1946).

The chemical changes occurring in this condition are indistinguishable from those observed in many patients with extrahepatic biliary obstruction.

The cause of the increase in serum alkaline phosphatase activity occurring in patients suffering from biliary obstruction has provoked much discussion. The liver appears to be able to remove phosphatase from blood plasma and excrete it in the bile. However, hepatectomized animals show, at most, a moderate rise in phosphatase activity of serum (Freeman, 1951; Flock *et al.*, 1952). This suggests that failure of the liver to excrete phosphatase produced in other organs is responsible only to a limited extent. Histochemical studies show high concentrations of phosphatase in the cholangiolar epithelium (Burke, 1950) in cholangiolitic hepatitis. Sherlock and Walshe (1947) found increased amounts in the hepatic cells and nuclei in hepatitis and in bile-duct obstruction. The amount in the sinusoidal walls also was found increased. Thus it appears possible that the excess phosphatase in plasma may have several sources. The predominant source may be the cholangiolar epithelium in biliary-tract disease and the liver parenchyma in hepatitis. Rosenthal and associates (1952) have shown that regenerating liver parenchyma is very rich in phosphatase. Roche and Sarles (1954) describe experiments that suggest that the liver regulates concentrations of alkaline phosphatase activities of serum.

Applications of phosphatase-activity measurements include not only the detection of involvement of the biliary tract but also the evaluation of the clinical course of patients with such lesions. Ulevitch *et al.* (1951) have pointed out that phosphatase activity and serum bilirubin may change independently and that phosphatase activity is the more sensitive indicator of change in degree of biliary obstruction.

Bile-Pigment Metabolism

Jaundice is such a conspicuous sign of liver damage or bile duct blockage that it has attracted more than its share of attention, often to the neglect of other and more important aspects of liver or biliary tract disease. A number of excellent reviews of bile pigment chemistry and metabolism have appeared within the last few years (Watson, 1946; Lemberg and Legge, 1949; Gray, 1953; Lathe, 1954; Gray, 1954). With the evidence provided by McNee (1913) in Aschoff's laboratory, Whipple and Hooper (1913), and Mann (1921) demonstrated that the major site of bilirubin formation from hemoglobin was the Kupffer cells of the reticuloendothelial system throughout the body. [*See* Lathe (1954) for the history of these developments.)

Certain peculiarities in the behavior of bilirubin suggest that it may exist in serum in two forms. These are readily differentiated by means of their rates of reaction with diazotized sulfanilic acid (Hijmans van den Bergh and Müller, 1916). A rapidly reacting form of bilirubin (direct or prompt reacting bilirubin) is considered to have been secreted into the bile by the parenchymal cells and subsequently to have returned to the blood stream because of disruption of the liver structure by parenchymal disease or because of biliary obstruction. This form of bilirubin (cholebilirubin) is distinguished from a second (hemobilirubin) considered to be in transport from extrahepatic sites of hemoglobin breakdown to the liver. The latter reacts with the diazo reagent slowly and yields additional color after alcohol, caffeine, or other catalysts are added to the reaction mixture.

All the bilirubin in serum is bound to protein, chiefly albumin, but it is possible that a portion is more firmly bound. Plasma protein fractionation by Cohn (1948) and his associates has yielded an alpha-globulin which, it is stated, binds bilirubin firmly and specifically. Martin (1949) has described its characteristics, among them a delaying action on the diazo reaction of bilirubin bound by it. Attempts to establish a structural change in the bilirubin molecule that might provide a basis for the observed difference have led to negative or equivocal results. However, Najjar (1952) recently described the preparation from serum of two bilirubins differing in crystal form and solubility and in their reactivity with the diazo reagent. Other factors influencing the rate of reaction include the concentration of bilirubin and its degree of dispersion. There is reason to believe that the serum lipid may be involved. For a review of the various hypotheses concerning the diazo reaction of serum bilirubin the reader is referred to Gray (1953) Chapter VIII, also Lathe (1954).

Cole and Lathe (1953) succeeded in separating serum bilirubin into two components by means of reverse phase chromatography using silicone-treated kieselguhr as adsorbent. A rapidly moving type is more soluble in water and gives the direct diazo reaction (without addition of alcohol). The other is more soluble in organic solvents and reacts only in presence of alcohol. The latter is thought to be bilirubin. The nature of the fast-moving component is not established, but it predominates in serum in obstructive jaundice and in bile. In hemolytic jaundice the slower component predominates. No protein was present in the extracts of serum studied, hence Cole and Lathe conclude that differing degrees of association of bilirubin with protein cannot be responsible for the differences in behavior of various serums with the diazo reagent. The presence of several pigments in bile, some of which do not react with the diazo reagent, was demonstrated.

The direct reacting pigment found in serum of patients with obstructive jaundice and in bile was separated in turn, into two pigments by Cole, Lathe, and Billing (1954), each giving the direct reaction. They differ from bilirubin in their much greater solubilities in water, and in their absorption spectra. The latter have a maximum at 419 mμ in contrast to bilirubin which had a maximum at 454 mμ.

Lathe (1954) believes that bilirubin is first converted to Pigment I (see below) by the liver, since it appears in blood in substantial amounts after injection of bilirubin whereas there is little Pigment II. The latter, however, is more abundant in bile.

Sera obtained from patients ill with hemolytic anemias or pernicious anemia when tested with the diazo reagent produce relatively little color in 1 minute compared to that produced after addition of methanol. This is true also after administration of aged or incompatible blood and the serum of newborn. On the other hand, approximately 50 per cent of the total color appears in 1 minute when the sera of patients with biliary obstruction or moderate to severe parenchymal damage are tested. Kernicterus, an intense pigmentation of the basal ganglia associated with jaundice of the brain, occurs occasionally in newborn infants. Some impairment of bilirubin excretion during the first days of life appears to be a general occurrence in all newborn and if rapid blood destruction occurs at this time, such as that produced by erythroblastosis due to development of anti-Rh agglutinin in the mother, very high serum-bilirubin concentrations may occur. Either because of this or because of associated changes in the brain, permanent injury to the brain or death may result. The nature and significance of the brain pigmentation is discussed by Claireaux *et al.* (1953), Vogel (1953), and Day (1954). The attending pediatrician may be guided in his treatment of the newborn by the height of the serum bilirubin, in relation to other factors, and his decisions will be influenced also by the rate of increase in its postnatal concentration. Replacement of the infant's blood by means of exchange transfusion is a commonly accepted therapeutic approach.

The need for bilirubin determinations in these circumstances is such that the laboratory should be prepared to do them immediately. A series of measurements usually are required.

The serum bile-pigment concentration of normal 3629-Gm. (8-lb.) babies is usually less than 3–5 mg. per 100 ml., according to Lathe (1954); that of 1814-Gm. (4-lb.) babies is much higher and may rise to 10 to 15 mg. per 100 ml.

Another abnormality of bile-pigment metabolism has been described recently by Dubin and Johnson (1954a and b). Its symptoms are chronic jaundice, abdominal pain, and fatigue. The outstanding feature is the presence of large amounts of an unidentified granular brown pigment in the liver.

Methods for Measurement of Concentration of Bilirubin in Serum

Methods for measurement of bilirubin concentration of serum include the direct comparison of the yellow color of diluted serum with that of 0.01% potassium dichromate, the "icterus index" of Meulengracht (1921). This crude method is remarkable only because it serves so much better than one would anticipate in view of the many sources of error to which it is susceptible. Henry *et al.* (1953) have described methods for avoiding some of the errors. It is quite unreliable unless serum bilirubin concentrations are elevated. Spectrophotometric measurement of bilirubin is feasible provided appropriate corrections are made for heme pigments and opalescence of the serum. However, the diazo reagent is by far the most generally used.

There has been confusion about the mechanism of the reaction of bilirubin with this reagent which Lathe (1954) has helped to clarify. He cites the work of Fischer and Haberland (1935) as demonstrating that the bilirubin molecule is split into two dipyrroles, neo- and isoneoxanthobilirubinic acid. In this way, the alpha position (adjacent to the nitrogen in the pyrrole ring) of one of the dipyrroles becomes available for coupling to the diazo reagent. The other dipyrrole would not react because the methylene group of the bridge would remain as hydroxymethyl. Presumably some of the bilirubin would split on one side and some on the other side of the methylene carbon. In this way a mixture of two diazo pigments—one the diazo derivative of neo- and the other of isoneoxanthobilirubinic acid—is formed. However, each molecule of bilirubin gives rise to only one diazo derivative. The remaining "half" is present as an unreactive alcohol.

Evaluation of the speed of the reaction of bilirubin with the diazo reagent, formerly judged by the eye, has been replaced by photometric measurement of the color formed 30 minutes (Malloy and Evelyn, 1937) or 1 minute (Ducci and Watson, 1945) after adding the reagent. Billing (1954) found a "reasonable correlation between the percentage of direct-reacting pigments found chromatographically and that obtained by the Malloy and Evelyn method at 30 minutes." However, the method of Ducci and Watson has proven to be the more useful clinically. Kingsley *et al.* (1953) have described the technic of the latter with an improved method for standardization. Shinowara (1954) has described the determination of bilirubin and hemoglobin with the aid of the spectrophotometer. Moreland *et al.* (1950) substitute sulfanilamide for sulfanilic acid in the diazo reaction.

The factors affecting serum bilirubin determinations have been discussed by Proffitt and Morrison (1949). *p*H and nitrite concentration are critical. White and Duncan (1952) report that bilirubin added to serum gives less color than it does in chloroform-ethanol solution, and that Beer's law is not obeyed when determinations are done by the Malloy and Evelyn method (1936) if the concentration exceeds 15 mg. per 100 ml.

A micro technic for measurement of serum bilirubin has been described by Hsia *et al.* (1952).

Berman *et al.* (1954) have discussed the relationship of xanthochromia of cerebrospinal fluid to serum bilirubin and have described a method for measurement of bilirubin in cerebrospinal fluid. [*See also* Amatuzio, Weber, and Nesbitt (1953).]

Interpretation

Total serum bilirubin of 95 per cent of healthy individuals is below 1.10 mg. per 100 ml. of serum. Occasionally persons who appear to be in good health will have concentrations as high as 1.50 mg./100 ml.

The direct reacting, "1-minute" bilirubin reading estimates bilirubin reacting with the Ehrlich diazo reagent promptly in the absence of ethanol, methanol, or other catalyst. This fraction represents 10 to 20 per cent of the total bilirubin of normal serum. In 95 per cent of healthy individuals it does not exceed 0.18 mg./100 ml. and in 99 per cent is below 0.25 mg./100 ml. In the presence of hyperbilirubinemia due to any cause other than increased hemolysis, the 1-minute direct reading increases to approximately 50 per cent of the total, and ranges from 30 to 70 per cent. The direct bilirubin may be elevated in serum of some patients whose serum total bilirubin is within normal limits, and it is somewhat superior to the latter for detection of liver involvement. When hemolysis occurs with severity sufficient to cause hyperbilirubinemia, the total serum bilirubin consistently is elevated to a greater degree than is the prompt reacting portion. However, the behavior of the serum bilirubin in jaundice caused by biliary obstruction does not differ from that occurring in jaundice caused by injury to the hepatic parenchymal cells, at least not to an extent that enables conclusions to be reached in a given patient regarding the etiology of the jaundice. Measurement of the rate of the diazo reaction of bilirubin adds little of value for differential diagnosis because hemolytic jaundice, the one condition that it distinguishes generally can be recognized by other more specific findings. The significance of serum-bilirubin determinations with special reference to the 1-minute reading has been discussed by Zieve *et al.* (1951) and Klatskin and Drill (1950).

Studies of total serum bilirubin are useful for following the clinical course of a patient. Rising serum-bilirubin concentrations in general have unfavorable implications; falling values are characteristic of remission of liver disease or biliary obstruction. A stabilized serum-bilirubin concentration is considered a highly desirable prerequisite to operation for relief of biliary obstruction. ACTH and cortisone given to patients with increased serum bilirubin cause a marked decrease in bilirubin concentration of serum.

Tests for Bilirubin in Urine

Many of the procedures widely used for detection of bilirubin in urine are not sufficiently sensitive to be useful for detection of early hepatitis or moderate liver damage. Foord and Baisinger (1940) compared many of the commonly used procedures and found that the Harrison-Fouchet method as described by Godfried (1934) was one of the most dependable, and the experience of many workers has confirmed the value of this procedure. Several modifications of this method in which the reagents are applied to paper strips (Watson and Hawkinson, 1946) or to tablets of plaster of Paris have proven to be convenient although less sensitive than the original Harrison-Fouchet method. The latter concentrates the bilirubin in urine by adsorption on freshly precipitated barium phosphate and sulfate. The blue-green color produced by treating the precipitate with acid ferric chloride is quite specific for bilirubin and closely related pigments. Urobilinogen or urobilin do not react.

Other methods for testing urine for bilirubin include the methylene blue test which depends upon the extinction by additional methylene blue of the green color produced by interaction of bilirubin and methylene blue (Reinhold and Fowler, 1947). This test is easily applied, but it measures also other yellow pigments that may be present. It gives a roughly quantitative estimate of bilirubin concentration.

Recently, Free and Free (1953) described a rapid and sensitive diazo test for bilirubin which appears to compare favorably with the Harrison-Fouchet method and which may prove to be superior (Klatskin and Bungards, 1953; Sobotka *et al.*, 1953; Giordano and Winstead, 1953; Tallach and Sherlock, 1954).

Bilirubin is present in the urine of healthy persons in concentrations so low that it is not detected by ordinary methods. Positive tests for bilirubin in urine thus indicate the existence of liver damage or biliary obstruction. They occur, at times, before serum bilirubin is elevated. It is for this reason that urine bilirubin tests are useful for the detection of acute viral hepatitis in its early stages (Neefe *et al.*, 1944; Swift *et al.*, 1950). Later in this disease, urine bilirubin tests may become negative while the disease is still active and serum-bilirubin concentrations remain above normal limits. The means by which bilirubin passes the renal barrier is far from clear, since it is firmly bound to protein in serum and nondiffusible or only slightly so. Some may enter the urine combined with protein which is a fairly regular constituent of urine of patients suffering from hepatitis. The remainder must be split from protein by a renal mechanism still unknown. An investigation of the relationship of the bilirubin in urine to the new pigments discovered by Cole *et al.* (1954) obviously is needed.

Shutkin and Caine (1955) report the detection of bilirubin in urines of 11 patients with subclinical liver disease out of 1000 routine tests of urines of hospital patients. The "Bilazo" test of Free and Free (1953) was used.

After the presence of liver disease has been established and if serum-bilirubin concentrations are being measured, urine bilirubin tests offer little useful information.

Urobilinogen in Urine and Feces

Urobilinogen is normally present in urine. It is formed by reduction of bilirubin by bacterial action in the cecum and colon. Urobilinogen is reabsorbed from the intestine and excreted mainly by way of the bile. Impaired excretory ability of the liver leads to an increase in its output in the urine. Thus, measurement of urobilinogen concentration in urine is a test of liver function. However, when the liver is damaged to such an extent that the secretion of bile is suppressed, no urobilinogen will be formed or detected. It is absent also if obstruction of the bile ducts prevents entry of bile into the intestine. Patients receiving (a) certain diets not conducive to maintenance of the usual bacterial flora, (b) antibiotics, or (c) other substances altering the bacterial flora of the intestine may excrete little or no urobilinogen in feces or urine.

Urobilin is formed by oxidation of urobilinogen. Whereas urobilinogen is colorless, urobilin is yellow. Urobilinogen is converted to urobilin on standing in the presence of oxygen, or by oxidizing agents. This change is delayed by protecting urine from light and air and by alkaline reactions. Urobilin may be reconverted to urobilinogen by treatment with ferrous sulfate and sodium hydroxide.

The presence of increased amounts of urobilinogen in urine is a characteristic finding in patients with disease of the parenchymal cells of the liver. At times it may offer the only conclusive evidence of the existence of liver disease. Changes in urine urobilinogen excretion are likely to occur independently of changes in other tests, and for this reason it is desirable to include it in a battery of such tests.

For more detailed information about urobilinogen and related pigments, the recent review of Gray (1954) may be consulted. Watson *et al.* (1954) have studied the formation and interrelationship of urobilinogens by administration of bilirubin labeled with N^{15}. Under special conditions dextrorotatory urobilin (*d*-urobilin) may be formed in the intestine.

Two procedures are widely used for estimation of the urobilinogen excretion in urine. One is the simplified quantitative Ehrlich reaction of Watson, Schwartz, Sborov, and Bertie (1944), as modified by Watson and Hawkinson (1947). This method is designed for use as a routine or screening test and for most purposes is capable of supplying the information sought. However, it may be necessary to apply in special circumstances a method yielding more specific data, and for this reason the quantitative method of Schwartz, Sborov, and Watson (1944) is recommended. Balikov (1953) has improved the technic of the latter.

Interpretation

The excretion of urobilinogen in urine by healthy persons averages 0.64 mg. in 24 hours. Only 2.5 per cent excrete more than 1.56 mg. and only 0.5 per cent more than 2.1 mg. in 24 hours. Patients with disease of the liver may excrete amounts of urobilinogen greatly exceeding these limits —up to 100 mg. or more in a 24-hour urine collection—although values ranging from 2 to 10 mg. are more usual. However, the excretion may fall within normal limits in patients with severe liver damage owing to the small amount of bile pigment reaching the intestine of such patients. Thus high values may be encountered following the onset of jaundice, to be followed by a period in which the output is within normal limits. This may persist for only a day or two or may continue for 1 or more weeks. It, in turn, is followed by a second period of elevated excretions which gradually return to normal limits as the illness improves.

Urobilinogen (Stercobilinogen) in Feces

The urobilinogen of feces consists of several closely related compounds differing in minor details of structure. The principal one is stercobilinogen which is distinguished from urobilinogen by measurement of optical rotation. Stercobilinogen reacts with Ehrlich's aldehyde reagent and the procedures for its determination are similar to those described for urine. Measurement of stercobilinogen output provides useful information to the clinician concerning (1) the rate of hemoglobin destruction and (2) the completeness of obstruction of the bile ducts. Such information may contribute substantially to the correct evaluation of the patient with jaundice. Knowledge of the rate at which hemoglobin is destroyed is of great value also in study of anemias.

Interpretation

Healthy persons excrete 100 to 350 Ehrlich units per 100 Gm. of feces, or 40 to 280 mg. as stercobilinogen. As much as 2000 mg. may be excreted each day by patients suffering from hemolytic anemia. Transfusion of blood often is followed by an increased excretion of stercobilinogen in feces, and may obscure interpretation of the findings.

Obstruction of the bile ducts caused by neoplastic or other growths is characterized by complete or nearly complete interruption of the flow of bile into the intestine. The daily excretion of stercobilinogen by such patients is only 1 or 2 Ehrlich units (or milligrams) and infrequently exceeds 5 Ehrlich units. Obstruction caused by calculi interferes less with excretion of bile and the daily output of stercobilinogen in feces will exceed 10 Ehrlich units. It is important to keep in mind, however, that either parenchymal or cholangiolitic disease of the liver, if severe, may suppress secretion of bile or otherwise prevent its entry into the intestine. As a result, stercobilinogen outputs as low as those found in obstruction due to neoplastic growth may be encountered in hepatitis, cirrhosis, or cholangitis. The low outputs are generally transitory in the latter, in contrast to the persistently low values characteristic of complete mechanical obstruction.

Measurement of Excretory Capacity of the Liver

Bile acids and various other substances, among them a number of dyes, are taken up by the liver and rapidly secreted into the bile. In liver disease the rate of excretion may be lowered, and because of this the use of certain of these substances has been of great value in measurement of liver function. Disodium phenoltetrabromophthalein sulfonate (sulfobromophthalein, sodium; bromsulfalein), introduced by Rosenthal and White (1925), has proved to be superior to numerous other substances tested for this purpose.

The diversion of much of the blood that ordinarily would flow through the liver into collateral channels is an important cause for delayed removal of injected bromsulfalein from the blood stream. As already mentioned, such a diversion becomes a major factor in cirrhosis, but it may be significant also when the liver is injured by viral or chemical agents and in patients with heart failure. A second important factor is the decreased mass of functioning liver cells, and a third may be inability of damaged liver cells to transport the dye into the bile. It was believed for a long time that the Kupffer cells were mainly responsible for removal of bromsulfalein from the blood stream. Mendeloff (1949 a and b) compared the activities of hepatic polygonal cells in removing Rose Bengal, a dye closely resembling bromsulfalein in its behavior, from the circulation. Fluorescence microscopy demonstrated no dye in Kupffer cells, while the polygonal cells contained large amounts. Brauer and Pessotti (1948) found that bromsulfalein was taken up by slices of liver but not by splenic or lymph node slices.

The belief, formerly widely held, that the reticuloendothelial cells were primarily responsible for removal of bromsulfalein from the circulation was based mainly on experiments in which India ink was injected into the blood stream. When bromsulfalein was injected following India ink, removal of the dye was delayed presumably because of blockade of the reticuloendothelial system by the carbon particles in the ink. However, Shore and Zilversmit (1953) and Zilversmit and Shore (1954) have demonstrated in convincing experiments that carbon suspensions are without effect on bromsulfalein excretion, whereas a carbon-free filtrate of India ink was sufficiently toxic to the liver to cause the delay in dye excretion.

Although up to 95 per cent of the bromsulfalein injected into healthy persons is rapidly removed from the circulation, only a small amount appears in the urine. The proportion excreted in the urine becomes much larger (Norcross *et al.*, 1951) in the presence of liver damage. Lattanzi (1950) reports 20 to 48 per cent excretion in 24 hours by patients suffering from liver disease.

Retention of bromsulfalein in patients with jaundice due to hepatitis or biliary obstruction may be prolonged for as much as 29 days (Giges, 1951). Patients with cirrhosis did not show this tendency. It is doubtful whether application of the bromsulfalein test to the study of jaundiced patients provides information not readily obtainable by other means. The prolonged retention of dye remaining in the circulation after previous tests and the complications introduced by the presence of bilirubin in measurement of dye retention make it essential to collect a control sample of blood before such a test is done. Zieve *et al.* (1951) have derived a correction to be applied to results of bromsulfalein tests if total bilirubin in serum exceeds 2 mg./100 ml.

A recent report by Brauer *et al.* (1955) suggests that the fate of bromsulfalein in the body may not be merely one of excretion in bile and urine. After bromsulfalein labeled with S^{35} was administered, the bile always contained more total S^{35} than the bromsulfalein. This apparently was not due to desulfonation.

The use of actual instead of ideal weight in calculating dosages of dye to be injected may cause erroneous results, especially in the presence of ascites, edema, or adiposity.

Rosenthal and White (1925) used 2.0 mg. per Kg. of body weight. The 5 mg. per Kg. dosage, however, has been adopted widely and provides a more sensitive and more precise test. The existence of an enterohepatic circulation of bromsulfalein (Lorber and Shay, 1952) does not appear to influence the results sufficiently to necessitate a return to the original dosage (Owen, 1951).

[Note: It is advisable to question the patient concerning sensitivities to drugs. Reactions to bromsulfalein are rare but a few individuals do not tolerate it, and it may have effects so severe as to constitute a medical emergency. A preliminary skin test may be done. Obviously, the injection of bromsulfalein should be done only by a physician or under his immediate supervision.]

The time at which the postinjection blood specimen is collected is not of great importance, provided that appropriate standards of normal for that time are used. Mateer *et al.* (1943) introduced the 45-minute sampling time and it has proved to be satisfactory. Calculation of the rate of disappearance of bromsulfalein by means of multiple specimens collected at 5- to 15-minute intervals after the injection has been advocated. The liver removes a constant fraction of the bromsulfalein remaining in the circulating blood during any time interval (Bradley, 1949) and by collecting a series of blood specimens the accuracy of the estimate of the bromsulfalein retained is improved. For a description of "clearance" studies of patients the reader is referred to papers by Deutsch (1941), Lewis (1948), Lavers *et al.* (1949), Goodman (1952), Goodman and Kingsley (1953), Neumayr *et al.* (1954), and Nadeau (1954).

Interpretation

Healthy persons after injection of 5 mg. of bromsulfalein per Kg. of body weight retain less than 10 per cent at 30 minutes and 7.0 per cent at 45 minutes. At 60 minutes, no dye is retained.

Bromsulfalein retention is generally accepted as the most sensitive and dependable among the laboratory procedures currently used to demonstrate involvement of the liver. It is especially helpful for evaluating suspicious or positive results obtained by means of flocculation tests in the absence of hyperbilirubinemia. The bromsulfalein test outscores all others in the proportion of positive tests found in Laennec's cirrhosis. It has been among the most useful for following recovery from viral hepatitis and for detecting residual liver damage from this disease. It is probably the only procedure capable of detecting fatty liver, although it cannot be depended upon to do so consistently.

Retention of bromsulfalein in the blood stream may occur because of spasm of the sphincter of Oddi caused by morphine (Burnett, 1954), the mechanism being similar to that causing serum amylase to rise under similar conditions. Burnett (1954) reports that bromsulfalein was retained to an abnormal extent in 22 of 23 patients suffering from inflammatory disease of the gall bladder.

Miscellaneous Tests

Serum-Cholinesterase Activity

Serum-cholinesterase activity is usually lowered in the presence of atrophy of or damage to the liver parenchyma. Similar changes have been reported for serum esterase and lipase. Depression of serum cholinesterase activity closely follows changes in serum albumin concentrations. However, severe liver damage is not consistently accompanied by significantly lowered cholinesterase activity. Serial measurement of cholinesterase activity appears to provide a useful method for following the course of liver disease. It is of special value for study of the liver damage associated with deficient diets. Current articles dealing with its application to the study of liver disease include those of Mann *et al.* (1952), Fremont-Smith *et al.* (1952), Wilson *et al.* (1952), and Vorhaus and Kark (1953). Molander *et al.* (1954) have studied the effects of neoplastic disease involving the liver on serum-cholinesterase activity. Markedly depressed values were observed.

Serum cholinesterase may be measured conveniently by the method of Michel (1949) or by a photometric adaptation of it (Reinhold *et al.*, 1953).

Coproporphyrin in Urine

The output of coproporphyrin in urine rises markedly in patients suffering from various types of liver disease (Watson, Hawkinson, *et al.*, 1949; Watson, Sutherland, and Hawkinson, 1951). Measurement of coproporphyrin excretion provides a sensitive and valuable method for detecting liver damage that may escape detection by other methods. The excretion of coproporphyrin generally is within normal limits in patients who have biliary-tract lesions, but high values occur with sufficient frequency to impair its usefulness for differential diagnosis. Care must be used also to exclude other causes of increased porphyrin excretion; for example, various drugs and intoxicants. An idiopathic coproporphyrinuria has been described (Watson, Schwartz, *et al.*, 1949).

A simplified technic for determination of coproporphyrin has been described recently (Schwartz, Zieve, and Watson, 1951). The small amounts of coproporphyrin in many samples of urine require the use of a highly sensitive fluorimeter for dependable measurements. The high cost of such instruments has been a deterrent to the wider use of porphyrin analysis. The improved methods now available give much higher results than those formerly used mainly because of the detection of porphyrin precursors in urine and their inclusion in the assay (Watson, Pimenta de Mello, *et al.*, 1951).

Watson and his associates (see references above) have shown that the type of coproporphyrin excreted is related to the cause of liver damage. Thus Type I coproporphyrin predominates in the urine of patients ill with viral hepatitis, whereas Type III predominates in cirrhosis of "alcoholic" origin.

Increased excretion of uroporphyrin in urine has been observed in patients with liver disease. Porphobilinogen excretion in urine also may be increased sufficiently to give a positive test in urine in the presence of liver disease (Watson *et al.*, 1954).

Combined Intravenous Bromsulfalein-Hippuric Acid-Galactose Test

Zieve, Hill, and Nesbitt (1950) have devised a procedure for administration of the three substances simultaneously. They find that simultaneous administration does not alter the behavior of the test substances.

Peptidase Activity of Human Serum

Fleisher and Butt (1953) have found tripeptidase activity to be increased in serum of patients with liver disease or with obstruction of the bile ducts. Bile shows marked tripeptidase activity. Hydrolysis of several dipeptides is decreased in liver disease, according to these authors.

Protein-Bound Iodine of Serum in Liver Disease

Kydd and Man (1951) found sharply increased concentrations of protein-bound iodine in serum during earlier stages of viral hepatitis. On the other hand, cirrhotic patients tended to have subnormal or low normal concentrations.

SELECTION OF PROCEDURES

The choice of methods to be applied in the study of a patient with disease of the liver or biliary tract will vary according to the type of information sought. The following outline shows the principal purposes for which chemical methods are applied together with a list of the procedures likely to prove useful.

Detection of subclinical liver disease in absence of jaundice: urine bilirubin, bromsulfalein retention, direct and total bilirubin, flocculation tests (cephalin-cholesterol flocculation, thymol turbidity and flocculation, zinc turbidity), urine urobilinogen, zone electrophoresis protein pattern.

Studies designed for the purpose of investigating the presence of residual viral hepatitis in veterans by Zieve *et al.* (1953) and Neefe *et al.* (1955) illustrate one problem to which this group of tests has been applied. Another is the testing of blood donors for the purpose of detecting certain carriers of viral hepatitis who appear to have subclinical liver disease (Reinhold, 1955).

Detection of residual liver damage, "recovery" stages of hepatitis, chronic passive congestion, portal cirrhosis: bromsulfalein, direct and total bilirubin, flocculation tests, serum albumin and globulin, or electrophoretic protein pattern, prothrombin, serum cholinesterase, urine urobilinogen and coproporphyrin [*see* Kunkel *et al.* (1947)].

Evaluation of the course of the jaundiced patient suffering from parenchymatous liver disease: serum direct and total bilirubin, flocculation tests, serum albumin and globulin, prothrombin. In addition, if severe, serum esterified cholesterol or cholinesterase. Blood urea N or NPN, glucose, and serum electrolytes also are important [*see* Kimmel, *et al.* (1954)].

Jones (1955) mentions an abrupt or steady rise in serum bilirubin, and declining serum albumin, cholinesterase, and prothrombin, together with decreasing urine output and rise in blood leukocyte count as evidence of deteriorating liver function.

Differentiation of jaundice due to biliary disease from that due to parenchymatous disease: serum alkaline phosphatase, cephalin-cholesterol flocculation, and thymol turbidity, serum mucoprotein, electrophoretic protein pattern, prothrombin response, repeated fecal urobilinogen tests.

Among the recent papers that discuss the differential diagnosis of jaundice are those of Mellinkoff *et al.* (1952), Popper and Schaffner (1952), Ricketts (1953), and Wang (1953).

Differentiation of extrahepatic biliary obstruction due to calculus from that due to neoplasm, stricture, etc.: fecal urobilinogen.

For following the course of the surgical patient with disease of the biliary tract: plasma prothrombin, phosphatase, serum direct and total bilirubin, albumin and globulin, electrolytes, blood urea N or NPN, and serum lipids.

Differentiation of hemolytic jaundice: serum direct and total bilirubin, fecal urobilinogen, erythrocyte fragility, reticulocyte count.

A decision regarding the number of tests to be used requires experience and judgment. The information gained increases as the number of tests increases but with rapidly diminishing returns beyond an optimum that will vary in different patients. Usually, the tests listed will suffice for an initial study, with additional requests to be made if further information is needed. To apply simultaneously the entire group of tests listed in any of the categories would seldom be justified.

Comparatively little has been done to evaluate the advantage gained by the use of two or more tests in combination. Gutman and Hanger (1941) found that serum phosphatase and cephalin-cholesterol flocculation supplemented each other for the diagnosis of common duct disease and that combining the findings of the two tests substantially improved the accuracy. Maclagan (1947) compared a number of tests singly and in pairs. Thymol turbidity alone gave correct diagnoses in 22 per cent of cases of liver disease that could be unequivocally classified as either obstruction or parenchymal. Serum alkaline phosphatase was correct in 46 per cent. However, a combination of thymol turbidity and alkaline phosphatase gave correct diagnoses in 79 per cent.

Wootton, King, and Maclean-Smith (1951) cite a statistical analysis by R. A. Fisher in which he used the method of discriminant functions to compare the effectiveness of four tests applied to jaundiced patients with that of two tests. The four-test group yielded only slightly more reliable information than a properly selected pair of tests. It is possible, therefore, to eliminate some procedures.

The practice in clinics where interest is centered on the study of liver disease, varies with respect to selection of the flocculation tests that are regularly used. Reliance on a single test is infrequent. Usually two or three tests are used. Probably the most frequent combination is the thymol test (Maclagan, 1944) and cephalin-cholesterol flocculation (Hanger, 1939). Often the zinc turbidity (Kunkel, 1947) or the ammonium sulfate turbidity (Huerga and Popper, 1949) are included. The colloidal red test (Ducci, 1947) gives results resembling closely those of the colloidal gold test applied to serum. The latter, according to Maclagan (1951), largely duplicates the results of simpler tests and thus no longer performs a useful service. Neefe *et al.* (1950) found no need for routine use of the colloidal red test in the study of viral hepatitis. A few clinics routinely use five or six tests, but this is done largely for the purpose of comparison and evaluation of the tests.

A comparison of a group of tests with respect to their behavior during the onset of viral hepatitis induced in volunteer subjects has been made by Neefe and Reinhold (1946). Seven tests were abnormal in 95 per cent or more of the patients. These were the 1-minute direct bilirubin, urine bilirubin by the Harrison spot method, cephalin-cholesterol flocculation, thymol turbidity, thymol flocculation, colloidal gold, and bromsulfalein retention. Thus any of the seven might have served. However, the study showed that these tests differed distinctly in the times at which they first became positive. The bromsulfalein test showed a striking advantage in this respect and urine bilirubin ranked second. Had the reliance been placed only upon the thymol test, the hepatitis of some of the individuals might have escaped detection.

The ranking of the same group of tests in the same subjects was distinctly different when they were evaluated according to their ability to disclose persistence of the disease or its sequelae. In general the order is now reversed with the tests depending on changes in serum proteins showing a greater tendency to persist than those based on excretory function. Again dependence on a single test of either group would have meant failure to detect change in some patients. Furthermore, bromsulfalein retention persisted in some patients long after flocculation tests had become normal, so that dependence on the latter alone may fail to demonstrate liver damage in these circumstances. It appears inadvisable, therefore, to curtail too severely the number of procedures used, particularly when a wide variety of clinical material is being studied.

Quite frequently patients are encountered with equivocal signs of involvement of the liver which cannot be conclusively demonstrated by either clinical examination or laboratory studies. In such circumstances biopsy of the liver done either in the course of surgical exploration or by needle is considered essential. Besides providing helpful information about such patients, the widespread use of liver biopsy has greatly increased the understanding of liver disease. It has also enabled correlations to be made between the results of laboratory studies and the appearance of the liver under the microscope. A number of such studies have shown that there is a general correlation between the severity of the changes in the liver and the degree of change in the chemical tests used.

Popper (1951) found that the cephalin-cholesterol flocculation, thymol turbidity, and serum albumin and globulin concentrations showed a statistically significant correlation between degree of liver cell damage and degree of chemical abnormality. No significant correlation was found with phosphatase, prothrombin activity, urine urobilinogen, serum total cholesterol, or blood sedimentation rate.

Moyer and Wurl (1951) found the bromsulfalein test to be most consistently correlated. Schneider *et al.* (1953) report a good correlation in portal cirrhosis between biopsy findings and serum-albumin concentration, cephalin-cholesterol flocculation, serum bilirubin, and bromsulfalein retention. Correlation with the thymol turbidity was poor.

At times the results of chemical studies will be within normal limits despite the existence of pathologic changes in the sample of liver tissue. Frequently, however, the results of the chemical studies will be abnormal in the absence of conclusive indications of abnormality in the liver sections (Christian, 1952).

There are a number of explanations for such discrepancies, among them the possibility of sampling errors in removing the 10 mg. (or less) sample of liver that a needle biopsy yields. It is probable also that methods of staining and examining sections of liver fail to demonstrate changes in cell function. The greatest utility of each method for the study of liver disease will be realized if liver biopsy and chemical studies are coordinated. In such a plan, chemical studies will serve for screening and evaluation of the patients and for following the clinical course. Liver biopsy will supplement such studies, particularly in patients who present diagnostic problems. The coordinated use of liver biopsy and biochemical studies is discussed by Popper and Schaffner (1952).

On rare occasions, chemical studies of patients with relatively substantial involvement of the liver may fail to demonstrate significant abnormalities (Ricketts, 1951). The use of chemical methods to study the clinical course also may have limitations. As an example, the patient studied by Flynn and Walshe (1951) before and after resection of about one sixth of the liver showed no change in serum bilirubin, prothrombin, bromsulfalein retention, hippuric-acid excretion, or alkaline-phosphatase activity. Some deterioration of the flocculation tests and an excessive output of urobilinogen in urine gave the only substantial evidence of altered status.

Another curious phenomenon, and one deserving more study, is the "hyperfunction" of the liver that may occur in mild forms of liver disease (Rosenberg and Soskin, 1941; Zieve and Hill, 1953).

Table 1 summarizes the prevailing response obtained when tests for the bile pigments and other procedures commonly used are applied in study of diseases of the liver parenchyma and the contrast in the response in disease of the biliary tract. Table 2 shows the response as reported in a variety of other diseases.

The causes of abnormal hepatic tests in these miscellaneous diseases are varied. Liver disease, antecedent to or not necessarily related to the disease diagnosed, may exist. Bogoch *et al.* (1955) found that 7 of 15 patients with diabetes mellitus had abnormal hepatic tests because of

Table 1. Prevailing Response of Hepatic Tests in Diseases of Liver and Biliary Tract

Syndrome	*Bilirubin and urobilinogen*	*Tests for parenchymal involvement*	*Tests for biliary-tract involvement*
Viral hepatitis without jaundice	May be present in urine and may increase slightly in serum. Urobilinogen may increase in urine.	BSF usually abnormal. CCF, TT, TF, ZT, one or more, may be abnormal.	Normal
Viral hepatitis with jaundice	Increased in serum and urine. Urobilinogen generally increased in urine and feces but may be absent.	Abnormal. Lowered mucoprotein.	Mainly normal but may be abnormal.
"Toxic" hepatitis: cholangiolitic jaundice	Increased in serum and urine.	CCF, TTT, TF, ZT may be normal or abnormal. A/G usually normal.	Increased serum phosphatase, lipid. Similar to extrahepatic obstruction.
Laennec's cirrhosis	May or may not be abnormal in serum and urine. Urobilinogen variable.	BSF abnormal. CCF, TT, TF, or ZT abnormal in about ¾. A/G abnormal.	Variable. Phosphatase may be high.
Extrahepatic obstruction			
Partial	Variable. Intermittent or continuous elevation.	Generally normal, but liver parenchyma may become injured and tests positive.	Variable but with elevated serum phosphatase and lipid prevalent. Good response to vitamin K.
Complete	Extreme elevation. Very low fecal urobilinogen.	Same as preceding.	Elevated serum phosphatase and lipid. Good response to vitamin K.
Biliary cirrhosis (Ahrens *et al.*, 1950; Ricketts *et al.*, 1950)	Bilirubin elevated. Urobilinogen variable.	BSF increased. A/G abnormal. TT increased. CCF increased about half.	Elevated phosphatase. Marked elevation of serum lipid, especially phospholipid.

BSF, bromsulfalein; CCF, cephalin-cholesterol flocculation; TF, thymol flocculation; TT, thymol turbidity; ZT, zinc turbidity; A, serum albumin; G, serum globulin.

liver disease not directly related to the diabetes. Abnormal turbidity and flocculation tests are easily explained by the occurrence in many diseases of changes in serum proteins, sufficiently like those occurring in liver disease to permit abnormal reactions to occur. Elevated alkaline-phospha-

Table 2. Prevailing Response of Hepatic Tests in Miscellaneous Diseases

Syndrome	*Bilirubin and urobilinogen*	*Tests for parenchymal involvement*	*Tests for biliary-tract involvement*
Hemolytic jaundice	Total serum bilirubin moderately elevated; 1-minute bilirubin normal or slightly increased. Urine bilirubin negative. Fecal urobilinogen increased urine urobilinogen often normal.	Seldom abnormal but may become so due to hypoxia or other complications.	Seldom abnormal. Pigment stones may cause biliary obstruction.
Amebic hepatitis (Heller *et al.*, 1953)	Bilirubin variable.	CCF abnormal. TT normal.	Normal
Amebic abscess (Brem, 1955)	..	Elevated TT in $2/8$. Elevated BSF in $4/8$. Lowered A in $3/8$.	Elevated phosphatase in $4/8$.
Amyloidosis, secondary (Wald, 1954)	..	Elevated CCF in $11/12$. BSF > 10% in $8/23$. Decreased cholesterol ester in $13/20$.	..
Lupus erythematosus (Kofman *et al.*, 1955)	Bilirubin elevated in 27%.	Elevated CCF in 70%. Elevated TT in 100% Elevated BSF in 47%.	Elevated phosphatase 31%.
Metastatic carcinoma of the liver (Thomas and Zimmerman, 1952)	..	Elevated CCF in $15/37$. Elevated TT in $8/37$. Elevated BSF in all.	..
(Simons, 1954)	Elevated	Elevated CCF in $19/56$. Elevated TT in $30/59$ upwards.	Elevated phosphatase in all.
(Rhees *et al.*, 1954)	Nonicteric	..	Elevated phosphatase in 68%. Elevated mucroprotein.
(Molander *et al.*, 1954)	..	Lowered cholinesterase.	..
Hepatocellular adenoma (1 case) (Stumpf and Liber, 1954)	Normal	CCF and TT elevated. BSF 32%.	Phosphatase markedly elevated.
Multiple myeloma (Walsh *et al.*, 1955)	..	Elevated CCF in 36%. Elevated TT in 15%.	..

(table continued on page 410)

Table 2—*Continued*

Syndrome	*Bilirubin and urobilinogen*	*Tests for parenchymal involvement*	*Tests for biliary-tract involvement*
Chronic congestive heart failure (Evans *et al.*, 1952)	Bilirubin increased in 1/4.	Floc. and turbidity tests 18–41% positive. BSF elevated in severe failure.	..
Obesity (Zelman, 1952)	Elevated urine urobilinogen in 6/19. Bilirubin increased in 2/20.	Elevated BSF in all. CCF abnormal in 4/20. TT in 10/20.	Elevated phosphatase in 5/19.
Infectious mononucleosis (Brown *et al.*, 1949)	..	Elevated CCF in 38/39. Elevated TT in 19/39.	..
Rheumatoid arthritis (Darby, 1953)	..	Elevated BSF in 23%. Elevated flocculation tests in 73%.	..
Injury to spinal cord (Cooper *et al.*, 1951)	Bilirubin increased in 1/8.	Increased BSF in 6/8. Increased CCF in 1/8.	..
Weil's disease (Chinn *et al.*, 1951)	Bilirubin increased in 5/6. Urobilinogen in 4/4.	Increased CCF in 5/6. Increased TT in 3/6.	Moderately increased phosphatase in 5/6.
Diabetes mellitus (Bogoch *et al.*, 1955)	Bilirubin normal.	Increased BSF in 4/8. Increased G 6/8. Decreased albumin in 5/8.	Slightly increased alk. phosphatase in 1/8.

BSF, bromsulfalein; CCF, cephalin-cholesterol flocculation; TF, thymol flocculation; TT, thymol turbidity; ZT, zinc turbidity; A, serum albumin; G, serum globulin.

tase activities may be a result of bone involvement—for example, osteitis deformans, a fairly frequent illness of older people. Some of the abnormalities in liver function reported in miscellaneous illness are the result of inadequately defined standards of normal. Insufficient attention has been given to factors such as age, sex, race, and diurnal variations. Faulty technic also may contribute. The use of actual instead of ideal weight in calculating bromsulfalein dosages is an example. Erroneously high retention may occur in adipose subjects. When all these possibilities are excluded, it remains well established that certain diseases are accompanied by significant involvement of the liver.

REFERENCES

1. Abell, L. L., Levy, B. B., Brodie, B. B., and Kendall, F. E., *J. Biol. Chem.* **195,** 357 (1952).
2. Adams, R. D., and Foley, J. M., *in* Merritt, H. H., and Hare, C. C., *Metabolic and Toxic Diseases of Nervous System.* Baltimore, Md., Williams & Wilkins (1953), p. 198.

3. Ahrens, E. H., Jr., Payne, M. A., Kunkel, H. G., Eisenmenger, W. J., and Blondheim, S. H., *Medicine* **29,** 299 (1950).
4. Aikawa, J. K., Felts, J. H., and Harrel, Jr., G. T., *Gastroenterology* **24,** 437 (1953).
5. Albertsen, K., Christoffersen, N. R., and Heintzelmann, F., *Acta Med. Scand.* **136,** 302 (1950).
6. Alexander, B., *New Eng. J. Med.* **252,** 526 (1955).
7. Alexander, B., and Goldstein, R., *J. Clin. Invest.* **29,** 795 (1950).
8. Almaden, P. J., and Ross, S. W., *Ann. Internal Med.* **40,** 146 (1954).
9. Althausen, T. L., *Am. J. Med.* **4,** 208 (1949).
10. Althausen, T. L., Lockhart, J. C., and Soley, M. H., *Am. J. Med. Sci.* **199,** 342 (1940).
11. Althausen, T. L., and Weaver, G. K., *Ann. Internal Med.* **12,** 674 (1938).
12. Amatuzio, D. S., and Nesbitt, S., *J. Clin. Invest.* **29,** 1486 (1950).
13. Amatuzio, D. S., Stutzman, F. L., Shrifter, N., and Nesbitt, S., *J. Lab. Clin. Med.* **39,** 26 (1952).
14. Amatuzio, D. S., Weber, L. J., and Nesbitt, S., *J. Lab. Clin. Med.* **41,** 615 (1953).
15. Armas-Cruz, R., Lobo-Parga, G., and Madrid, M., *J. Lab. Clin. Med.* **39,** 533 (1952).
16. Artman, E. L., and Wise, R. A., *Am. J. Med.* **15,** 459 (1953).
17. Babb, W., and Pedrazzini, A., *Schweiz. med. Wochschr.* **79,** 167 (1949).
18. Balch, H. E., Michaels, G. D., and Smyrl, S., *Am. J. Med.* **17,** 117 (1954).
19. Balfour, W. M., *Gastroenterology* **9,** 686 (1947).
20. Balikov, B., *The Clinical Chemist* **5,** 89 (1953). Reprinted in *Clin. Chem.* **1,** 264 (1955).
21. Barkan, G., and Walker, B. S., *J. Biol. Chem.* **135,** 37 (1940).
22. Bartels, E. C., *Ann. Internal Med.* **12,** 577 (1938).
23. Bateman, J. C., Shorr, H. M., and Elgvin, T., *J. Clin. Invest.* **28,** 539 (1949).
24. Bauer, R., *Wien. med. Wochschr.* **56,** 2538 (1906).
25. Bearn, A. G., *Am. J. Med.* **15,** 442 (1953).
26. Bearn, A. G., and Kunkel, H. G., *J. Clin. Invest.* **33,** 400 (1954a).
27. Bearn, A. G., and Kunkel, H. G., *Proc. Soc. Exp. Biol. Med.* **85,** 44 (1954b).
28. Berman, L. B., Lapham, L. W., Pastore, E., *J. Lab. Clin. Med.* **44,** 273 (1954).
29. Bernhart, F. W., and Schneider, R. W., *Am. J. Med. Sci.* **205,** 606 (1943).
30. Bessman, S. P., and Bessman, A. N., *J. Clin. Invest.* **34,** 622 (1955).
31. Billing, B. H., *Biochem. J.* **56,** XXX (1954).
32. Billing, B. H., Haslam, R. M., Hein, D. E., Conlon, H. J., Hamilton, D. L., Mindrum, G. M., and Schiff, L., *J. Lab. Clin. Med.* **45,** 363 (1955).
33. Bjorneboe, M., Gormsen, H., and Lundquist, F., *J. Immunol.* **55,** 121 (1947).
34. Bogenhard, H., *Klin. Wochschr.* **32,** 697 (1954).
35. Bogoch, A., Casselman, W. G. B., Kaplan, A., and Bockus, H. L., *Am. J. Med.* **18,** 354 (1955).
36. Bollman, J. L., *Transactions of the Ninth Conference on Liver Injury.* (F. W. Hoffbauer, Ed.) New York, Macy (1950).
37. Bongiovanni, A. M., Eberlein, W. R., Grumbach, M. M., Van Wyk, J. J., and Clayton, G., *Proc. Soc. Exp. Biol. Med.* **87,** 282 (1954).
38. Borsook, H., and Dubnoff, J. W., *J. Biol. Chem.* **168,** 397 (1947).
39. Bradley, S. E., *New Eng. J. Med.* **240,** 456 (1949).
40. Bradley, S. E., Ingelfinger, F. J., Bradley, G. P., and Curry, J. J., *J. Clin. Invest.* **24,** 890 (1945).
41. Brante, G., *Scand. J. Clin. & Lab. Invest.* **4,** 293 (1952).
42. Brauer, R. W., and Pessotti, R. L., *Federation Proc.* **7,** 207 (1948).
43. Brem, T. H., *Am. J. Med. Sci.*, **229,** 155 (1955).
44. Brown, H., Willardson, G. H., Samuels, L. T., and Tyler, F. H., *J. Clin. Invest.* **33,** 1524 (1954).
45. Brown, J. W., Sims, J. L., White, E., and Clifford, J. E., *Am. J. Med.* **6,** 321 (1949).

46. Bruns, F., and Hinsberg, K., *Biochem. Z.* **325,** 532 (1954).
47. Bruns, F., and Jacob, W., *Klin. Wochschr.* **32,** 1041 (1954).
48. Bruns, F., and Puls, W., *Klin. Wochschr.* **32,** 656 (1954).
49. Bunker, J. P., Stetson, J. B., Coe, R. C., Guillo, H. C., and Murphy, A. J., *J. Am. Med. Assoc.* **157,** 1361 (1955).
50. Burke, J. O., *Gastroenterology* **16,** 660 (1950).
51. Burnett, W., *Lancet* **266,** 488 (1954).
52. Campbell, J. A., and Tagnon, H. J., *New Eng. J. Med.* **234,** 216 (1946).
53. Cantarow, A., Paschkis, K. E., Williams, T. L., and Havens, W. P., Jr., *Federation Proc.* **10,** 23 (1951).
54. Carne, H. O., *The Clinical Chemist* **5,** 76 (1953).
55. Carter, A. B., and Maclagan, N. F., *Brit. Med. J.* **2,** 80 (1946).
56. Carter, J. R., *Am. J. Pathol.* **25,** 309 (1949).
57. Cartwright, G. E., and Wintrobe, M. M., *J. Clin. Invest.* **28,** 86 (1949).
58. Cayer, D., and Cornatzer, W. E., *Gastroenterology* **14,** 1 (1950).
59. Charlwood, P. A., *Biochem. J.* **56,** 480 (1954).
60. Chart, J. J., and Shipley, E. S., *J. Clin. Invest.* **32,** 560 (1953).
61. Chinn, A. B., Roth, H. P., and Moore, R. D., *Am. J. Med. Sci.* **222,** 530 (1951).
62. Christian, E. R., *Am. J. Med.* **13,** 689 (1952).
63. Christian, E. R., *A.M.A. Arch. Internal Med.* **94,** 22 (1954).
64. Claireaux, A. E., Cole, P. G., and Lathe, G. H., *Lancet* **2,** 1226 (1953).
65. Cohen, P. P., and Thompson, F. L., *J. Lab. Clin. Med.* **32,** 475 (1947).
66. Cohn, E. J., *Blood* **3,** 478 (1948).
67. Colcher, H., Patek, A. J., Jr., and Kendall, F. E., *J. Clin. Invest.* **27,** 768 (1946).
68. Cole, P. G., and Lathe, G. H., *J. Clin. Pathol.* **6,** 99 (1953).
69. Cole, P. G., Lathe, G. H., and Billing, B. H., *Biochem. J.* **57,** 514 (1954).
70. Colwell, A. P., *Ann. Internal Med.* **41,** 963 (1954).
71. Conn, J. W., Newburgh, L. W., Johnston, M. W., and Sheldon, J. M. *Arch. Int. Med.* **62,** 765 (1938).
72. Conway, E. J., *Biochem. J.* **29,** 2755 (1935).
73. Conway, E. J., and Cooke, R., *Biochem. J.* **33,** 457 (1939).
74. Cook, J. L., and Dounce, A. L., *Proc. Soc. Exp. Biol. Med.* **87,** 349 (1954).
75. Cooper, I. S., Rynearson, E. H., McCarty, C. S., *J. Lab. Clin. Med.* **38,** 689 (1951).
76. Darby, P. W., *J. Clin. Pathol.* **6,** 331 (1953).
77. Day, R. L., *Proc. Soc. Exp. Biol. Med.* **85,** 261 (1954).
78. Deiss, W. P., and Cohen, P. P., *J. Clin. Invest.* **29,** 1014 (1950).
79. Deiss, W. P., and Musser, M. J., *J. Lab. Clin. Med.* **36,** 815 (1950).
80. Dekema, H., *Ned. Tijdschr. Geneesk.* **95,** 3774 (1951).
81. Denny-Brown, D., *in* Merritt, H. H., and Hare, C. C., *Metabolic and Toxic Diseases of Nervous System.* Baltimore, Md., Williams & Wilkins (1953), pp. 190–97.
82. Denny-Brown, D., and Porter, H., *New Eng. J. Med.* **245,** 917 (1951).
83. Dent, C. E., and Walshe, J. M., *Brit. Med. Bull.* **10,** 247 (1954).
84. Dent, C. E., and Walshe, J. M., *in* Sherlock, S., and Wolstenholme, G. E. W., *Liver Disease*, Philadelphia, Blakiston (1951).
85. Desmond, M. M., Zimmerman, H. J., Sweet, L. K., and Thomas, L. J., *Pediatrics* **3,** 49 (1949).
86. Deutsch, E., *New Eng. J. Med.* **225,** 171 (1941).
87. Dible, J. H., *Brit. Med. J.* **1,** 833 (1951).
88. Dohan, C. G., Richardson, E. G., Bluemle, W. L., and Gyorgy, P., *J. Clin. Invest.* **31,** 481 (1952).
89. Dreyfus, J.-C., Schapira, G., and Schapira, F., *J. Clin. Invest.* **33,** 794 (1954).
90. Dubin, I. N., and Johnson, F. B., *Am. J. Med.* **16,** 906 (1954a).

91. Dubin, I. N., and Johnson, F. B., *Medicine* **33,** 155 (1954b).
92. Ducci, H., *Gastroenterology* **15,** 628 (1950).
93. Ducci, H., *J. Lab. Clin. Med.* **32,** 1273 (1947).
94. Ducci, H., *in* Sherlock, S., and Wolstenholme, G. E. W., *Liver Disease.* Philadelphia, Blakiston (1951).
95. Ducci, H., and Watson, C. J., *J. Lab. Clin. Med.* **30,** 293 (1945).
96. Dunn, M. S., Akawaie, S., Yeh, H. L., and Martin, H., *J. Clin. Invest.* **29,** 302 (1950).
97. Ehrich, W. E., *in* Tullis, J. L., *Blood Cells and Plasma Proteins.* New York, Acad. Press, (1953).
98. Eisenmenger, W. J., Ahrens, E. A., Blondheim, S. H., and Kunkel, H. G., *J. Lab. Clin. Med.* **34,** 1029 (1949).
99. Elias, H., *Am. J. Anat.* **84,** 311 (1949).
100. Elias, H., *Am. J. Anat.* **85,** 379 (1949).
101. Elias, H., *Transactions of the Eleventh Conference on Liver Injury.* (F. W. Hoffbauer, Ed.) New York, Macy (1953).
102. Elias, H., and Sokol, A., *Anat. Rec.* **115,** 71 (1953).
103. Emmrich, R., *Klin. Wochschr.* **26,** 659 (1948) (*Chem. Abstr.* **44,** 8492).
104. Evans, J. M., Zimmerman, H. J., Wilmer, J. G., Thomas, L. J., and Etheridge, C. B., *Am. J. Med.* **13,** 704 (1952).
105. Eversole, W. J., and Giere, F. A., *Am. J. Physiol.* **167,** 282 (1951).
106. Fagreus, A., *Acta Med. Scand.* **Suppl. 130,** 204 (1948).
107. Fairlie, C. W., Baros, T. P., French, A. B., Jones, C. M., and Beacher, H. K., *New Eng. J. Med.* **244,** 615 (1951).
108. Farquhar, J. W., *Am. J. Med. Sci.* **218,** 291 (1949).
109. Fischer, H., and Haberland, H. W., *Hoppe-Seyler's Z. physiol. Chem.* **232,** 236 (1935).
110. Fitch, D. R., Watanabe, R. K., Kassouny, D., Neefe, J. R., Reinhold, J. G., and Norris, R. F., *Am. J. Clin. Pathol.* **25,** 158 (1955).
111. Fleisher, G. A., and Butt, H. R., *J. Clin. Invest.* **32,** 674 (1953).
112. Flock, E. V., Block, M. A., Bollman, J. L., and Mann, F. C., *Am. J. Physiol.* **170,** 467 (1952).
113. Flock, E. V., Bollman, J. L., Grindlay, J. H., and Mann, F. C., *Federation Proc.* **12,** 203 (1953).
114. Flood, C. A., Gutman, E. B., and Gutman, A. B., *Arch. Internal Med.* **59,** 981 (1937).
115. Flynn, F. V., and Walshe, J. M., *Brit. Med. J.* **1,** 1484 (1951).
116. Foord, A. G., and Baisinger, C. F., *Am. J. Clin. Pathol.* **10,** 238 (1940).
117. Foster, D. P., and Whipple, G. H., *Am. J. Phys.* **58,** 365 (1922).
118. Franklin, E. C., and Bauman, A., *Am. J. Med.* **15,** 450 (1953).
119. Franklin, M., Bean, W. H., Paul, W. D., Routh, J. I., de la Huerga, J., and Popper, H., *J. Clin. Invest.* **30,** 729 (1951).
120. Frederickson, D. S., Loud, A. V., Hinkelman, B. T., Schneider, H. S., and Frantz, I. D., Jr., *J. Exp. Med.* **99,** 43 (1954).
121. Free, A. H., and Free, H. M., *Gastroenterology* **24,** 414 (1953).
122. Freeman, S., *Am. J. Physiol.* **164,** 792 (1951).
123. Fremont-Smith, K., Volwiler, W., and Wood, P. A., *J. Lab. Clin. Med.* **40,** 692 (1952).
124. Fuld, H., *Klin. Wochschr.* **12,** 1364 (1933).
125. Gabuzda, G. J. Jr., Eckhardt, R. D., and Davidson, C. S., *J. Clin. Invest.,* **31,** 1015 (1952).
126. Gabuzda, G. J., Jr., Phillips, G. B., and Davidson, C. S., *New Eng. J. Med.* **246,** 124 (1952).
127. Gabuzda, G. J., Jr., Traeger, H. S., and Davidson, C. S., *J. Clin. Invest.* **33,** 780 (1954).
128. Gaffney, G. W., Schreier, K., diFerrante, N., and Altman, K. I., *J. Biol. Chem.* **206,** 695 (1954).

129. Geill, T., *Nord. Med.* **19,** 1599 (1943).
130. Gellis, S. S., and Hsia, D. Y. Y., *New Eng. J. Med.* **249,** 400 (1953).
131. Geschwind, I. I., and Li, C. H., *Endocrinology* **50,** 226 (1952).
132. Giges, B., *J. Lab. Clin. Med.* **38,** 210 (1951).
133. Gilder, H., Redo, F., Burr, D., and Child, C. G., III, *J. Clin. Invest.* **33,** 555 (1954).
134. Giordano, A. S., and Winstead, M., *Am. J. Clin. Pathol.* **23,** 610 (1953).
135. Gitlow, S. E., Beyers, M. R., and Colmore, J. P., *J. Lab. Clin. Med.* **40,** 541 (1952).
136. Glazebrook, A. J., *Edinburgh Med. J.* **52,** 83 (1945).
137. Godfried, E. G., *Biochem. J.* **28,** 2056 (1934).
138. Goodman, R. D., *J. Lab. Clin. Med.* **40,** 531 (1952).
139. Goodman, R. D., and Kingsley, G. R., *J. Am. Med. Assoc.* **153,** 462 (1953).
140. Gordon, E. E., Freeman, S., and Farmer, C. J., *Federation Proc.* **11,** 56 (1952).
141. Graff, M. M., Greenspan, E. M., Lehman, I. R., and Holecheck, J. J., *J. Lab. Clin. Med.* **37,** 736 (1951).
142. Grassmann, W., Hannig, K., and Knedel, M., *Deut. med. Wochschr.* **76,** 333 (1951).
143. Gray, C. H., *The Bile Pigments,* New York, Wiley (1953).
144. Gray, C. H., *in* Williams, R. T., *The Biochemical Society (London) Symposium No. 12.* Cambridge, England, University Press (1954).
145. Gray, S. H., Probstein, J. G., and Heifetz, C. J., *Arch. Internal Med.* **67,** 805 (1941).
146. Greenman, L., *J. Biol. Chem.* **183,** 577 (1950).
147. Greenspan, E. M., *A.M.A. Arch. Internal Med.* **93,** 863 (1954).
148. Greenspan, E. M., *J. M. Sinai Hosp.* **21,** 270, 279 (1955).
149. Greenspan, E. M., and Dreiling, P. A., *Arch. Internal Med.* **91,** 474 (1953).
150. Greenspan, E. M., Tepper, B., Tepper, L. L., and Schoenbach, E. B., *J. Lab. Clin. Med.,* **39,** 44 (1952).
151. Grindlay, J. H., and Bollman, J. L., *Surg., Gynecol. Obstet.,* **94,** 491 (1952).
152. Gross, J. B., Comfort, M. W., Wollaeger, E. E., and Power, M. H., *Gastroenterology* **16,** 140 (1950a); **16,** 157 (1950b).
153. Gutman, A. R., and Hanger, F. M., *Med. Clin. North Amer.* **25,** 845 (1941).
154. Hanger, F. M., *J. Clin. Invest.* **18,** 261 (1939).
155. Hanger, F. M., *Trans. Assoc. Am. Physicians* **60,** 82 (1947).
156. Hare, M. L. C., *Biochem. J.* **22,** 968 (1928).
157. Harrington, W. J., Manheimer, R. H., Desforges, J. F., Minkel, H. P., Brocon, C. B., and Stohloon, F., *Bull. New Eng. Med. Center* **12,** 121 (1950).
158. Hartmann, F., *Z. klin. Med.* **147,** 551 (1951).
159. Havens, W. P., Jr., *Medicine* **11,** 279 (1948).
160. Havens, W. P., Jr., and Williams, T. L., *Acta Med. Scand.* **Suppl. 136,** 141 (1949).
161. Heller, P., Korn, R. J., and Zimmerman, H. J., *New Eng. J. Med.* **249,** 596 (1953).
162. Helve, O., *Acta Med. Scand.* **125,** 505 (1946).
163. Henry, C. J., Golub, O. J., Berkman, S., and Segalove, M., *Am. J. Clin. Pathol.* **23,** 841 (1953).
164. Hepler, O. E., and Gurley, H., *J. Lab. Clin. Med.* **27,** 1593 (1942).
165. Hijmans van den Bergh, A. A., and Müller, P., *Biochem. Z.* **77,** 90 (1916).
166. Hillman, R. W., *J. Lab. Clin. Med.* **34,** 1279 (1949).
167. Hoagland, C. L., and Shank, R. E., *J. Am. Med. Assoc.* **130,** 618 (1946).
168. Hoffbauer, F. W., Rames, E. D., and Meinert, J. K., *J. Lab. Clin. Med.* **34,** 1259 (1949).
169. Holly, H. L., and McLester, J. S., *J. Am. Med. Assoc.* **145,** 392 (1951).
170. Holmberg, C. G., and Laurell, C. B., *Acta Chem. Scand.* **1,** 944 (1947).
171. Howard, R. B., *J. Clin. Invest.* **29,** 824 (1950).
172. Howard, R. B., Balfour, W. M., and Cullen, R., *J. Lab. Clin. Med.* **43,** 848 (1954).
173. Hoyer, G., and Jorgensen, J., *Scand. J. Clin. & Lab. Invest.* **4,** 319 (1952).
174. Hsia, D. Y. Y., and Gellis, S. S., *J. Clin. Invest.* **33,** 1603 (1954).

175. Hsia, D. Y. Y., Hsia, H. H., and Gellis, S. S., *J. Lab. Clin. Med.* **40,** 610 (1952).
176. de la Huerga, H., and Popper, H., *J. Lab. Clin. Med.* **34,** 877 (1949).
177. de la, Huerga, H., Yesinick, C., and Popper, H., *Am. J. Clin. Pathol.* **23,** 1163 (1953).
178. Jacob, W., and Neuhaus, J., *Klin. Wochschr.* **32,** 923 (1954).
179. Jager, B. V., and Nickerson, M., *J. Biol. Chem.* **173,** 683 (1948).
180. Jennings, E. R., Cherney, P., and Zak, B., *Am. J. Clin. Pathol.* **23,** 1173 (1953).
181. Jones, C. M., *in* Panel on Liver Disease, *J. Am. Med. Assoc.* **158,** 116 (1955).
182. Karmen, A., Wróblewski, F., and La Due, J. S., *J. Clin. Invest.* **34,** 126 (1955).
183. Katz, E. J., Hasterlik, R. J., and Snapp, F. E., *J. Lab. Clin. Med.* **44,** 353 (1954).
184. Kibrick, A. C., Rodgers, H. E., and Skupp, S. J., *Am. J. Clin. Pathol.* **22,** 698 (1952).
185. Kimbel, K. H., *Klin. Wochschr.* **32,** 566 (1955).
186. Kimmel, J. R., Burns, T. W., Harper, H. A., Dirstine, P. H., and Higgins, A. R., *Gastroenterology* **26,** 723 (1954).
187. Kingsley, G. R., Getchell, G., and Schaffert, R. R., *in Standard Methods of Clinical Chemistry.* (M. Reiner, Ed.) New York, Acad. Press (1953), Vol. 1.
188. Kinsell, L. W., Harper, H. A., Barton, H. C., Hutchin, M. E., and Hess, J. R., *J. Clin. Invest.* **27,** 677 (1948).
189. Kinsell, L. W., Harper, H. A., Giese, G. K., Margen, S., and Hess, J. R., *J. Clin. Invest.* **28,** 1439 (1949b).
190. Kinsell, L. W., Michaels, G. D., Barton, H. C., and Weiss, H. A., *Ann. Internal Med.* **29,** 881 (1948).
191. Kinsell, L. W., Michaels, G. D., Weiss, H. A., and Barton, H. C., Jr., *Am. J. Med. Sci.* **217,** 554 (1949).
192. Kirk, E., *Amino Acid and Ammonia Metabolism in Liver Disease.* Copenhagen, Denmark (1936).
193. Kirsner, J. B., Sheffner, A. L., Palmer, W. L., and Bergeim, O., *J. Lab. Clin. Med.* **36,** 735 (1950).
194. Kitzes, G., Elvehjem, C. A., and Schuette, H. A., *J. Biol. Chem.* **155,** 653 (1944).
195. Klatskin, G., and Bungards, L., *New Eng. J. Med.* **248,** 712 (1953).
196. Klatskin, G., and Drill, V. A., *J. Clin. Invest.* **29,** 660 (1950).
197. Kleckner, M. S., Jr., Kark, R. M., Baker, L. A., Chapman, A. Z., and Kaplan, E., *J. Am. Med. Assoc.* **157,** 1471 (1955).
198. Klein, B., Gordon, B. S., and Graef, I., *Clin. Chem.* **1,** 118 (1955).
199. Knedel, M., *Med. Monatsschr.* **5,** 707 (1951).
200. Knisely, M. H., *in Transactions of the Tenth Conference on Liver Injury.* (F. W. Hoffbauer, Ed.) New York, Macy (1951).
201. Koch-Weser, D., de la Huerga, J., and Popper, H., *J. Lab. Clin. Med.* **24,** 49 (1951).
202. Kofman, S., Johnson, G. C., and Zimmerman, H. J., *A.M.A. Arch. Internal Med.* **95,** 669 (1955).
203. Kunkel, H. G., *Proc. Soc. Exp. Biol. Med.* **67,** 217 (1947).
204. Kunkel, H. G., Ahrens, E. H., and Eisenmenger, W. J., *Gastroenterology* **11,** 499 (1948).
205. Kunkel, H. G., Ahrens, E. H., Eisenmenger, W. J., Bongiovani, W. J., and Slater, E. J., *J. Clin. Invest.* **30,** 654 (1951).
206. Kunkel, H. G., and Hoagland, C. L., *J. Clin. Invest.* **26,** 1060 (1947).
207. Kunkel, H. G., Lably, D. H., and Hoagland, C. L., *Ann. Internal Med.* **27,** 202 (1947).
208. Kydd, D. M., and Man, E. B., *J. Clin. Invest.* **30,** 874 (1951).
209. Lamberg, B. A., and Gordin, R., *Acta Endocrinol.* **15,** 82 (1954). See also *Chem. Abstr.* **48,** 5364 (1954).
210. Landau, G., *Deut. med. Wochschr.* **79,** 948 (1954).
211. Lathe, G. H., *in* Williams, R. T., *The Biochemical Society (London) Symposium No. 12*, Cambridge, England, University Press (1954).

212. Latner, A. L., and Pendleton, G. B., *Biochem. J.* **44,** 32 (1949).
213. Lattanzi, A., *Riv. gastroenterol.* **2,** 311 (1950).
214. Lavers, G. D., Cole, W. H., Keeton, R. W., Kepart, M. C., and Syniewics, J. M., *J. Lab. Clin. Med.* **34,** 965 (1949).
215. Lemberg, R., and Legge, J. W. *Hematin Compounds and Bile Pigments.* New York, Interscience (1949).
216. Lewis, A. E., *Am. J. Clin. Pathol.* **18,** 789 (1948).
217. Lewis, A. E., *Am. J. Physiol.* **163,** 54 (1950).
218. Lewis, L. A., Page, I. H., and Thomas, C., *Am. J. Physiol.* **172,** 83 (1953).
219. Lichtman, S. S., *Am. J. Digest. Diseases Nutrition* **108,** April 1954.
220. Linder, H. K., Bruger, M., and Green, C. H., *N. Y. State J. Med.* **48,** 1371 (1948).
221. Lloyd, C. W., and Williams, R. H., *Am. J. Med.* **4,** 315 (1948).
222. Loftus, L. R., Huizenga, K. A., Stauffer, M. H., Rome, H. P., and Cain, J. C., *J. Am. Med. Assoc.* **157,** 1286 (1955).
223. Lorber, S., and Shay, H., *Gastroenterology* **20,** 262 (1952).
224. Lord, J. W., Jr., and Andrus, W. D., *Arch. Internal Med.* **68,** 199 (1941).
225. Luetscher, J. A., and Johnson, B. B., *J. Clin. Invest.* **33,** 1441 (1954).
226. McDermott, W. V., Jr., and Adams, R. D., *J. Clin. Invest.* **33,** 1 (1954).
227. McDermott, W. V., Jr., Adams, R. D., and Riddell, A. G., *Proc. Soc. Exp. Biol. Med.* **88,** 380 (1955).
228. Machella, T. E., Helm, J. D., and Chornock, F. W., *J. Clin. Invest.* **21,** 763 (1942).
229. McIver, M. A., *Surgery* **12,** 654 (1942).
230. Maclagan, N. F., *Brit. J. Exp. Pathol.* **25,** 234 (1944).
231. Maclagan, N. F., *Biochem. J.* **42,** xli (1948).
232. Maclagan, N. F., and Bunn, D., *Biochem. J.* **41,** 580 (1947).
233. Maclagan, N. F., *Brit. Med. J.* **2,** 197 (1947).
234. Maclagan, N. F., Martin, N. H., and Lunnon, J. G., *J. Clin. Pathol.* **5,** 1 (1952).
235. Maclagan, N. F., and Rundle, F. F., *Quart. J. Med.* **9,** 215 (1952).
236. McNee, J. W., *J. Pathol. Bacteriol.* **18,** 315 (1913).
237. Malloy, H. T., and Evelyn, K. A., *J. Biol. Chem.* **119,** 481 (1936).
238. Man, E. B., Kartin, B. L., Durlacher, S. H., and Peters, J. P., *J. Clin. Invest.* **24,** 623 (1945).
239. Mann, F. A., Shonzo, E. S., and Mann, F. C., *Am. J. Physiol.* **164,** 111 (1951).
240. Mann, F. C., *Am. J. Med. Sci.* **161,** 37 (1921).
241. Mann, F. C., *Medicine* **6,** 419 (1927).
242. Mann, J. D., Bollman, J. L., Huizenga, K. A., Farrar, T., and Grindlay, J. H., *Gastroenterology* **27,** 399 (1954).
243. Mann, J. D., Mandel, W. I., Eichmann, P. L., Knowlton, M. A., and Sborov, V. M., *J. Lab. Clin. Med.* **39,** 543 (1952).
244. Marrack, J. R., Johns, R. G. S., and Hoch, H., *Brit. J. Exp. Pathol.* **31,** 36 (1950).
245. Martin, N. H., *J. Am. Chem. Soc.* **71,** 1230 (1949).
246. Martin, N. H., *J. Clin. Pathol.* **2,** 275 (1949).
247. Martin, N. H., *in* Sherlock, S., and Wolstenholme, G. E. W., *Liver Disease,* Philadelphia, Blakiston (1951).
248. Martin, N. H., *Nature* **162,** 145 (1948).
249. Matassarin, B. M., and Delph, M. H., *Am. J. Med. Sci.* **224,** 622 (1952).
250. Mateer, J. G., Baltz, J. I., Comanduras, P. D., Steele, H. H., Brouwer, S. W., and Yagle, E. M., *Gastroenterology* **8,** 52 (1947).
251. Mateer, J. G., Baltz, J. L., Marion, D. F., and MacMillan, J. M., *J. Am. Med. Assoc.* **121,** 723 (1943).
252. Mellinkoff, S. M., and Tumulty, P. A., *New Eng. J. Med.* **247,** 745 (1953).
253. Mellinkoff, S. M., Tumulty, P. A., and Harvey, A. M., *New Eng. J. Med.* **246,** 729 (1952).

254. Mellinkoff, S. M., Venden, D. J., and Frankland, M., *A.M.A. Arch. Internal Med.* **94**, 604 (1954).
255. Mendeloff, A. I., *Bull. New Eng. Med. Center* **11**, 163 (1949a).
256. Mendeloff, A. I., *Proc. Soc. Exp. Biol. Med.* **70**, 556 (1949b).
257. Metcoff, J., Nobuyuki, N., and Rance, C. P., *J. Clin. Invest.* **33**, 665 (1954).
258. Meulengracht, E., *Deut. Ark. klin. Med.* **137**, 38 (1921).
259. Michel, H. O., *J. Lab. Clin. Med.* **34**, 1564 (1949).
260. Miller, L. L., American Gastroenterological Society 1953 Meeting, Atlantic City, N. J.
261. Miller, L. L., and Axelrod, L. R., *Metabolism, Clin. and Exp.* **3**, 438 (1954).
262. Miller, L. L., Bly, C. G., Watson, M. L., and Bale, L. F., *J. Exp. Med.* **94**, 431 (1951).
263. Mitchell, R. G., Butt, H. R., and Code, C. F., *J. Clin. Invest.* **33**, 1199 (1954).
264. Molander, D. W., Friedman, M. M., LaDue, J. S., *Ann. Internal Med.* **41**, 1139 (1954).
265. Moore, D. B., Pierson, D. S., Hanger, F. M., and Moore, D. H., *J. Clin. Invest.* **24**, 292 (1945).
266. Moreland, F. B., O'Donnell, W. W., and Gast, J. H., *Federation Proc.* **9**, 207 (1950).
267. Moses, C., *J. Lab. Clin. Med.* **30**, 267 (1945).
268. Moyer, J. H., and Wurl, O. A., *Am. J. Med. Sci.* **221**, 28 (1951).
269. Musser, M. J., Deiss, W. P., Jr., and Lorenz, T. H., *J. Lab. Clin. Med.* **45**, 357 (1955).
270. Nadeau, G., *Am. J. Clin. Pathol.* **24**, 740 (1954).
271. Najjar, V. A., *Pediatrics* **10**, 1 (1952).
272. Neefe, J. R., *Gastroenterology* **7**, 1 (1946).
273. Neefe, J. R., Gambescia, J. L., Gardner, H. T., and Knowlton, M., *Am. J. Med.* **5**, 600 (1952).
274. Neefe, J. R., Gambescia, J. M., Kurtz, C. H., Smith, H. D., Williams, S. C., Reinhold, J. G., Beebe, G., Jablon, S., and Lucke, M., *Ann. Internal Med.* In press (1955).
275. Neefe, J. R., and Reinhold, J. G., *Gastroenterology* **7**, 397 (1946).
276. Neefe, J. R., and Reinhold, J. G., *Science* **100**, 83 (1944).
277. Neefe, J. R., Stokes, J. H., Reinhold, J. G., and Lukens, F. W., *J. Clin. Invest.* **23**, 836 (1944).
278. Nelson, W. P., Rosenbaum, J. D., and Strauss, M. B., *J. Clin. Invest.* **30**, 738 (1951).
279. Neumayr, A., Parzer, O., and Vetter, H., *Deut. med. Wochschr.* **79**, 1039 (1954).
280. Nikkila, E., *Scand. J. Clin. & Lab. Invest.* **Suppl. to Vol. 5**, 25 (1953).
281. Nolf, P., and Adant, M., *Le Sang* **22**, 257 (1951).
282. Norcross, J. W., White, R. M., and Bradley, R. J., *Am. J. Med. Sci.* **221**, 137 (1951).
283. Ottenberg, R. W., Wagreich, H., Bernstein, A., and Harrow, B., *Arch. Biochem.* **2**, 63 (1943).
284. Owen, C. A., Jr., *J. Lab. Clin. Med.* **38**, 583 (1951).
285. Parnas, J. K., and Klisiecki, A., *Biochem. Z.* **173**, 224 (1926).
286. Patek, A. J., Jr., Segal, D., and Bevans, M., *Am. J. Med. Sci.* **221**, 77 (1951).
287. Persky, H., Grinker, R. R., and Mirsky, I. A., *J. Clin. Invest.* **29**, 110 (1950).
288. Peters, T. Jr., and Apt, L., *Clin. Res. Proc.* **3**, 93 (1955).
289. Peterson, R. E., *J. Lab. Clin. Med.* **39**, 225 (1952).
290. Peterson, R. E., Guerra, S., and Sborov, V., *J. Lab. Clin. Med.* **43**, 59 (1954).
291. Peterson, U. P., *Acta Med. Scand.* **144**, 333, 345 (1953).
292. Pierce, F. T., Jr., and Gofman, J. W. *Circulation* **4**, 25 (1951).
293. Popper, H., *in Transactions Ninth Conference on Liver Injury.* (F. W. Hoffbauer, Ed.) New York, Macy (1951).
294. Popper, H., *Am. J. Med.* **16**, 98 (1954).
295. Popper, H., and Rosenbaum, J. D., *J. Lab. Clin. Med.* **40**, 523 (1952).
296. Popper, H., and Schaffner, F. W., *J. Am. Med. Assoc.* **150**, 1367 (1952).
297. Popper, H., Steigman, F., Dyniewicz, H., and Dubin, A., *J. Lab. Clin. Med.* **33**, 1630 (1948).
298. Proffitt, B. K., and Morrison, D. B., *Federation Proc.* **8**, 239 (1949).

299. Quick, A. J., *Am. J. Med. Sci.* **185,** 630 (1933).
300. Quick, A. J., *Am. J. Clin. Pathol.* **10,** 222 (1940).
301. Ralli, E. P., Leslie, S. H., Stueck, G. H. Jr., and Laken, B. *Am. J. Med.* **11,** 1579 (1951).
302. Ralli, E. P., Leslie, S. H., Stueck, G. H. Jr., Shorr, H. E., Robson, J. S., Clarke, D. H., and Laken, B., *Medicine* **28,** 301 (1949).
303. Ratnoff, O. D., *J. Lab. Clin. Med.* **42,** 933 (1953).
304. Ravdin, I. S., Johnston, C. G., Reigel, C., and Wright, S. L., *J. Clin. Invest.* **12,** 659 (1933).
305. Recant, L., *J. Lab. Clin. Med.* **44,** 917 (1954).
306. Reinhold, J. G., *The Clinical Chemist* **5,** 82 (1953).
307. Reinhold, J. G., *in* Reiner, M., *Standard Methods of Clinical Chemistry.* New York, Acad. Press (1953).
308. Reinhold, J. G., *Clin. Chem.* **1,** 3 (1955).
309. Reinhold, J. G., and Fowler, C. B., *J. Biol. Chem.* **167,** 401 (1947).
310. Reinhold, J. G., and Gentzkow, C. J., *in* Simmons, J. S., and Gentzkow, C. J., *Laboratory Methods; Public Health and General.* Philadelphia, Lea & Febiger (1955).
311. Reinhold, J. G., Rawnsley, H. M., and Yonan, V. L., *Proceedings of the Third International Congress of Biochemistry*, Brussels, Belgium, 1955.
311a. Reinhold, J. G., Tourigny, L. G., and Yonan, V., *Am. J. Clin. Pathol.* **23,** 645 (1953).
312. Rhees, M. C., Ellerbrook, L. D., and Lippincott, S. W., *Am. J. Clin. Pathol.* **24,** 774 (1954).
313. Ricketts, W. E., *Am. J. Med. Sci.* **221,** 287 (1951).
314. Ricketts, W. E., *Gastroenterology* **23,** 391 (1953).
315. Ricketts, W. E., Kirsner, J. B., Palmer, W. L., *Gastroenterology* **16,** 404 (1950).
316. Riddell, A. G., and McDermott, W. V., *Lancet* **1,** 263 (1954).
317. Roberts, S., *J. Biol. Chem.* **200,** 77 (1953).
318. Roberts, S., and Brunish, R., *Federation Proc.* **12,** 259 (1953).
319. Roberts, W. M., *Brit. Med. J.* **1,** 734 (1933).
320. Robertson, T., *Am. J. Med.* **9,** 315 (1950).
321. Roche, J., and Sarles, H., *Bull. soc. chim. biol.* **36,** 501 (1954).
322. Rosenberg, D. H., and Soskin, S., *Am. J. Digest. Diseases* **8,** 421 (1941).
323. Rosenman, R. H., Friedman, M., and Byers, S., *Federation Proc.* **11,** 132 (1952).
324. Rosenthal, O., Fahl, J. C., and Vars, H. M., *Am. J. Physiol.* **171,** 604 (1952).
325. Rosenthal, S. M., and White, E. C., *J. Am. Med. Assoc.* **84,** 112 (1925).
326. Rothman, M. M., Meranze, D. R., and Meranze, T., *Am. J. Med. Sci.* **192,** 526 (1936).
327. Saifer, A., *Am. J. Med.* **13,** 730 (1952).
328. Saifer, A., *J. Clin. Invest.* **27,** 737 (1948).
329. Saltzman, A., and Caraway, W. T., *J. Clin. Invest.* **32,** 711 (1953).
330. Satoskar, R. S., Lewis, R. A., and Gaitonde, B. B., *J. Lab. Clin. Med.* **44,** 349 (1954).
331. Schachter, D., and Taggart, J. V., *J. Biol. Chem.* **203,** 925 (1953).
332. Schedl, H. P., Ditto, K., and Bean, W. B., *J. Lab. Clin. Med.* **42,** 116 (1953).
333. Scheinberg, I. H., and Gitlin, D., *Science* **116,** 484 (1952).
334. Schneider, E. M., Berman, J. R., Gall, E. A., and Schiff, L., *Am. J. Med.* **15,** 207 (1953).
335. Schreier, K., *Deut. med. Wochschr.* **76,** 868 (1951).
336. Schwartz, R., Phillips, G. B., Gabuzda, G. J., and Davidson, C. S., *J. Lab. Clin. Med.* **42,** 499 (1953).
337. Schwartz, R., Phillips, G. B., Seegmiller, J. E., Gabuzda, G. J., and Davidson, C. S., *New Eng. J. Med.* **251,** 685 (1954).
338. Schwartz, S., Sborov, V., and Watson, C. J., *Am. J. Clin. Pathol.* **14,** 598 (1944).
339. Schwartz, S., Zieve, L., and Watson, C. J., *J. Lab. Clin. Med.* **37,** 843 (1951).
340. Seligson, D. L., *in* H. R. Butt, *Panel on Hepatic Coma*, American Gastroenterological Association, 1953.

341. Seligson, D. L., McCormick, G. J., and Sborov, V., *J. Clin. Invest.* **31**, 661 (1952).
342. Selman, D., *Gastroenterology* **22**, 244 (1952).
343. Sérégé, H., *J. med. Bordeaux* **31**, 271, 291, 312 (1901). Cited by Wakim.
344. Shank, R. E., and Hoagland, C. L., *J. Biol. Chem.* **162**, 133 (1946).
345. Shapiro, S., and Richards, R. K., *Ann. Internal Med.* **22**, 841 (1945).
346. Sharnoff, J. G., Budnick, M., and Jakab, G., *Am. J. Clin. Pathol.* **21**, 234 (1951).
347. Shay, H., Berk, J. E., and Siplet, H., *Gastroenterology* **9**, 644 (1947).
348. Shay, H., and Siplet, H., *J. Lab. Clin. Med.* **43**, 741 (1954).
349. Sherlock, S., and Walshe, V., *Clin. Sci.* **6**, 223 (1948).
350. Sherlock, S., and Walshe, V., *J. Pathol. Bacteriol.* **59**, 615 (1947).
351. Shore, M. L., and Zilversmit, D. B., *Federation Proc.* **12**, 131 (1953).
352. Shorr, E., Zweifach, B. W., Furchgott, R. F., and Baez, S., *Circulation* **3**, 42 (1951).
353. Simons, R. L., *Am. J. Med. Sci.* **228**, 312 (1954).
354. Sjöström, P. M., *Acta Chir. Scand.* **77**, 505 (1936).
355. Sjöström, P. M., *Acta Chir. Scand.* **Suppl. 49** (1937).
356. Smith, L. H., Ettinger, R. H., and Seligson, D., *J. Clin. Invest.* **32**, 273 (1953).
357. Snapper, I. H., and Saltzman, A., *Arch. Biochem.* **24**, 1 (1949).
358. Snell, A. M., and Roth, G. M., *J. Clin. Invest.* **11**, 957 (1932).
359. Sobotka, H., Luisada-Opper, A. V., and Reiner, M., *Am. J. Clin. Pathol.* **23**, 607 (1953).
360. Sperry, W. M., and Brand, F. C., *J. Biol. Chem.* **213**, 68 (1955).
361. Sperry, W. M., and Webb, M., *J. Biol. Chem.* **187**, 97 (1950).
362. Stefanini, M., *Am. J. Med.* **14**, 64 (1953).
363. Stefanini, M., *Federation Proc.* **8**, 255 (1949).
364. Stein, W. H., Bearn, A. G., and Moore, S., *J. Clin. Invest.* **33**, 410 (1954).
365. St. George, S., and Friedman, M., *Federation Proc.* **14**, 146 (1955).
366. Strub, I. H., Talso, P. J., and Kirsner, J. B., *Gastroenterology* **28**, 163 (1955).
367. Stumpf, H. H., and Liber, A. F., *Am. J. Med.* **17**, 887 (1954).
368. Stutzman, F. L., and Amatuzio, D. S., *J. Lab. Clin. Med.* **41**, 215 (1953).
369. Swift, W. E., Miller, W. N., Streitfield, F. H., and Knowlton, M., *Am. J. Med.* **8**, 581 (1950).
370. Tallach, J. A., and Sherlock, S., *Brit. Med. J.* **2**, 212 (1954).
371. Teilum, G., *Am. J. Pathol.*, **24**, 389, 489 (1948).
372. Thomas, L. J., and Zimmerman, H. J., *J. Lab. Clin. Med.* **39**, 882 (1952).
373. Traeger, H. S., Gabuzda, G. J., Jr., Ballou, A. N., and Davidson, C. S., *Metabolism, Clin. and Exp.* **3**, 99 (1954).
374. Ulevitch, H., Gall, E. A., Hoxworth, P. I., Schiff, V., and Craller, D. L., *J. Lab. Clin. Med.* **38**, 693 (1951).
375. Uzman, L., and Denny-Brown, D., *Am. J. Med. Sci.* **215**, 599 (1948).
376. Ventura, S., *J. Clin. Pathol.* **5**, 271 (1952).
377. Viollier, G., *Helv. Med. Acta* **17**, 354 (1950).
378. Vogel, F. S., *J. Exp. Med.* **98**, 509 (1953).
379. Voight, G., *Klin. Wochschr.* **29**, 356 (1951).
380. Vorhaus, L. U., and Kark, R. M., *Am. J. Med.* **14**, 707 (1953).
381. Wagreich, H., Bernstein, A., Pader, M., and Harrow, B., *Proc. Soc. Exp. Biol. Med.* **46**, 582 (1941).
382. Waife, S. O., Brenner, L. O., and Thompson, C. M., *Gastroenterology* **17**, 236 (1951).
383. Wakim, K. G., *Am. J. Med.* **14**, 256 (1954).
384. Wald, M. H., *J. Lab. Clin. Med.* **44**, 946 (1954).
385. Walsh, J. R., Humoller, F. L., and Zimmerman, H. J., *J. Lab. Clin. Med.* **45**, 253 (1955).
386. Walshe, J. M., *Quart. J. Med.* **22**, 483 (1953).
387. Walshe, J. M., and Senior, B., *J. Clin. Invest.* **34**, 302 (1955).
388. Wang, I., *Brit. Med. J.* **2**, 471 (1953).

389. Waterlow, J., Transactions of the Eleventh Conference on Liver Injury. (F. C. Hoffbauer, Ed.) New York, Macy (1953).
390. Watson, C. J., *Blood* **1,** 99 (1946).
391. Watson, C. J., and Hawkinson, V., *Am. J. Clin. Pathol.* **17,** 108 (1947).
392. Watson, C. J., and Hawkinson, V., *J. Lab. Clin. Med.* **31,** 914 (1946).
393. Watson, C. J., Hawkinson, V., and Bossemaier, I., *Arch. Internal Med.* **93,** 643 (1954).
394. Watson, C. J., Hawkinson, V., Capps, R. B., and Rappaport, A. M., *J. Clin. Invest.* **28,** 621 (1949).
395. Watson, C. J., and Hoffbauer, F. G., *Ann. Internal Med.* **25,** 195 (1946).
396. Watson, C. J., Lowry, P., Collins, S., Graham, A., and Ziegler, N. R., *Trans. Assoc. Am. Physicians* **67,** 242 (1954).
397. Watson, C. J., Pimenta de Mello, R., Schwartz, S., and Hawkinson, V., *J. Lab. Clin. Med.* **38,** 831 (1951).
398. Watson, C. J., Schwartz, S., Sborov, V., and Bertie, E., *Am. J. Clin. Pathol.* **14,** 605 (1944).
399. Watson, C. J., Schwartz, S., Schulz, W., Jacobson, L. A., and Zagaria, R., *J. Clin. Invest.* **28,** 465 (1949).
400. Watson, C. J., Sutherland, D., and Hawkinson, V., *J. Lab. Clin. Med.* **37,** 8 (1951).
401. West, C. D., *Endocrinology* **49,** 467 (1951).
402. West, C. D., *J. Clin. Endocrinol.* **11,** 897 (1951).
403. Whipple, G. H., and Hooper, C. W., *J. Exp. Med.* **17,** 593 (1913).
404. White, F. D., and Duncan, D., *Can. J. Med. Sci.* **30,** 552 (1952).
405. White, L. P., Phear, E. A., Sherlock, S. P. V., and Summerskill, W. H. J., *J. Clin. Invest.* **34,** 158 (1955).
406. Wilson, A., Calvert, R. J., and Geoghagan, H., *J. Clin. Invest.* **31,** 815 (1952).
407. Wolfson, W. Q., Cohn, C., Calvery, E., and Zebuta, F., *Am. J. Clin. Pathol.* **18,** 733 (1948).
408. Wootton, I. D. P., King, E. J., and Maclean-Smith, J., *Brit. Med. Bull.* **7,** 307 (1951).
409. Wroblewski, F., and LaDue, J. S., *J. Lab. Clin. Med.* **44,** 958 (1954).
410. Yonan, V. L., and Reinhold, J. G., *Am. J. Clin. Pathol.* **24**. 232 (1954).
411. Zatuchni, J., and Miller, G., *New Eng. J. Med.* **251,** 1003 (1954).
412. Zelman, S., *Arch. Internal Med.* **90,** 141 (1952).
413. Zieve, L., *J. Lab. Clin. Med.* **42,** 134 (1953).
414. Zieve, L., and Hanson, M., *J. Lab. Clin. Med.* **42,** 872 (1953).
415. Zieve, L., Hanson, M., and Hill, E., *J. Lab. Clin. Med.* **37,** 40 (1951).
416. Zieve, L., and Hill, E., *J. Lab. Clin. Med.* **42,** 705 (1953).
417. Zieve, L., Hill, E., Hanson, M., Falcone, A. B., and Watson, C. J., *J. Lab. Clin. Med.* **38,** 446 (1951).
418. Zieve, L., Hill, E., and Nesbitt, S., *J. Lab. Clin. Med.* **36,** 705 (1950).
419. Zilversmit, D. B., and Davis, A. K., *J. Lab. Clin. Med.* **35,** 155 (1950).
420. Zilversmit, D. B., and Shore, M. L., *Proc. Soc. Exp. Biol. Med.* **86,** 442 (1954).
421. Zimmerman, H. J., Heller, P., and Hill, R. P., *New Eng. J. Med.* **244,** 245 (1951).

Addenda

Bassir, O., and Hall, J., *Biochem. J.* **60,** XX (1955).
Bollman, J. L., and Mann, F. D., *Am. J. Physiol.* **92,** 92 (1930).
Brauer, R. W., Pessotti, R. L., and Krebs, J. S., *J. Clin. Invest.* **34,** 35 (1955).
Byers, S. O., Friedman, M., and Michaelis, F., *J. Biol. Chem.* **188,** 637 (1951).
Friedman, M., and Byers, S. O., *J. Clin. Invest.* **34,** 1369 (1955).
Kassouny, D. Y., Norris, R. F., Reinhold, J. G., and Neefe, J. R. To be published.
LaDue, J. S., Wróblewski, F., and Karmen, A., *Science* **120,** 497 (1954).
Mandel, E. E., Gorsuch, T. L., and Cooper, G. E., *Clin. Chem.* **1,** 221 (1955).

Murphy, T. L., Chalmers, T. C., Eckhardt, R. D., and Davidson, C. S., *New England J. Med.* **239,** 605 (1949).
Myers, J. D., Brannon, E. S., and Holland, B. C., *J. Clin. Invest.* **29,** 1069 (1950).
Nelson, R. M., and Seligson, D., *Surgery* **34,** 1 (1953).
Shetlar, M. R., *Anal. Chem.* **24,** 1844 (1952).
Schulz, F. H., *Das Fibrinogen: Seine Bestimmung, seine physiologischen und pathologischen Veranderungen, seine biologische Bedeutung, und seine Entstehungsort,* Leipzig, Germany, Thieme, (1953).
Shinowara, G. Y., *Am. J. Clin. Path.* **24,** 696 (1954).
Shutkin, M. W., and Caine, D., *Am. J. Gastroenterol.* **23,** 235 (1955).
Pierce, F. T., Jr., Kimmel, J. R., Burns, T. W., *Metabolism, Clin. and Exp.* **3,** 229 (1954).

Erratum

On page 320 (Vol. 1, 1955), the second and third sentences in the last paragraph should read, "It is interesting that most of the values are quite low. Among the few high values is Number 8, a man about 45 years old who proved to be an alcoholic and may have had some liver dysfunction."

the Clinical Chemist

MINUTES OF THE MEETING OF THE AACC EXECUTIVE COMMITTEE

The National Executive Committee of the American Association of Clinical Chemists met in Minneapolis, Minn., on September 14, 1955. Those present were: Otto Schales (President), Max M. Friedman (National Secretary), Louis B. Dotti (National Treasurer), Monroe E. Freeman, Joseph H. Gast, Samuel Natelson, Margaret M. Kaser (Alternate for Icie M. Hoobler), Joseph I. Routh (Alternate for William G. Goldwater), Hugh J. McDonald (by invitation), Albert E. Sobel (by invitation), and David Seligson (by invitation).

Appointments

Committees of the Association were continued, with the following new appointments:

Program Committee: Joseph H. Gast, Chairman.

Standard Methods: David Seligson, Chairman; Joseph H. Gast, Margaret M. Kaser, Miriam Reiner, John G. Reinhold, and Joseph I. Routh.

Clinical Chemistry

Harold D. Appleton submitted a statement on behalf of the Board of Editors of CLINICAL CHEMISTRY. Manuscripts are being received in such quality and quantity that there is no problem in meeting the present page allotments. Thought is already being given to the expansion of the present journal. Advertising support is encouraging, and as of September 1, 1955, subscriptions have exceeded 2100.

Louis B. Dotti submitted a Treasurer's report showing a substantial increase in assets since one year ago. The report which follows does not include royalties for 1955 accruing from CLINICAL CHEMISTRY. The items for the Association's former publication, *The Clinical Chemist* refer to the last three issues in 1954.

Treasurer's Report

JULY 1, 1954 TO JUNE 30, 1955

Income

Membership dues	$6602.12
Royalties from Academic Press	303.42
Bank interest	71.04
Directory	90.00
The Clinical Chemist	350.42
Membership certificates	32.00
Subscriptions to CLINICAL CHEMISTRY	15.20
TOTAL	$7464.20

Expenses

CLINICAL CHEMISTRY subscriptions	$3600.00
CLINICAL CHEMISTRY	125.75
The Clinical Chemist	1399.70
Section allotments	257.60
Certificates	5.10
Directory	166.86
National Secretary	389.96
National Treasurer	106.40
Membership Committee	91.85

Subscriptions to CLINICAL CHEMISTRY		15.40
Refund to members		67.60
TOTAL		$6226.22
Total income	$7464.20	
Total expenses	6226.22	
Balance	$1237.98	
Bank balance July 1, 1954	2518.13	
Bank balance July 1, 1955	$3756.11	

Ernst Bischoff Award

The Executive Committee recommended that nominations for the Ernst Bischoff Award be expedited by requiring the nominator to give only a brief resume of the nominee, including only his important contributions. It was felt that heretofore members refrained from submitting nominations because of the amount of time required. It was also recommended that a nomination may be renewed for a following year merely upon the request of the nominator.

International Participation

Monroe E. Freeman, the Association's representative to the Commission on Clinical Chemistry and the International Federation of Clinical Chemistry, reported on the Commission meetings in Zurich, Switzerland, July 21–27, 1955.

Albert E. Sobel discussed the plans for the International Congress on Clinical Chemistry to be held in New York City during the week of September 9, 1956, under the auspices of the American Association of Clinical Chemists. Approval was given for making available the sum of $3000.00 for expenses incidental to the International Congress, these funds to be released at the discretion of the National Treasurer. It was moved, seconded, and passed that Sobel be authorized to appoint all the necessary committees for the International Congress, subject to approval by the President of the Association.

Standard Methods

David Seligson reported for the Editorial Committee of *Standard Methods*. This committee had met the previous evening and submitted a prospectus for Volume II. After detailed discussion of the form that *Standard Methods* should take, the Executive Committee voted that the series be composed of individual volumes, rather than continuous revised editions.

David Seligson also reported on the project of standard samples, to be carried out by the same editorial committee. It was proposed that a study be made to establish standard samples for certified constituents, this certification to be made by the American Association of Clinical Chemists. It was further proposed that secondary standards be established for such methods as required turbidity measurements. This study would assemble data for statistical variations and "normal" ranges and correlate them with *Standard Methods*. Various sources of financial support were indicated.

Investment Program and Budget Committee

It was moved, seconded, and approved that the Association purchase a $500.00 savings bond as a start for an investment program. It was also voted that the National Treasurer be bonded for $10,000, to conform with legal requirements.

It was moved, seconded, and passed that a budget committee be appointed, this committee to approve all expenditures not previously allocated by the Executive Committee. This budget committee will consist of Louis B. Dotti, Max M. Friedman, and one additional member yet to be designated.

Membership and Dues

It was moved, seconded, and passed that the Executive Committee recommend to the membership that dues for 1956 be kept at $11.00 for members and $7.50 for associate members. (This was subsequently voted at the membership meeting held on September 15, 1955.)

Since the dues of associate members are below the subscription rates of the journal they receive, and furthermore part of those dues is returned as section allotments, it was moved, seconded, and passed that beginning with January 1, 1958, those associate members who will have been at that time associate members for a period of 4 years shall be assessed full member dues. After that date *newly elected* associate members shall be permitted 4 years at the reduced dues. Assessment to full member dues shall not be construed as promotion to full membership.

MAX M. FRIEDMAN
National Secretary

SEVENTH ANNUAL MEETINGS

The annual meetings of the American Association of Clinical Chemists in Minneapolis were held September 12–16, 1955, in conjunction with the meetings of the American Chemical Society. The program and accounts of the sessions have been detailed in recent issues of *Chemical and Engineering News*.

There were 195 papers given in the Division of Biological Chemistry, most of which were of interest also to clinical chemists. Also included were two sessions devoted to clinical chemistry and a symposium on "Newer Techniques Applicable in Clinical Chemistry."

The social highlight, as usual, was the annual dinner at which Otto Schales, President of the AACC, presented the Ernst Bischoff Award.

The exact attendance at the seventh annual meetings is not known, since registration was through the American Chemical Society, but the large numbers who attended the sessions on clinical chemistry attest to the increasing interest in this chemical specialty.

ERNST BISCHOFF AWARD

The fourth Ernst Bischoff Award was presented at the annual dinner of the Association in Minneapolis, Minn., on September 15, 1955. The recipient was Michael X. Sullivan, Professor of Biochemistry at Georgetown University, Washington, D. C. The ceremonies were presided over by Otto Schales, President of the AACC, and

Sullivan was cited "for his contributions to clinical chemistry as the author of numerous analytical methods in the field of biochemistry, for his devoted efforts in the instruction and education of biochemists, and for his contributions to the progress of the knowledge of proteins and especially of sulfur compounds."

Doctor Sullivan accepted the Award with an address on "Highly Specific Tests in Clinical Chemistry." This was enthusiastically received by an audience that included several of his former students.

The Ernst Bischoff Award is given annually by the American Association of Clinical Chemists to a scientist for his outstanding contributions to clinical chemistry. The Award consists of a scroll, a medal, and an honorarium of $500.00. The recipient is selected by the Honorary Members of the Association from a list of nominees submitted by the membership at large.

Members are urged to forward nominations as soon as possible for the 1956 Ernst Bischoff Award, which will be presented during the International Congress in New York City to be held during the week of September 9, 1956. The brief should be sent in triplicate, typewritten, to Professor Joseph H. Roe, George Washington University, School of Medicine, Washington, D. C.

ASSOCIATE MEMBERS

The minutes of the Executive Committee meeting in Minneapolis includes a change of the dues status of associate members, to begin on January 1, 1958. The dues for that membership category are now less than the subscription to the Association's journal, which all members receive, and part of the dues is returned to the local section as section allotments.

After January 1, 1958, an associate member will be permitted 4 years of reduced dues, following which the dues will be the same as for full members. At that date this regulation will become retroactive for all members.

Increase of dues to full membership rates shall not be construed as promotion to full membership. An associate member may at any time request upgrading by writing to the Committee on Membership to that effect and submitting, in justification of such a request, data additional to those concerning the original application. The national office does not have the facilities for automatic periodic review of the status of all members as has been suggested. It therefore becomes the responsibility of each associate member individually to request such a review.

Any associate member desiring such a change in status should address a communication to that effect to Dr. Harry Sobotka, The Mount Sinai Hospital, New York 29, N. Y. A list of requirements for full membership will be sent on request.

INTERNATIONAL CONGRESS ON CLINICAL CHEMISTRY

Plans are now moving ahead in preparation for the International Congress on Clinical Chemistry to be held in New York City during the week of September 9, 1956. A large and enthusiastic audience is anticipated. This will be the first opportunity for clinical chemists from abroad to visit the United States during a formal conclave on clinical chemistry. There will be the added advantage in that the American Chemical Society meetings are to be held in Atlantic City during the week of September 16, 1956. This will permit attendance at both meetings with little additional travel expense.

At this writing it is not yet possible to give the details of the program for the International Congress. There will, however, be several days of scientific sessions, and chemists are advised to submit abstracts as soon as possible. Symposia are being organized by invitation. A social and ladies' program will of course be included.

NEWS FROM THE SECTIONS

Chicago Section

The present officers of the Chicago Section are as follows:

Chairman: A. Dubin (Director of Chemistry, Hektoen Institute, Cook County Hospital)

Vice-Chairman: G. S. Stewart (Department of Biochemistry, Presbyterian Hospital)

Secretary: H. Feinberg (Cardiovascular Department, Medical Research Institute, Michael Reese Hospital)

Treasurer: A. Kaplan (Department of Biochemistry, Medical Research Institute, Michael Reese Hospital)

Executive Committee at Large:

C. Chen (Department of Biochemistry, Northwestern Medical School)

H. J. McDonald (Department of Biochemistry, Stritch School of Medicine, Loyola University)

H. F. Weisberg (Department of Biochemistry, Mt. Sinai Hospital)

Midwest Section

As prescribed by Section By-Laws, an election of officers was held in the Midwest Section at the last meeting of the spring session. The new officers for the coming year are:

Chairman: Robert L. Dryer

Vice Chairman and Program Director: Kurt M. Dubowski

Secretary-Treasurer: Robert S. Melville

Throughout this past year the Section held meetings at various locations, including the Mayo Clinic in Rochester, Minn., the State Univesity of Iowa in Iowa City, and the Medical Associates Clinic in Dubuque, Iowa.

Of outstanding interest was the first Annual Instrument Clinic and demonstration held at the State University of Iowa on March 31 and April 1. A wide variety of instruments and equipment of optical, physiological, microchemical, radioisotopic, and general analytical interest was displayed.

Plans are being made for even more extensive clinics to be held in the future. The purpose of these clinics is to acquaint workers in various fields with available instruments and to give them an opportunity to discuss their problems with the appropriate technical representatives of the instrument industry.

The American Association of Clinical Chemists

Program of the Annual Meeting

To Be Held in Conjunction with the National Meetings of the American Association for the Advancement of Science, Atlanta, Georgia

December 26, 1955, 2 p.m., Dixie Ballroom, Henry Grady Hotel

Symposium: **Recent Concepts in Clinical Chemistry**

ALBERT E. SOBEL, *Presiding*

1. Opening Remarks. ALBERT E. SOBEL, The Jewish Hospital of Brooklyn, Brooklyn, N. Y.
2. Role of the Clinical Chemist in the Hospital. JOSEPH H. GAST, Baylor University, College of Medicine, Houston, Texas
3. New Concepts in Acid-Base Balance. SAMUEL NATELSON, Rockford Memorial Hospital, Rockford, Ill.
4. Studies on Lipid Metabolism. D. B. ZILVERSMIT, Department of Physiology, University of Tennessee, Memphis, Tenn.
5. Blood Proteins. HENRY G. KUNKEL, Rockefeller Institute for Medical Research, New York, N. Y.

AACC Dinner

7 p.m., Dixie Ballroom, Henry Grady Hotel

December 27, 1955, 9 a.m., Room B, Henry Grady Hotel

Analytical Methods

I. J. GREENBLATT, *Presiding*

1. The Use of Infrared Spectroscopy in Clinical Chemistry. DIETRICH E. BEISCHER, U.S. Naval School of Aviation Medicine, Pensacola, Fla.
2. Cyanomethemoglobin "Certified Hemoglobinometry Standards" as a Reference in Other Spectrophotometric Procedures. EUGENE W. RICE, Clinical Laboratories, Presbyterian and Women's Hospitals, and Department of Pathology, School of Medicine, University of Pittsburgh, Pittsburgh, Pa.
3. An Ultra Micro Method for the Determination of Proteins in Biological Fluids. GEORGE R. KINGSLEY and GLORIA GETCHELL, Department of Physiological Chemistry, School of Medicine, University of California at Los Angeles, and the Clinical Biochemistry Laboratory, Veterans Administration Center, Los Angeles, California.
4. The Effect of High Salt Concentration on Color Production of the Protein-Biuret Reaction. HAROLD L. ROSENTHAL and TOYOKO

KAWAKAMI, Division of Chemistry, Clinical and Pathological Laboratories, Rochester General Hospital, Rochester, N. Y.

5. A Simplified and Safer Urea Determination. AARON S. GOLDBERG, Department of Chemistry, Bronx Hospital, New York, N. Y.
6. A Simplified Device for the Estimation of Urea. R. L. DRYER, J. I. ROUTH, and A. R. TAMMES, Clinical Biochemistry Laboratory, State University of Iowa, Iowa City, Iowa.
7. The Distribution of C^{14}-Labeled Salicylic Acids in Animal Tissues. R. W. KNOUSE, J. I. ROUTH, and W. D. PAUL, Clinical Biochemistry Laboratory, State University of Iowa, Iowa City, Iowa.

December 27, 1955, 2 p.m., Room B, Henry Grady Hotel

Metabolism and Analytical Methods

SAMUEL NATELSON, *Presiding*

8. The Determination of Oxalate in Urine. ESTELLE R. HAUSMAN, JOHN S. MCANALLY, and GEORGE T. LEWIS, Department of Biochemistry, School of Medicine, University of Miami, Coral Gables, Fla.
9. Glycogenesis in the Liver Following Parenteral Administration of Fructose, Glucose, and Invert Sugar. JOSEPH H. ROE, ROBERT W. LONGLEY, and OLAF ALVIG, Department of Biochemistry, School of Medicine, George Washington University, Washington, D. C.
10. Elevation of Rabbit Blood Glycogen Following Parenteral Prednisone. I. J. GREENBLATT, A. S. WATNICK, R. WAYNE, and H. ALBAUM, Beth-El Hospital, and Brooklyn College, Brooklyn, N. Y.
11. Vitamin A Absorption in Mongolism. ALBERT E. SOBEL, M. STRAZZULIA, B. S. SHERMAN, B. ELKAN, S. W. MORGENSTERN, N. MARIUS, and A. MEISEL, Departments of Biochemistry and Pediatrics, The Jewish Hospital of Brooklyn, Brooklyn, N. Y.
12. Serum Iron in Liver Disease. EMANUEL E. MANDEL and LEONA NIESPODZANY, The Chicago Medical School, Chicago, Ill., and the Communicable Disease Center, U. S. Public Health Service, Atlanta, Ga.
13. The System of Analysis on the Essential Blood Electrolytes and Distribution of Sodium and Potassium in Plasma and Erythrocytes. V. M. SYCHEFF, The French Hospital Clinical Laboratory, San Francisco, Calif.
14. A Comparative Study of the Estimation of Vitamin B_{12}. H. BAKER, H. SOBOTKA, I. PASHER, and S. H. HUTNER, The Mount Sinai Hospital, Department of Chemistry, and Haskins Laboratory, New York, N. Y.

Index to Volume 1

Abnormalities in blood clotting, in liver disease, 379
Absorption, fat, 98
Adlersberg, David: Electrophoresis and Monomolecular Layer Studies with Serum Lipoproteins, 18
Akerson, Irving B., see Gottfried, S. P.
Albumin, serum, denaturation of, 181
American Board of Clinical Chemistry, 137, 277
Amylase: Turbidimetric method, 159
A New Journal: Appleton, H. D., 1
A Note on Quantitative Urobilinogen Determinations: Balikov, B., 264
Anderson, J. T., see Keys, A.
Appleton, Harold D.: A New Journal, 1
A Practical Manual of Medical and Biological Staining Techniques: Gurr, E. (Book Review), 81
Arginase: Blood, method, 110
Balikov, Bernard: A Note on Quantitative Urobilinogen Determinations, 264
Becker, E., see Friedman, M. M.
Beer's Law: for stained protein patterns on filter paper, 329
Beher, W. T., see Gaebler, O. H.
Berger, Eugene Y.: Calcium Determination in Biologic Material, 249
Bile-pigment metabolism, 391
Bischoff, Ernst, Award, 72, 346, 423, 424
Bluemle, Dolores B., see Singer, R. B.
Bossak, E. T., see Adlersberg, D.
Brown, Herman, see Samson, M.
Brown, Ray K.: Serum Lipoproteins, Chemical and Enzymatic Studies, 83
Butt, Arthur J., see Leonard, R. H.
Calcium: EDTA method, 125: cerate oxidimetry method, 250
Calcium Determination in Biologic Material: Berger, E. Y., 249
Calculi, Quantitative method for urinary, 241
Cannan, R. Keith: Proposal for the Distribution of a Certified Standard for Use in Hemoglobinometry, 151
Carbohydrate metabolism in liver disease, 359
Carbon Monoxide, blood, micro-method, 170
Cell Volume, Blood, micro-method, 299
Cephalin-Cholesterol Flocculation Test, 377
Chemical Abnormalities in Blood Serum Associated with the Carrier State of Viral Hepatitis: Reinhold, J. G., 3
Chemical Evaluation of the Functions of the Liver, (Revised): Reinhold, J. G., 351
Chemical Physiology of Liver Disease, 358
Chemotherapy of Infections: Collier, H. O. J., (Book Review), 81
Cholesterol: Determination with p-toluenesulfonic acid, 345: Effect of Diet on blood, 34
Clinical Chemistry in Practical Medicine: Stewart, C. P. and Dunlop, D. M., (Book Review), 80
Clinical Significance of the Magnesium: Calcium Ratio; Technic for the determination of Magnesium and Calcium in Biologic Fluids: Friedman, H. S. and Rubin, M. A., 125
Coco, S., see Mason, W. B.
CO_2 Content, micro-determination, 293
Code of Ethics of the American Association of Clinical Chemists, 203
Colorimetric Determination of Blood Arginase: Friedman, M. M. and Becker, E., 110
Convenient Apparatus for the Continuous Dehydration of Histologic Material: Nadeau, G. and Joly, L. P., 190
Cooper, Gerald E., see Mandel, E. E.
Copper and diseases of the liver, 387
Cross-Contaminator Exclusion Test for Dry-Ashing Determination of Protein-Bound Iodine: Samson, M., Brown, H. and Eichen, S., 269
De Lalla, L. S., see Brown, R. K.
Detoxification reactions of the liver, 387
Digestion, fat, 93
Di Mauro, S., see Gottfried, S. P.
Diseases of the liver and biliary tract, 354
Disturbances of water and electrolyte balances in liver diseases, 384
Effect of Shaking on the Accuracy of Salt

Fractionation Methods for Serum Albumin: Saifer, A. and Zymaris, M. C., 180
Effects of Diet on Blood Lipids in Man: Keys, A., Anderson, J. T., Fidanza, F., Keys, M. H. and Swahn, B., 34
Eichen, S., see Samson, S.
Electrometric pH Determinations: Theory and Practice: Bates, R. G. (Book Review), 149
Electrophoresis and Monomolecular Layer Studies with Serum Lipoproteins: Adlersberg, D., Bossak, E. T., Sher, I. H. and Sobotka, H., 18
Estimation of Hydrocortisone Secretion: Silber, R. H., 234
Estimation of Lipid Fractions of Blood Plasma; System Using the Allen Volumetric Method: Kibrick, A. C. and Skupp, S. J., 317
Fatty Acids: Blood, Iodine numbers, 324: Blood plasma, 320: Blood, thiocyanogen numbers, 324
Fidanza, F., see Keys, A.
Freeman, Monroe E: President's Address, 68
Friedman, Howard S.: Clinical Significance of the Magnesium: Calcium Ratio, 125
Friedman, Max, M.: Colorimetric Determination of Blood Arginase, 110
Friedman, Nathan, H., see Gottfried, S. P.
Gaebler, O. H.: Reproducibility and Validity of Sodium Sulfate Fractionation of Proteins in Plasma and Knee Joint Fluid, 105
Galpin, R. R., see Gaebler, O. H.
Gordon, B. S., see Klein, B.
Gorsuch, T. L., see Mandel, E. E.
Gottfried, Sidney P.: Serum Beta-Lipoproteins of Normal, Atherosclerotic and Lipemic Individuals, 253
Graef, I., see Klein, B.
Green, D. E.: Oxidation and Synthesis of Fatty Acids in Soluble Enzyme Systems of Animal Tissues, 53
Hemochromatosis: 118
Hemoglobin: cyanmethemoglobin standard, 153: method, 153
Hepatic tests: evaluation of, 8: on blood donors, 10
Hepatitis: 3
Hormone metabolism in liver disease, 382
Human Biochemistry: Kleiner, I. S., (Book Review), 82
Hydrocortisone: method for calculation of secretion, 235
Iodine and Thiocyanogen Numbers of the Fatty Acids of Blood Plasma: Kibrick, A. C. and Skupp, S. J., 324
Improved Methods of Analysis for Oxygen, Carbon Monoxide and Iron on Fingertip Blood: Natelson, S. and Menning, C. M., 165
Iron: Blood, micro-method, 172: tissues, 118
Iron Content of Tissues in Exogenous and Endogenous Hemochromatosis: Klein, B., Gordon, B. S. and Graef, I., 118
Joly, L. P., see Nadeau, G.
Jones, Betty Jo: p-Toluenesulfonic Acid, Cholesterol Determination, and Explosions, 345
Kauffman, D. L., see Brown, R. K.
Keys, Ancel: Effect of Diet on Blood Lipids In Man; particularly Cholesterol and Lipoproteins, 34
Keys, M. H., see Keys, A.
Kibrick, Andre C.: Estimation of Lipid Fractions of Blood Plasma, 317
Kibrick, Andre C.: Iodine and Thiocyanogen Numbers of the Fatty Acids of Blood Plasma, 324
Klein, Bernard: Iron Content of Tissues in Exogenous and Endogenous Hemochromatosis, 118
Laboratory Instructions in Biochemistry: Kleiner, I. S. and Dotti, L. B., (Book Review), 82
Laurence, D. J. R., see Rees, V. H.
Legal Medicine, Pathology and Toxicology: Gonzales, T. A., Vance, M., Helpern, M. and Umberger, C. J., (Book Review), 148
Legislation, Clinical Chemistry, 347
Leonard, Reid H.: Quantitative Identification of Urinary Calculi, 241
Lipids: Fractions in blood plasma, method, 318: in liver disease, 360
Lipids, The: Their Chemistry and Biochemistry: Deuel, H. J., Jr. (Book Review), 219
Lipoproteins: 18, alteration by enzymes, 86: beta, changes at 6.5° and 37.5°, 255: effect of diet, 34: in human disease, 26: in mammals, 22: preparation, 84: Monomolecular layer studies, 18
Magnesium: method for biologic fluids, 125

Mandel, Emanuel E.: Seromucoid in Hepatobiliary Disease, 221
Mason, W. Burkett: Purification of Chromium (VI) for Use in the PBI Determination, 117
Menning, C. M., see Natelson, S.
Monomolecular Layer Studies: Lipoproteins, 18
Moreland, Ferrin B., see Jones, B. J.
Nadeau, Guy: Convenient Apparatus for the Continuous Dehydration of Histologic Material, 190
Natelson, Samuel: Improved Methods of Analysis for Oxygen, Carbon Monoxide and Iron on Fingertip Blood, 167
Neutral Fats: plasma, 320
Nitrogen metabolism in liver disease, 364
Organic Analysis: Mitchell, J. Jr., Kolthoff, I. M., Proskauer, E. S., and Weissberger, A., (Book Review), 148
Oxidation and Synthesis of Fatty Acids in Soluble Enzyme Systems of Animal Tissues: Green, D. E., 53
Oxygen: blood micro-method for capacity and content, 166
Peralta, Oscar: Rapid Estimation of Amylase Activity of Serum by Turbidimetry, 157
pH: Blood micro-colorimetric determination, 288
Plasma proteins in liver disease, 368
Pope, R. H., see Gottfried, S. P.
Practical Clinical Biochemistry: Varley, Harold, (Book Review), 218
President's Address: Freeman, M. E., 68
Proposal for the Distribution of a Certified Standard for Use in Hemoglobinometry: Cannan, R. K., 151
Protein Bound Iodine, 117, 269
Proteins: plasma, 105: Knee joint fluid, 105
p-Toluenesulfonic Acid, Cholesterol Determinations and Explosions: Jones, B. J. and Moreland, F. B., 345
Purification of Chromium (VI) for use in the PBI Determination: Mason, W. B. and Coco, S., 117
Quantitative Identification of Urinary Calculi: Leonard, R. H. and Butt, A. J., 241
Rapid Estimation of Amylase Activity of Serum by Turbidimetry: Peralta, O. and Reinhold, J. G., 157
Recent Studies of Fat Digestion and Absorption: Reiser, R., 93
Recognition of Specialists in Other Fields: Turner, E. L., 196
Rees, V. H.: The Correspondence with Beer's Law for the Optical Density of Stained Protein Patterns on Filter Paper as a Function of Surface Protein Concentration, 329
Reiser, R., Recent Studies of Fat Digestion and Absorption, 93
Reinhold, John G.: Chemical Abnormalities in Blood Serum Associated with the Carrier State of Viral Hepatitis, 3
Reinhold, John G.: Chemical Evaluation of the Functions of the Liver (Revised), 351
Reinhold, John G., see Peralta, O.
Reproducibility and Validity of Sodium Sulfate Fractionation of Proteins in Plasma and Knee Joint Fluid: Gaebler, O. H., Beher, W. T., Sigler, J. W. and Galpin, R. R., 105
Rubin, M. A., see Friedman, H. S.
Saifer, Abraham: Effect of Shaking on the Accuracy of Salt Fractionation Methods for Serum Albumin, 180
Samson, Meyer: Cross-Contaminator Exclusion Test for Dry-Ashing Determination of Protein Bound Iodine, 269
Selection of procedures in liver disease, 403
Seromucoid in Hepatobiliary Disease: Mandel, E. E., Gorsuch, T. L. and Cooper, G. E., 221
Serum alkaline phosphatase, 390
Serum Beta-Lipoproteins of Normal, Atherosclerotic and Lipemic Individuals: Gottfried, S. P., Pope, R. H., Friedman, N. H., Akerson, I. B., and Di Mauro, S., 253
Serum iron in liver disease, 385
Serum Lipoproteins; Chemical and Enzymatic Studies: Brown, R. K., De Lalla, L. S. and Kauffman, D. L., 83
Sher, I. H., see Adlersberg, D.
Shohl, Jane, see Singer, R. B.
Sigler, J. W., see Gaebler, O. H.
Silber, Robert H.: Estimation of Hydrocortisone Secretion, 234
Simultaneous Determination of pH, CO_2 Content and Cell Volume in 0.1 ml. Aliquots of Cutaneous Blood; A Modification of the Shock and Hastings Technic:

Singer, R. B., Shohl, J. and Bluemle, D. B., 287
Singer, Richard G.: Simultaneous Determination of pH, CO_2 Content and Cell Volume in 0.1 ml. Aliquots of Cutaneous Blood, 287
Skupp, S. J., see Kibrick, A. C.
Sobotka, H., see Adlersberg, D.
Statistical Analysis in Chemistry and the Chemical Industry: Bennett, C. A., and Franklin, N. L., (Book Review), 81
Structure of the liver, 351
Sullivan, Michael X.: 1955 Ernst Bischoff Award, 346
Swahn, B., see Keys A.
The Correspondence with Beer's Law for the Optical Density of Stained Protein Patterns on Filter Paper as a Function of Surface Protein Concentration: Rees, V. H. and Laurence, D. J. R., 329
Thiocyanogen Numbers of Plasma Fatty Acids, 324
Thymol Flocculation Test, 376
Thymol Turbidity Test, 373
Turner, Edward L.: Recognition of Specialists in Other Fields, 196
Urobilinogen: erratum for page 265, 349: quantitative method, 264
Zymaris, M. C., see Saifer, A.